NEUROSCIENCE RESEARCH PROGRESS

THE CENTRAL CATECHOLAMINERGIC SYSTEM

ANATOMY, FUNCTIONS AND DISORDERS

NEUROSCIENCE RESEARCH PROGRESS

Additional books in this series can be found on Nova's website under the Series tab.

Additional e-books in this series can be found on Nova's website under the e-book tab.

NEUROSCIENCE RESEARCH PROGRESS

THE CENTRAL CATECHOLAMINERGIC SYSTEM

ANATOMY, FUNCTIONS AND DISORDERS

BERTALAN DUDÁS, M.D., PH.D.
EDITOR

NOVA BIOMEDICAL

New York

For permission to use material from this book please contact us:
Telephone 631-231-7269; Fax 631-231-8175
Web Site: http://www.novapublishers.com

Additional color graphics may be available in the e-book version of this book.

Library of Congress Cataloging-in-Publication Data

ISBN: 978-1-63117-937-2

Library of Congress Control Number: 2014938747

Published by Nova Science Publishers, Inc. † New York

To my son, Dominik

Contents

Preface

"Nothing has such power to broaden the mind as the ability to investigate systematically and truly all that comes under thy observation in life"
(Marcus Aurelius: Meditations, III, 11)

The catecholaminergic system is one of the most studied neurotransmitter systems. Since the original studies of Dahlström and Fuxe in the mid-60s, when they mapped the pattern of monoaminergic neurons using formaldehyde-induced flourescence technique developed by Falck and Hillarp, the distribution and the biological roles of catecholamines have been in the center of interest. It is clear now that catecholaminergic transmission not only plays a pivotal role in the modulation of stress response, but is also involved in numerous cortical functions, such as cognition, memory, learning, mood and behavior. Additionally, the catecholaminergic system appears to control vital hypothalamic functions. Several physiological processes, including growth, sexual regulation, and salt and water balance are regulated by catecholamines, either directly or via complex circuitries involving numerous neurotransmitter/neuroregulator systems. Both the involvement of catecholamines in Alzheimer's and Parkinson's diseases and their pivotal roles in schizophrenia and manic depression place these neurotransmitters in the focus of drug development that aims to address neurodegenerative disorders and psychiatric conditions.

Describing the morphology and functions of the central catecholaminergic system most certainly exceeds the scope of a single volume. Therefore, the goal of this book is not to compile our knowledge of the catecholamines, but rather to provide insight into the roles of these important neurotransmitters in vital central functions and pathological conditions, without placing a particular emphasis on their parts they play in the peripheral nervous system. I trust this volume will merit its place on the bookshelf of researchers in the field of catecholaminergic research.

Bertalan Dudás M.D., Ph.D.
2013 October

List of Contributors

Merouane Bencherif
Targacept Inc., Winston-Salem, NC, USA

Courtney Benson
Molecular and Structural Neurobiology & Gene Therapy Program,
Department of Pathology and Anatomical Sciences,
Western New York Stem Cell Culture and Analysis Center,
State University of New York at Buffalo, Buffalo, NY, USA

Martha C. Bohn
Lurie Children's Research Center
Feinberg School of Medicine
Northwestern University, Chicago, IL, USA

Thomas D. Corso
Department of Pharmaceutical Sciences
Lake Erie College of Osteopathic Medicine, Erie, PA, USA

Ryan Curl
Molecular and Structural Neurobiology & Gene Therapy Program,
Department of Pathology and Anatomical Sciences,
Western New York Stem Cell Culture and Analysis Center,
State University of New York at Buffalo, Buffalo, NY, USA

Bertalan Dudás
Neuroendocrine Organization Laboratory (NEO)
Lake Erie College of Osteopathic Medicine, Erie, PA, USA

George Grignol
Neuroendocrine Organization Laboratory (NEO)
Lake Erie College of Osteopathic Medicine, Erie, PA, USA

Aaron Kucinski
Department of Psychology
University of Michigan, Ann Arbor, MI, USA

Irene Lehner-Adam
University Hospital for Psychiatry and Psychotherapy
Paracelsus Medical University Salzburg, Austria
Christian Doppler University Clinic Salzburg
Salzburg, Austria

David G. Lichter
State University of New York at Buffalo
Buffalo, NY, USA

Istvan Merchenthaler
University of Maryland at Baltimore, School of Medicine
Baltimore, MD, USA

Robert S. Miletich
Department of Nuclear Medicine
State University of New York at Buffalo, Buffalo, NY, USA

Moritz Mühlbacher
University Hospital for Psychiatry and Psychotherapy
Paracelsus Medical University Salzburg, Austria
Christian Doppler University Clinic Salzburg
Salzburg, Austria

Sridhar Narla
Molecular and Structural Neurobiology & Gene Therapy Program,
Department of Pathology and Anatomical Sciences,
Western New York Stem Cell Culture and Analysis Center,
State University of New York at Buffalo, Buffalo, NY, USA

Michael S. Peroski
Neuroendocrine Organization Laboratory (NEO)
Lake Erie College of Osteopathic Medicine, Erie, PA, USA

Ewa K. Stachowiak
Molecular and Structural Neurobiology & Gene Therapy Program,
Department of Pathology and Anatomical Sciences,
Western New York Stem Cell Culture and Analysis Center,
State University of New York at Buffalo, Buffalo, NY, USA

Michal K. Stachowiak
Molecular and Structural Neurobiology & Gene Therapy Program,
Department of Pathology and Anatomical Sciences,
Western New York Stem Cell Culture and Analysis Center,
State University of New York at Buffalo, Buffalo, NY, USA

Scott Wersinger
Department of Psychology
State University of New York at Buffalo, Buffalo, NY, USA

In: The Central Catecholaminergic System
Editor: Bertalan Dudás
ISBN: 978-1-63117-937-2

Chapter 1

Anatomy of the Central Catecholaminergic System

Bertalan Dudás and Martha C. Bohn

Introduction

The human central catecholaminergic system is composed of dopaminergic, noradrenergic and adrenergic perikarya located mostly in the rhombencephalon, mesencephalon and diencephalon with fibers projecting into widespread areas of the brain and spinal cord. The distribution of the catecholaminergic elements has been extensively studied in numerous species including human, using formaldehyde-induced fluorescence as well as immunohistochemistry and *in situ* hybridization histochemistry. Since formaldehyde-induced fluorescence (Dahlstrom & Fuxe, 1964; Bjorklund et al., 1975; Bjorklund & Nobin, 1973; Axelsson et al., 1973) can differentiate only between dopamine and noradrenaline/adrenaline, but cannot be used to distinguish noradrenergic and adrenergic structures, immunohistochemistry and *in situ* hybridization histochemistry are frequently utilized to detect the key enzymes of the catecholamine synthesis. Tyrosine hydroxylase (TH), the key and rate-limiting enzyme of the catecholaminergic synthesis is present in all classes of catecholaminergic neurons (Dudás & Merchenthaler, 2001; Dudás & Merchenthaler, 2006; Hokfelt et al., 1976; Kitahama et al., 1987; Li et al., 1988; Panayotacopoulou et al., 1991; Panayotacopoulou et al., 2005; Zoli et al., 1993). Similarly, noradrenergic neurons cannot be distinguished from adrenergic neurons by either formaldehyde-induced fluorescence or by immunohistochemistry to dopamine-beta hydroxylase (DBH) which is expressed in both the noradrenergic and adrenergic neurons. Therefore, phenylethanolamine N-methyltransferase (PNMT), the rate limiting enzyme of the adrenaline synthesis, is widely used to identify the synthesis of adrenaline in the brain of several species including human by using immunohistochemistry (Ericson et al., 1989; Mezey, 1989; Palkovits et al., 1992; Bohn et al., 1986) and enzyme activity assays (Kopp et al., 1979; Lew et al., 1977; Nagatsu et al., 1977; Moreno et al., 1992). In addition, noradrenergic neurons can be identified by lacking PNMT and containing TH and DBH; in the similar manner, dopaminergic neurons are TH-positive but lack DBH and PNMT (Figure 1).

There are several excellent studies (Fallon et al., 1978; Fallon & Moore, 1978a; Fallon & Moore, 1978b; Felten et al., 1974; Felten & Sladek, Jr., 1983; Hokfelt et al., 1976; Moore & Bloom, 1978) and reviews (Nieuwenhuys, 1985) describing the anatomy of the catecholaminergic system in numerous species including human. Since the projections of the catecholaminergic pathways are generally based on animal studies and only few have been verified in human, some of the data we describe here are hypothetical. Nevertheless, the aim of the present chapter is to give a brief overview of our understanding of the human catecholaminergic system based on previous experimental findings and review volumes.

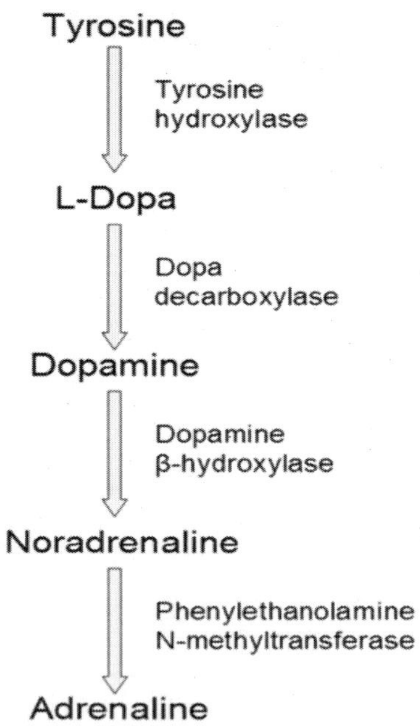

Figure 1. Enzymes of the dopamine, adrenaline and noradrenaline synthesis.

Part I: General Overview

Dopaminergic System

Dopaminergic neurons are widely distributed in the human brain and can be found in the mesencephalon, diencephalon and the telencephalon (Felten et al., 1974; Felten & Sladek, Jr., 1983; Moore & Bloom, 1978) [for a review see Nieuwenhuys (1985)]. The mesencephalic perikarya are clustered into three, more or less distinctive cell groups in the tegmentum, denoted A8, A9 and 10, arranged from lateral to medial, with A10 located at the midline (Figure 2). The most well-defined group is A9, which is formed by the compact part of the substantia nigra (Figure 3) and merges dorsolaterally with the group A8 that is located in the lateral tegmentum, caudal to the red nucleus (Nieuwenhuys, 1985). The ventral tegmental area contains the A10 cell group that is composed of perikarya accumulated in the midline medial to the substantia nigra.

In addition to the mesencephalic cell groups, the diencephalon contains four dopaminergic cell clusters, A11-A14 (Bjorklund & Nobin, 1973; Felten et al., 1974; Felten, 1976; Felten & Sladek, Jr., 1983; Ungerstedt, 1971). Group A11 is located in the caudal hypothalamus, around the mammillothalamic tract; this group is connected to the cell group A13 that extends into the caudomedial part of the zona incerta (Nieuwenhuys, 1985). The infundibular nucleus contains a relatively well-defined cell group, A12. Scattered in the periventricular area of the hypothalamus, primarily in the preoptic and tuberal region, dopaminergic cell bodies form group A14. In addition to these cell groups, additional subpopulations of dopaminergic perikarya have been described in the diencephalon in the paraventricular and supraoptic nuclei, as well as in the medial hypothalamus between the fornix and the optic tract (Dudás et al., 2010). The only telencephalic cell group, A15, is situated in the olfactory bulb (Nieuwenhuys, 1985).

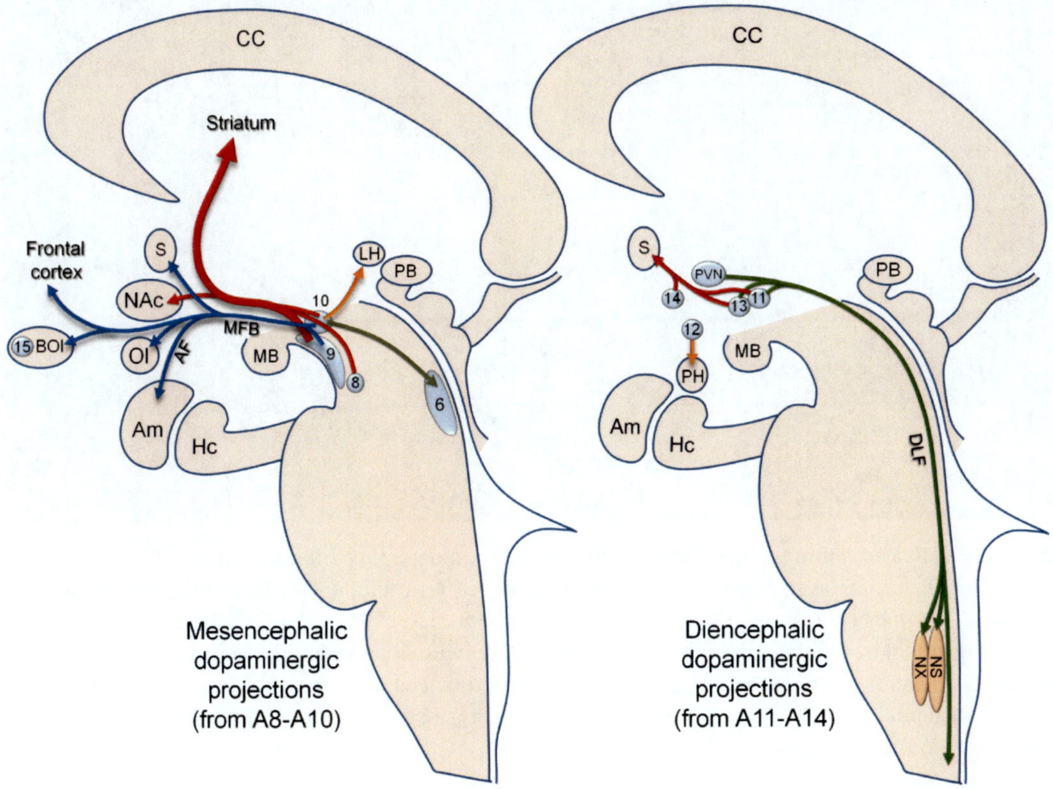

Figure 2. Schematic representation of the dopaminergic system in human. Catecholaminergic nuclei are illustrated in coerulean blue. Some of the connections are hypothetical and have not been confirmed in humans yet. The left side of the image depicts the mesencephalic dopaminergic projections from nuclei A8 (8), A9 or substantia nigra (9) and A10 (10); mesostriatal pathway is illustrated in red and mesolimbic and mesocortical pathway is depicted in blue. The right insert illustrates the diencephalic projections from nuclei A11-14 (11-14, respectively). Dopaminergic nucleus A15 is the only telencephalic cell group residing in the olfactory bulb (BOl). Mesostriatal pathway emerges from all of the mesencephalic dopaminergic nuclei which, apart from the corpus striatum, also innervate the nucleus accumbens (NAc). Dopaminergic fibers from A10 (10) and the medial part of the substantia nigra (9) project to the septum, (S), olfactory nuclei (Ol) and bulb BOl), bed nucleus of stria terminalis, amygdala (Am) via the amygdalofugal pathway and to the cingulate and frontal cortex. Dopaminergic neurons from A10 (10) also project to the lateral habenular nucleus (LH) and the locus coeruleus or A6 (6). Dopaminergic diencephalic projections include the tubero-infundibular pathway from A12 (12) located in the infundibular nucleus. Neurons located in A11 (11), A13 (13) and A14 (14) target the septal area (S) as well as hypothalamic areas (not shown). Dopaminergic cells from the paraventricular nucleus (PVN), A11 (11) and A13 form a descending pathway that targets spinal cord levels as well as the solitary nucleus (NS) and the dorsal vagal nucleus (NX). Abbreviations: Am, amygdala; Hc, hippocampus; CC, corpus callosum; PB, pineal body; MB, mammillary body. The nomenclature is adopted from Nieuwenhuys (1985).

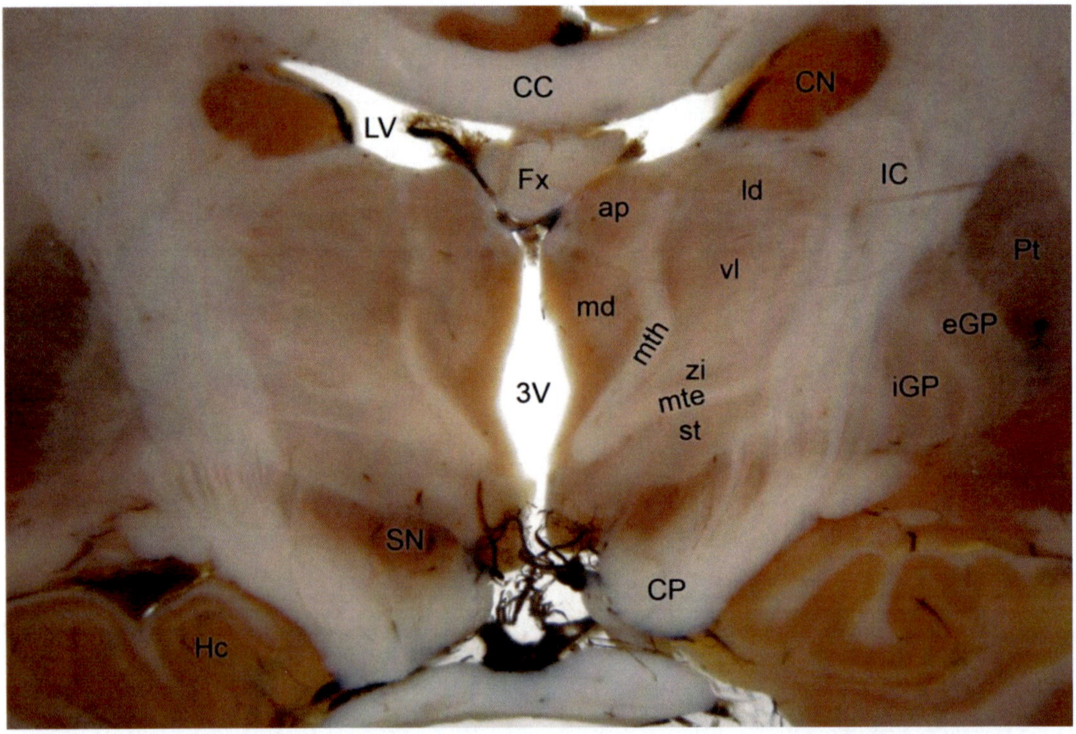

Figure 3. Plastinated, 5mm thick coronal section of the brain depicting substantia nigra (SN) and the surrounding diencephalic structures. Abbreviations: 3V, 3rd ventricle; ap, anteroprincipal thalamic nucleus; CC, corpus callosum; CP, cerebral peduncle; Fx, fornix; eGP, globus pallidus, external zone; iGP, globus pallidus, internal zone; Hc, hippocampus; IC, internal capsule; ld, laterodorsal thalamic nucleus; LV, lateral ventricle; md, medial dorsal thalamic nucleus; mte, mammillotegmental tract; mth, mammillothalamic tract; Pt, putamen; SN, substantia nigra; st, subthalamic nucleus; vl, ventrolateral thalamic nucleus; zi, zona incerta.

Additional groups of dopaminergic subpopulations have also been described, mainly in rats. Dopaminergic cells have been found in the dorsal vagal nucleus (Armstrong et al., 1982), although other authors reported that these cells appear to lack DOPA decarboxylase (Jaeger et al., 1984) hence they may not be dopaminergic. Dopaminergic neurons have also been described in the dorsal raphe nucleus of rat (Hokfelt et al., 1976; Lindvall & Bjorklund, 1974; Ochi & Shimizu, 1978) and cat (Miachon et al., 1984).

Although the projections of dopaminergic neurons have been extensively studied in rats, there are relatively few studies confirming these pathways in human. There is a general consensus that mesencephalic dopaminergic neurons commonly project to the telencephalon, to striatal (putamen, caudate nucleus, nucleus accumbens), limbic (olfactory nuclei and bulb, septum, bed nucleus of stria terminalis, amygdala, cingulate cortex) and other cortical areas including the frontal lobe cortex (Fig.2). Mesolimbic and mesocortical projections via the medial forebrain bundle originate from A10 and the medial zone of substantia nigra, while mesostriatal pathways appear to project from all of the mesencephalic dopaminergic cell groups A8, A9 and A10 (Nieuwenhuys, 1985). In addition to the telencephalic projections, mesencephalic dopaminergic neurons also project to the lateral habenular nucleus (Skagerberg et al., 1984; Swanson, 1982), subthalamic nuclei (Lindvall et al., 1983; Nobin &

Bjorklund, 1973), the locus coeruleus and probably the lateral parabrachial nuclei (Swanson, 1982). Diencephalic dopaminergic projections include the tubero-infundibular pathway, mostly from the cell group A12 located in the infundibular nucleus. Indeed, previous studies reported that the posterior hypophysis contains TH-IR fibers only without any detectable DBH-IR in pig (Leshin et al., 1996). The septal area is targeted by fibers from A11, A13 and A14; this pathway supply hypothalamic areas as well, including the paraventricular, supraoptic and dorsomedial nuclei (Lindvall & Stenevi, 1978; Lindvall et al., 1984). In addition, dopaminergic fibers project to spinal levels via the dorsal longitudinal fasciculus (Lindvall et al., 1983; Skagerberg et al., 1982), particularly from cell group A11 in rat (Bjorklund & Skagerberg, 1979; Hokfelt et al., 1979) and A13 in rabbit (Blessing and Chalmers, 1979). These fibers also innervate the solitary and the dorsal vagal nuclei.

Noradrenergic System

The noradrenergic system is composed of perikarya constrained to the pons and medulla oblongata (Figure 4). These neurons are clustered into seven cell groups in rodents, A1-A7, whose ascending and descending fibers innervate essentially all regions of the central nervous system (Dahlstrom & Fuxe, 1964; Nobin & Bjorklund, 1973; Olson et al., 1973a; Olson et al., 1973b). These cell groups, with the exception of A3, which lies dorsal to the inferior olivary complex in rodents, have been identified in primates including humans [for a review see Nieuwenhuys (1985)]. The most well-defined noradrenergic cell group, A6, is composed of densely packed, pigmented perikarya located in the locus coeruleus (Figure 4), representing about 50% of the central noradrenergic neurons (Nieuwenhuys, 1985). Due to its fundamental role in the central noradrenergic innervation, locus coeruleus has also been suggested as a central equivalent of a sympathetic ganglion (Amaral & Sinnamon, 1977). Group A1 is located in the lower medulla oblongata surrounding the lateral funiculus (Nieuwenhuys, 1985); group A2 is at the same level extending from the solitary nucleus to the dorsal vagal nucleus and area postrema (Armstrong et al., 1982). Group A4 neurons are scattered along the superior cerebellar peduncle just under the ependymal surface, while group A5 perikarya are situated in the tegmentum of the pons, in the close proximity of the facial nucleus and the superior olivary complex (Nieuwenhuys, 1985). Rostral pons contains the A7 group, located at the lateral zone of reticular formation. Groups A1, A5 and A7 are located along a line extending from the medulla to the rostral pons and form a caudorostral continuum (Nieuwenhuys, 1985).

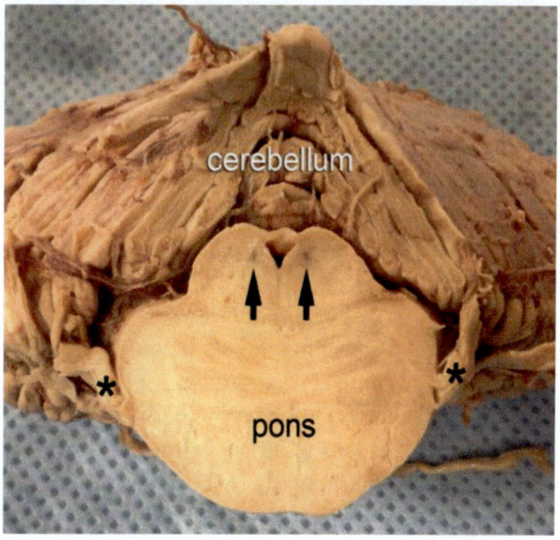

Figure 4. Pigmented neurons of the locus coeruleus appear as dark areas in the pons (arrowheads). Trigeminal nerve is labeled with the asterisk.

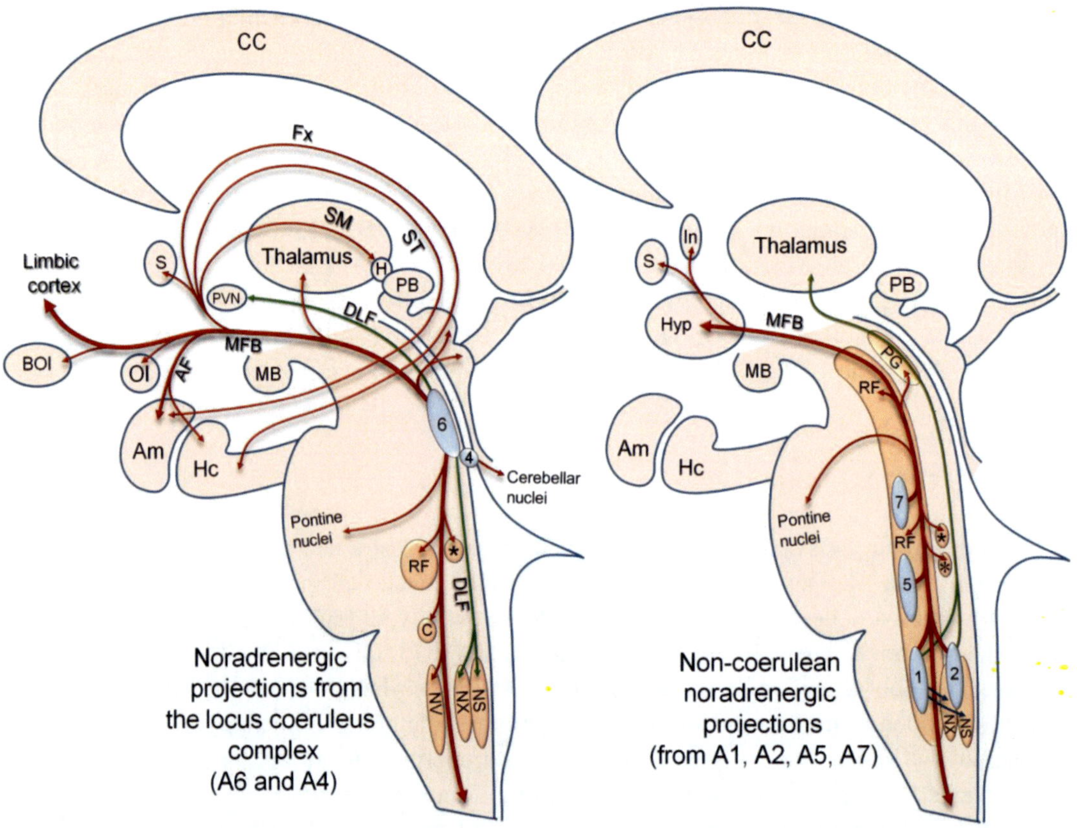

Figure 5. Schematic illustration of the noradrenergic system in humans. Catecholaminergic nuclei are illustrated in coerulean blue. Some of the connections are hypothetical and have not been confirmed in human yet. The left side of the image depicts the noradrenergic projections from the locus coeruleus or A6 (6), while the right insert demonstrates the non-coerulean projections from nuclei A1, A2, A5, A7 (1,2,5,7, respectively). Ascending pathways from locus coeruleus (6) run mainly in the medial forebrain bundle (MFB) and project to thalamus, limbic cortex, olfactory nuclei (Ol) and bulb (BOl). These fibers also target the amygdala (Am) via the amygdalofugal pathway (AF) and stria terminalis (ST), the hippocampus (Hc) via the fornix (Fx) the habenular nuclei (H) via the stria medullaris (SM) and the superior and inferior colliculi. Additionally, cerulean fibers target the hypothalamus, particularly the paraventricular nucleus (PVN) via the dorsal longitudinal fasciculus (DLF). Locus coeruleus and the adjacent adrenergic cell group A4 (4) project to the cerebellar nuclei. Descending cerulean pathways target the solitary nucleus (NS) and the dorsal vagal nucleus (NX) via the DLF as well as other pontine, myelencephalic and spinal levels including the reticular formation (RF), spinal trigeminal nucleus (NV), cochlear nuclei (C) and the principal sensory trigeminal nucleus (five-pointed asterisk in the left insert). Ascending non-coerulean pathways from nuclei A1, A2, A5, A7 (1,2,5,7, respectively) project the interstitial nucleus of stria terminalis (In) as well as to hypothalamic (Hyp) and septal areas (S) via the median forebrain bundle (MFB); these fibers also innervate the pontine nuclei, periventricular grey matter (PG) and the mesencephalic reticular formation (RF). Descending fibers target the trigeminal motor nucleus (five-pointed asterisk in the right insert), facial nucleus (six-pointed asterisk), pontine and myelencephalic reticular formation (RF), and spinal levels. Solitary nucleus and dorsal vagal nucleus receive noradrenergic fibers from cell cluster A1 (1). Abbreviations: Am, amygdala; CC, corpus callosum; Hc, hippocampus; MB, mammillary body, PB, pineal body. The nomenclature is adopted from Nieuwenhuys (1985).

Perikarya from the locus coeruleus project to the lower regions of the brainstem and to all segments of the spinal cord via the ill-defined bundle of the coeruleo-spinal fibers running in the reticular formation. The solitary nucleus and the dorsal vagal nucleus are innervated by cerulean neurons via the dorsal longitudinal fasciculus of Schütz. Noradrenergic neurons from locus coeruleus also project rostrally via the medial forebrain bundle that is a rather elusive, poorly defined network of fibers running antero-posteriorly through the lateral hypothalamus, or via the dorsal longitudinal fasciculus and its diencephalic continuation, the periventricular fiber system. These fibers innervate numerous mesencephalic, diencephalic, telencephalic and cerebellar areas.

Hypothalamic noradrenergic fibers originate mostly from the A1, A2, A5 and A7 cell groups and reach the hypothalamus primarily via the medial forebrain bundle (Figure 5; Nieuwenhuys, 1985). The hypothalamic DBH-IR axonal varicosities, which are believed to represent mostly noradrenergic elements due to the relative scarcity of PNMT-IR structures in the human hypothalamus (Dudás et al., 2010), form a moderately dense network in the PVN, SON and in the basal part of the infundibulum that includes the infundibular nucleus (Jansen et al., 2003; Dudás et al., 2010). Since the posterior hypophysis contains dopaminergic, TH-IR fibers that lack DBH in pigs (Leshin et al., 1996), infundibular noradrenergic fibers may target the adenohypophysis. Additionally, these axonal varicosities often surround portal vessels, suggesting the release of norepinephrine to the portal circulation (Dudás et al., 2010).

Non-coerulean noradrenergic fibers also innervate a broad spectrum of diencephalic and telencephalic areas including the septal region, the bed nucleus of stria terminalis, nucleus of the diagonal band of Broca (Lindvall & Stenevi, 1978; Moore, 1978), the amygdala via the ventral amygdalofugal pathway (Fallon et al., 1978) as well as the spinal cord.

Adrenergic System

Biochemical techniques identifying adrenaline or PMNT have revealed generally more adrenergic sites in the brain than the ones visualized by PMNT immunohistochemistry (Van den Gugten, 1976, Lew, 1977, Saavedra 1974). Although adrenaline is widely distributed in the brain (Mefford, 1988), there is a general consensus that most of the adrenergic structures are fiber varicosities supplied by cell groups mainly restricted to the myelencephalon (Figure 6). These neurons are clustered into three cell groups, C1, C2 and C3 (Astier et al., 1987; Dahlstrom & Fuxe, 1964; Kitahama et al., 1986; Kitahama et al., 1988; Cunningham, Jr. et al., 1990; Sawchenko & Bohn, 1989). Group C1 is by far the largest and it is located between the inferior olivary complex and the nucleus funiculi lateralis (Nieuwenhuys, 1985). Group C2 lies in the close proximity of the solitary nucleus, while group C3 is situated laterally to the dorsal raphe nuclei. According to several authors, groups C1 and C2 may be identical to catecholaminergic clusters A1 and A2, respectively (Dahlstrom & Fuxe, 1964) or they are at least close in proximity to them (Howe et al., 1980). Fibers from these adrenergic cell groups ascend and eventually reach diencephalic structures mainly via the medial forebrain bundle; these fibers terminate primarily in the locus coeruleus, periaqueductal grey and the thalamus (Hokfelt et al., 1973; Nieuwenhuys, 1985). Fibers from C2 also target the solitary nucleus and the dorsal vagal nucleus.

The presence of adrenaline in the hypothalamic regions has been identified mainly by measuring PNMT enzyme activity (Kopp et al., 1979; Nagatsu et al., 1977; Lew et al., 1977). Although adrenergic fibers are relatively abundant in the rat hypothalamus (Palkovits et al., 1992), and certain regions, including PVN appear to receive dense adrenergic innervations in the rat (Hokfelt, 1974b), only small number of fibers can be detected in the hypothalamus in humans (Dudás et al., 2010). Previous studies also described adrenergic cell bodies in the posterior hypothalamus of the rat (Foster et al., 1985a; Ruggiero et al., 1985), however, no apparent hypothalamic perikarya were detected in the human hypothalamus by others (Dudás et al., 2010), suggesting discernible species differences regarding the distribution of the adrenergic structures. These findings are in general consensus with previous studies reporting significantly smaller epinephrine content in the human hypothalamus comparing to that of other species (Mefford, 1988). Additional PNMT-IR perikarya have also been described in the limbic system (Mezey, 1989). Descending adrenergic fibers, predominantly from group C1, terminate in the intermediolateral cell column of the spinal cord synapsing directly on preganglionic neurons which innervate the adrenal medulla (Bernstein-Goral & Bohn, 1989).

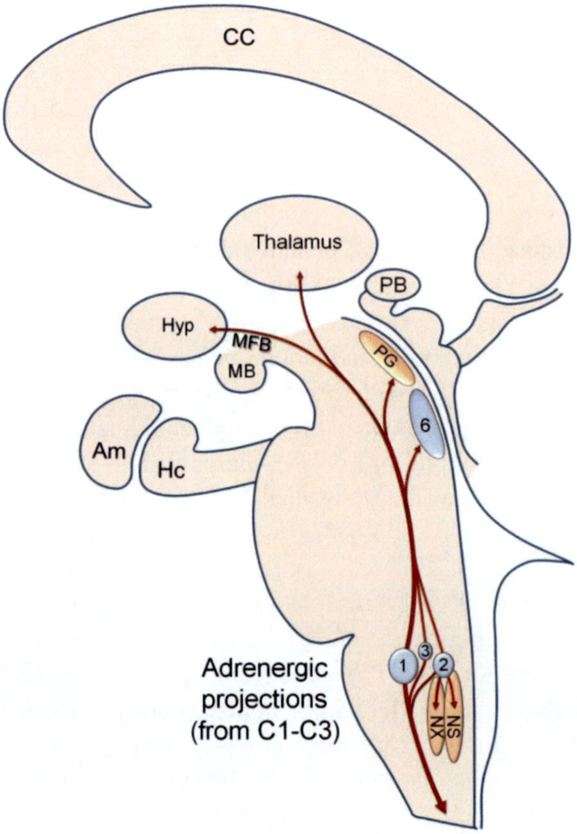

Figure 6. Schematic depiction of the human adrenergic system. Many of the connections are hypothetical and have not been confirmed in humans yet. Catecholaminergic nuclei are illustrated in coerulean blue. Ascending and descending connections mostly originate from adrenergic nucleus C1 (1), while C2 (2) and C3 (3) contribute less. Ascending pathways project to the A6, locus coeruleus (6), into the periaqueductal grey (PG), to the thalamus and via the median forebrain bundle (MFB) into the hypothalamus (Hyp). Adrenergic nucleus C2 (2) also projects to the solitary nucleus (NS) and the dorsal vagal nucleus (NX). Descending pathways, mostly from C1 (1) target the intermediolateral cell column of the spinal cord. Abbreviations: Am, amygdala; CC, corpus callosum; Hc, hippocampus; MB, mammillary body, PB, pineal body. The nomenclature is adopted from Nieuwenhuys (1985).

Part II: Catecholamines in the Human Hypothalamus

Introductory Remarks

The hypothalamus is a particularly complex part of the brain; it represents only a fragment of the brain volume and yet it is considered as one the most important regions involved in maintaining homeostasis and in the resulting survival of the individual. Consequently, the organization of the hypothalamus is extremely complex; this relatively small brain region comprises numerous nuclei, some of which are well–defined, while others are rather brain areas without definite boundaries comprising loosely organized network of neurons. These nuclei are responsible for a number of functions, including temperature regulation, control of feeding, metabolism, growth, reproduction, and circadian rhythms. Moreover, since the hypothalamus is often described as the chief effector of the limbic system, it can be considered as the main regulatory center of mood and behavior, the link between cortical areas and the distal autonomic regions as well as the hormonal systems, the switchboard between conscious and vegetative. In the next chapters we review the catecholaminergic regulation of major hypothalamic functions; therefore, along with a general overview of the catecholaminergic elements in the central nervous system, it is necessary to provide a detailed description of the catecholaminergic elements in the human hypothalamus.

Hypothalamic Adrenergic System

Immunohistochemical (Ericson et al., 1989; Mezey, 1989; Palkovits et al., 1992; Bohn et al., 1986a) and biochemical (Kopp et al., 1979; Lew et al., 1977; Nagatsu et al., 1977; Moreno et al., 1992) detection of PNMT, the rate limiting enzyme of the adrenaline synthesis, has been commonly used to identify the adrenergic neural elements in the brain of several species including humans. Although adrenaline is widely distributed in the brain (Mefford, 1988), and PNMT-IR perikarya have been described in the limbic system (Mezey, 1989) and the posterior hypothalamus of rats (Ruggiero et al., 1985), there is a common consensus that most of the hypothalamic adrenergic fiber varicosities are supplied by C1 and C2 cell groups located in the medulla oblongata (Astier et al., 1987; Dahlstrom & Fuxe, 1964; Kitahama et al., 1986; Kitahama et al., 1988; Cunningham, Jr. et al., 1990; Sawchenko & Bohn, 1989). Most of these studies also described adrenergic elements in the rat hypothalamus (Ericson et al., 1989; Lew et al., 1977; Moreno et al., 1992; Ruggiero et al., 1985; Mezey, 1989; Palkovits et al., 1992). Due to the lack of commercially available PNMT antibodies that consistently work in human tissue, only the presence of adrenaline in the human hypothalamic regions has been identified mainly by measuring PNMT enzyme activity (Kopp et al., 1979; Nagatsu et al., 1977; Lew et al., 1977). However, with the development of a reliably working PNMT antiserum, the immunohistochemical detection and the subsequent morphological analysis of adrenergic elements became feasible in humans (Dudás et al., 2010).

Recent studies revealed exceptionally small number of thin, PNMT-IR, adrenergic fibers in the human hypothalamus without any detectable perikarya by using immunohistochemistry combined with either silver intensification or tyramide signal amplification (TSA™) methods (Dudás et al., 2010)(Figures 7,8). These axonal varicosities are located mainly in the basal part of the infundibular area oriented parallel with the surface of the 3rd ventricle (Figures 7I-L;8A,C). More superiorly, the PNMT-IR fibers appear to form two distinct subdivisions. [1] Periventricularly arranged PNMT-IR fibers oriented parallel to, but not directly under the ependymal layer, are more abundant in the basal part of the periventricular area, while negligible amount of PNMT-IR fibers can be found in the paraventricular nucleus (PVN). Superiorly to the fornix, PNMT-IR axonal varicosities can be observed in the medial hypothalamic zone (Figure 7I-L). [2] PNMT-IR axons are also present in the basal part of the medial hypothalamus, in the infundibular region. These fibers appear to target the basal infundibulum, and they are generally arranged either parallel with the surface of the 3rd ventricle reaching the infundibulum superiorly to the perifornical area or parallel with the basal surface of the hypothalamus, directly under the pia mater (Figure 7I-L). In the basal part of the lateral hypothalamus, few PNMT-IR axons can be detected, several of them appear to be rostrocaudally arranged (Figure 7J-L).

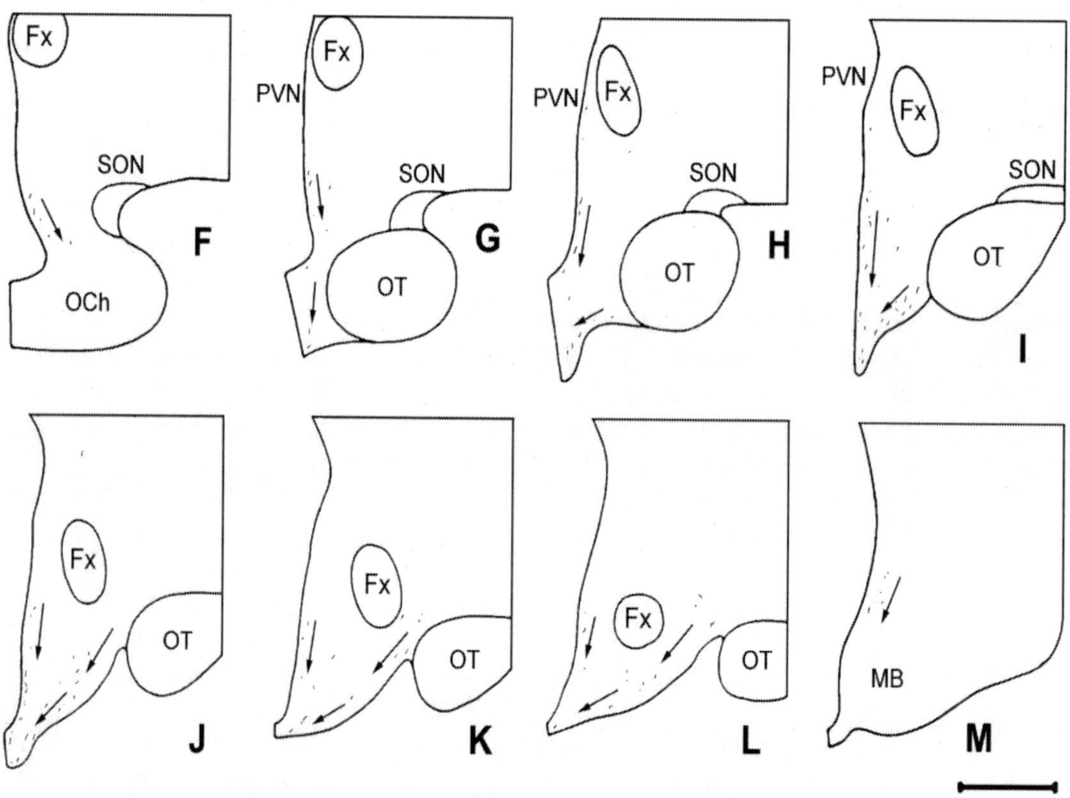

Figure 7. Adrenergic, phenylethanolamine N-methyltransferase-immunoreactive (PNMT-IR) elements are represented by extremely few axonal varicosities without observable perikarya in the human hypothalamus. Each slide (F-M) is the superimposition of eight 30 μm thick sections. Arrows denote the major directions of the PNMT-IR fibers. Abbreviations: AC, anterior commissure; Fx, fornix; MB, mammillary body; OCh, optic chiasm; OT, optic tract; PVN, paraventricular nucleus; SON, supraoptic nucleus. Scale bar: 5000 μm. Reprinted with permission from Elsevier (Dudás et al., 2010).

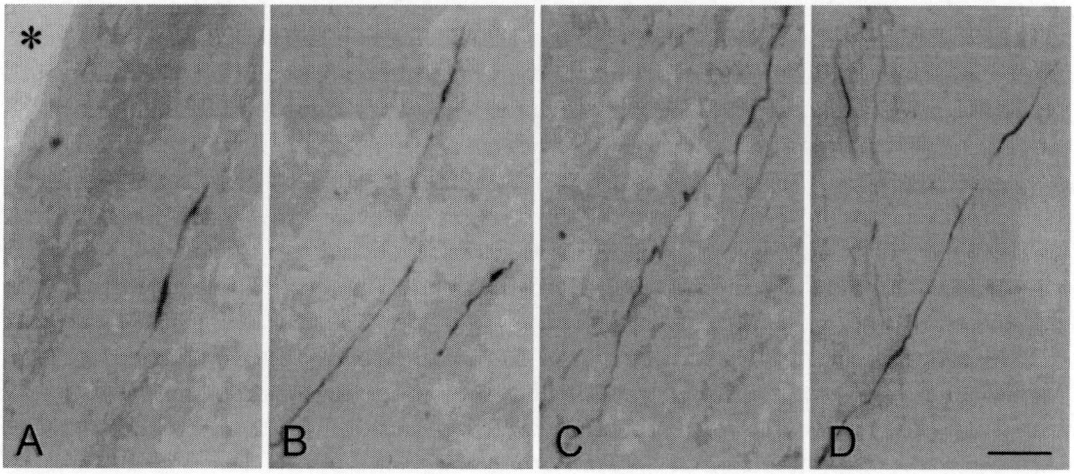

Figure 8. Adrenergic, phenylethanolamine N-methyltransferase-immunoreactive (PNMT-IR) neural elements in the human hypothalamus. Adrenergic axonal varicosities are located mainly in the basal part of the periventricular area adjacent to but not directly under the ependymal layer (A), basal part of the medial hypothalamus (B), and in the infundibular region that mostly correspond to the infundibular nucleus (C). The 3rd ventricle is denoted by the asterisk. For control, PNMT-IR fiber varicosities were detected in the human medulla oblongata using the same anti-PNMT antiserum as used for staining in the hypothalamus (D). Scale bar: 20 μm. Reprinted with permission from Elsevier (Dudás et al., 2010).

The small number of PNMT-IR, adrenergic fiber varicosities in the human hypothalamus (Figures 7,8) is in agreement with biochemical studies reporting significantly smaller adrenaline content in the human hypothalamus comparing to that of other species (Mefford, 1988). Although adrenergic cell bodies have been described in the posterior hypothalamus of the rat (Foster et al., 1985a; Ruggiero et al., 1985), only fiber varicosities without apparent perikarya can be observed in the human hypothalamus, suggesting discernible species differences regarding the distribution of the adrenergic structures. There is a general consensus that the source of the hypothalamic PNMT-IR fibers is the adrenergic C1 and C2 cell groups described in the rhombencephalon of several species (Foster et al., 1985b; Hokfelt et al., 1973; Howe et al., 1980; Ruggiero et al., 1985; Kitahama et al., 1985; Kitahama et al., 1986; Sawchenko & Bohn, 1989). Similarly to the noradrenergic system, these adrenergic axon varicosities are believed to reach the hypothalamus via the medial forebrain bundle, a rather elusive, poorly defined set of antero-posteriorly oriented fibers in the lateral hypothalamus. Indeed, immunohistochemical detection of the PNMT-IR fibers in humans suggests two major pathways that converge towards the medial forebrain bundle. [1] The periventricularly-arranged fibers seemingly targeting the infundibulum/median eminence appear to turn around the fornix superiorly and to run mediolaterally, while [2] fibers at the basal surface of the median eminence run parallel with the pial surface (Figure 8). Both fiber networks appear to converge at the basal part of the lateral hypothalamus suggesting that they may continue their path as part of the medial forebrain bundle.

The exact role of the adrenergic system in the regulation of hypothalamo-hypophyseal functions is yet to be understood. PNMT-IR fibers appear to converge towards the infundibulum and the hypophysial stalk (Figure 7,8C), indicating that these fibers [1] may modulate neurotransmitter systems in the periventricular area/infundibulum/infundibular nucleus, [2] may terminate around portal vessels and release adrenaline into the hypophysial portal blood and/or [3] may continue in the hypophysial stalk and terminate in the posterior hypophysis. Previous studies revealed no morphological associations between the adrenergic elements and other neurotransmitter systems including NPY (Ko et al., 2011) and GHRH (unpublished data). If these adrenergic fibers modulate hypothalamic functions, the phenotype of hypothalamic neurons innervated by them is yet to be identified. The presence of few PNMT-IR axons without well-defined terminal fields located in the superior part of the periventricular area and in the PVN (Figure 7) does not indicate significant adrenergic innervation in these areas. Moreover, the extremely small number of PNMT-IR axonal varicosities in the human hypothalamus suggests that, [1] the far majority of DBH-IR fibers represent noradrenergic structures, and [2] the volume of the hypothalamic structures innervated by the adrenergic system is rather limited, indicating that the adrenergic system does not play a significant role in the regulation of vital hypothalamic functions in humans.

DBH-IR Elements of the Diencephalon

The noradrenergic system in general is represented by neurons with perikarya restricted to A1-A7 cell groups located in the rhombencephalon. The ascending and descending fibers of these neurons innervate essentially all regions of the central nervous system (Dahlstrom & Fuxe, 1964; Nobin & Bjorklund, 1973; Olson et al., 1973a; Olson et al., 1973b). Since DBH is the key and rate-limiting enzyme of the synthesis of noradrenaline that later may be converted to adrenaline by PNMT, DBH is expressed both in the noradrenergic and adrenergic neurons. Moreover, adrenergic and noradrenergic elements can not be distinguished by formaldehyde-induced fluorescence. Thus, the detection of noradrenergic neurons is based on the concept that these structures are immunopositive for DBH but immunonegative for PNMT (note that TH is the rate limiting enzyme in all 3 types of catecholaminergic neurons). The hypothalamus is believed to receive ascending fibers from both adrenergic and noradrenergic neurons from the brain stem (Ericson et al., 1989; Swanson & Hartman, 1975) but these axonal varicosities have not been clearly distinguished from dopaminergic fibers.

Although previous studies reported about DBH-IR structures in the rat hypothalamus (Ericson et al., 1989; Jansen et al., 2003; Swanson & Hartman, 1975), the data describing the pattern of noradrenergic DBH-IR neural elements in humans, or the contribution of DBH-expressing adrenergic structures, are based mostly on detecting the DBH enzyme activity (Nagatsu et al., 1977; Jansen et al., 2003) and only few morphological studies do exist (Dudás et al., 2010). These reports revealed that, similarly to the adrenergic system, hypothalamic DBH-IR structures are represented by thin fiber varicosities; no perikarya can be detected in humans by immunohistochemistry combined with either silver intensification or tyramide signal amplification (TSA™) methods (Dudás et al., 2010)(Figures 9,10). However, the hypothalamic DBH-IR axonal varicosities are much more abundant in humans than the PNMT-IR fibers. The density of DBH-IR structures decreases from medial to lateral direction; the vast majority of them are located in the periventricular and medial hypothalamic zones of the preoptic and tuberal regions, and only a few DBH-IR axon varicosities can be observed in the lateral hypothalamic area. Similar pattern can be observed from anterior to posterior direction; the posterior hypothalamus contains only few DBH-IR fibers (Figure 9).

In front of the lamina terminalis, the number of axons arranged along the diagonal band of Broca gradually decreases laterally and inferiorly (Figure 9A-C). An additional set of fibers are located under the medial part of the anterior commissure (Figure 9A-D), while no substantial amount of axons can be seen in the lateral septal area. In the lamina terminalis itself, few DBH-IR axonal varicosities can be observed, generally oriented parallel with the surface of the 3rd ventricle (Figure 9D). A relatively dense fiber network with varicosities, commonly oriented supero-inferiorly, occupies the periventricular zone of the preoptic area (Figure 9E,F). In the tuberal region, the density of the DBH-IR axonal varicosities is decreasing from medial to lateral direction; fibers are located mostly in the periventricular and medial hypothalamic zones, generally stretched between the infundibulum and the PVN (Figure 9H-L). A dense fiber network, with axonal varicosities running in every direction, can be observed in the PVN, while more superiorly, the periventricular fibers are gradually decreasing in number (Figure 9G-I). The basal part of the infundibulum, including the infundibular nucleus, appears to receive a relatively dense innervation of DBH-IR axons, generally oriented parallel with the ependymal surface (Figure 9H-L). A relatively well-defined fiber network can be observed at the basal part of the medial hypothalamus below the fornix, at the lateral zone of the median eminence close to the optic tract (Figure 9J-L), and in the supraoptic nucleus (SON; Figure 9F-I). In contrast to the abundance of the DBH-IR axonal varicosities in the periventricular and medial hypothalamic areas, the fibers located in the medial part of the lateral hypothalamus are scarce, concentrated characteristically in the basal hypothalamic region and around the lateral side of the fornix (Figure 9E-L). Periventricularly arranged DBH-IR axonal varicosities can be observed in the posterior hypothalamus (Figure 9M-P). Scattered fibers are located medially and superiorly around the mammillary body, while no substantial amount of DBH-IR fibers can be detected in the mammillary nuclei, fornix and anterior commissure (Figure 9M-P).

Since the volume of the PNMT-IR fibers is rather limited in the human hypothalamus, it is conceivable that the vast majority of the DBH-IR fiber varicosities represent noradrenergic structures. The source of the hypothalamic noradrenergic fibers is believed to be the noradrenergic perikarya restricted to the pontine and medullary tegmental regions in several species, including humans. The ascending noradrenergic fibers, similarly to the adrenergic system, reach the hypothalamus most likely via the medial forebrain bundle running anteroposteriorly in the lateral hypothalamic region. Indeed, numerous DBH-IR fiber varicosities can be detected in the medial part of the lateral hypothalamus.

A relatively dense DBH-IR axonal network can be detected in the PVN (Jansen et al., 2003) and SON (Figure 9F-I) as well as in the basal part of the infundibulum that includes the infundibular nucleus (Dudás et al., 2010)(Figures 9I-L,10D). The abundance of the DBH-IR neuronal elements in these regions, although not comparable to the density of the TH-IR structures in the same areas, indicates that noradrenaline in DBH-IR fibers plays a significant regulatory role on neurotransmitter systems located in the PVN, SON and infundibulum. In addition, noradrenergic axonal varicosities may terminate around portal vessels or may continue in the hypophysial stalk and innervate hypophysial structures in human. If these descending fibers continue in the hypophysis, they probably target the adenohypophysis, since the posterior lobe of the hypophysis contains TH-IR fibers only without any detectable DBH-IR in pig (Leshin et al., 1996).

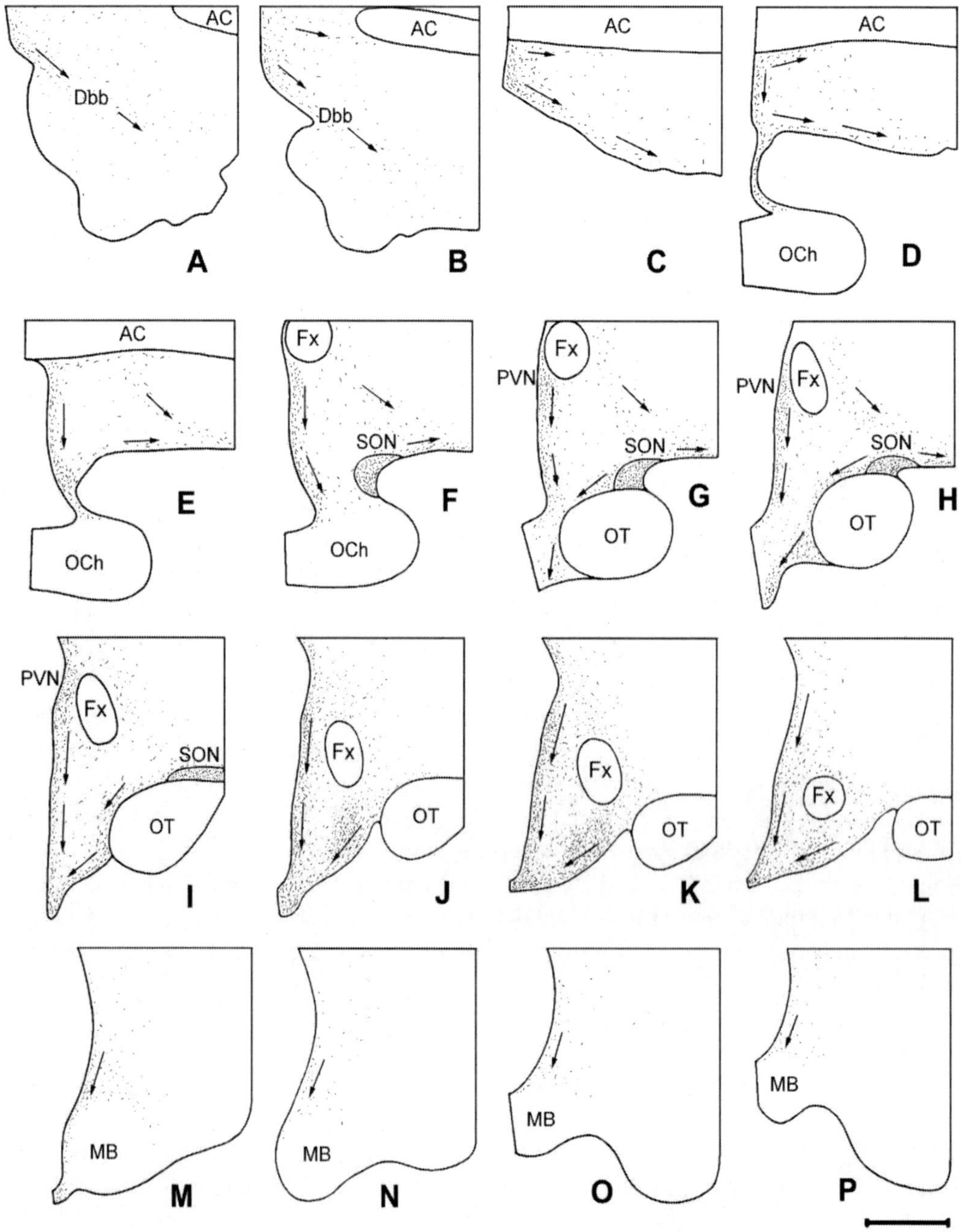

Figure 9. Noradrenergic or adrenergic, dopamine-beta hydroxylase-immunoreactive (DBH-IR) neural elements are represented exclusively by axonal varicosities in the human hypothalamus without discernible perikarya. Each slide (A-P) is the superimposition of eight 30 μm thick sections. Arrows denote the major directions of the DBH-IR fibers. Abbreviations: AC, anterior commissure; Dbb, diagonal band of Broca; Fx, fornix; MB, mammillary body; OCh, optic chiasm; OT, optic tract; PVN, paraventricular nucleus; SON, supraoptic nucleus. Scale bar: 5000 μm. Reprinted with permission from Elsevier (Dudás et al., 2010).

Since the PVN and SON contain an insignificant number of PNMT-IR axons, DBH-IR fibers in these regions appear to represent noradrenergic structures exclusively. Similarly, the diagonal band of Broca and the lamina terminalis contain a significant number of DBH-IR axonal varicosities, but no PNMT-IR structures, indicating that these fibers are indeed noradrenergic.

TH-IR Elements of the Diencephalon

The catecholaminergic, TH-IR system of the human hypothalamus is represented by both perikarya and axonal varicosities (Dudás & Merchenthaler, 2001; Dudás & Merchenthaler, 2006). Previous studies utilizing various techniques identified three catecholaminergic cell groups - A11, A12, A14 - in the hypothalamus (Bjorklund & Nobin, 1973; Felten et al., 1974; Felten, 1976; Felten & Sladek, Jr., 1983; Ungerstedt, 1971). Consequently, since no adrenergic and noradrenergic cell bodies can be detected in the human hypothalamus, it is plausible that the hypothalamic TH-IR cell bodies are all dopaminergic.

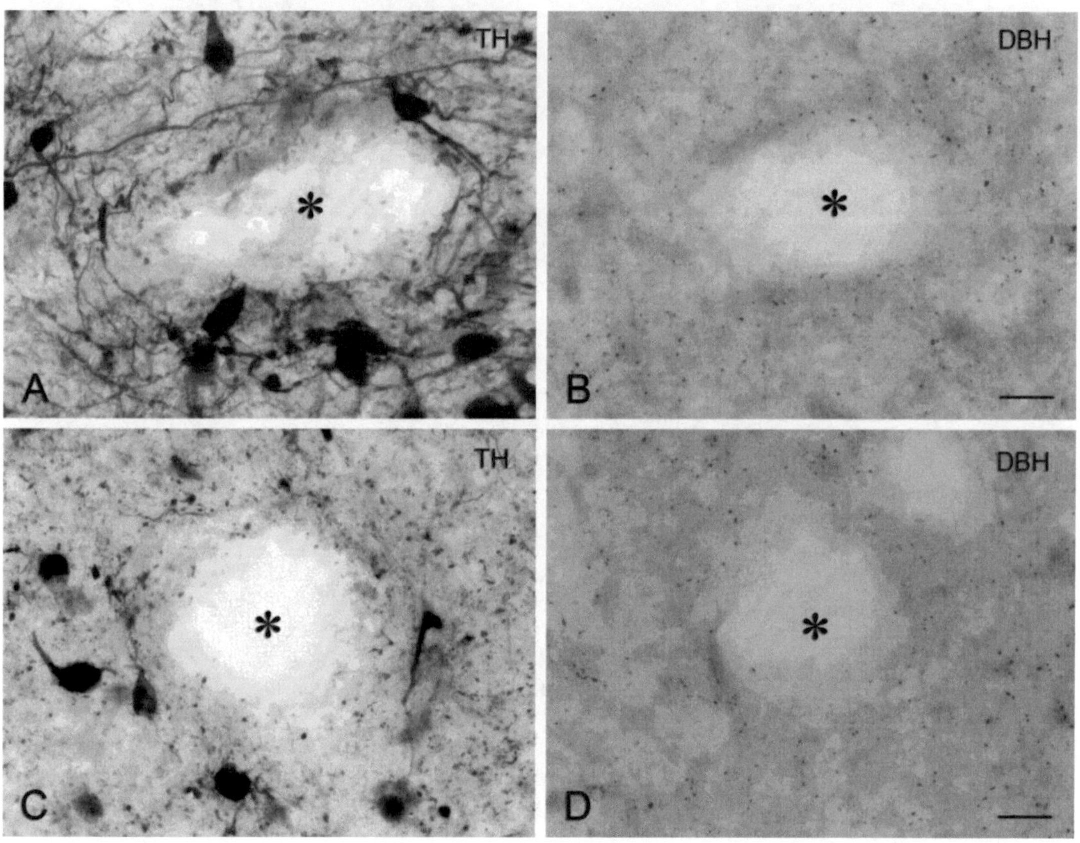

Figure 10. Consecutive sections show catecholaminergic, tyrosine hydroxylase (TH)-immunoreactive (IR)(A,C) and noradrenergic/adrenergic, dopamine-beta hydroxylase (DBH)-IR (B,D) neural elements in the PVN (A,B) and at the periventricular infundibular area (C,D) of the human hypothalamus. Inserts A-B and C-D illustrate catecholaminergic structures surrounding the same blood vessel (asterisk). Scale bar: 40 μm. Reprinted with permission from Elsevier (Dudás et al., 2010).

The majority of the TH-IR perikarya are located periventricularly in the preoptic and tuberal areas, and in the infundibulum/median eminence (Figures 10A,C,11); these perikarya correspond mostly to the previously described cell group A14 and A12, respectively. TH-IR perikarya are densely packed in the PVN and SON, while only a few TH-IR cell bodies are present in the caudal hypothalamus, corresponding to the posterior hypothalamic cell group A11 (Figure 11). In front of the lamina terminalis, a small number of immunoreactive cells can be observed at the medial-dorsal zone of the septal area; no perikarya can be found along the diagonal band of Broca and in the lamina terminalis itself. In the preoptic region, TH-IR neurons are arranged periventricularly and ventrally, with few perikarya located at the bottom of the optic recess on the dorsal surface of the optic chiasm (Figure 11).

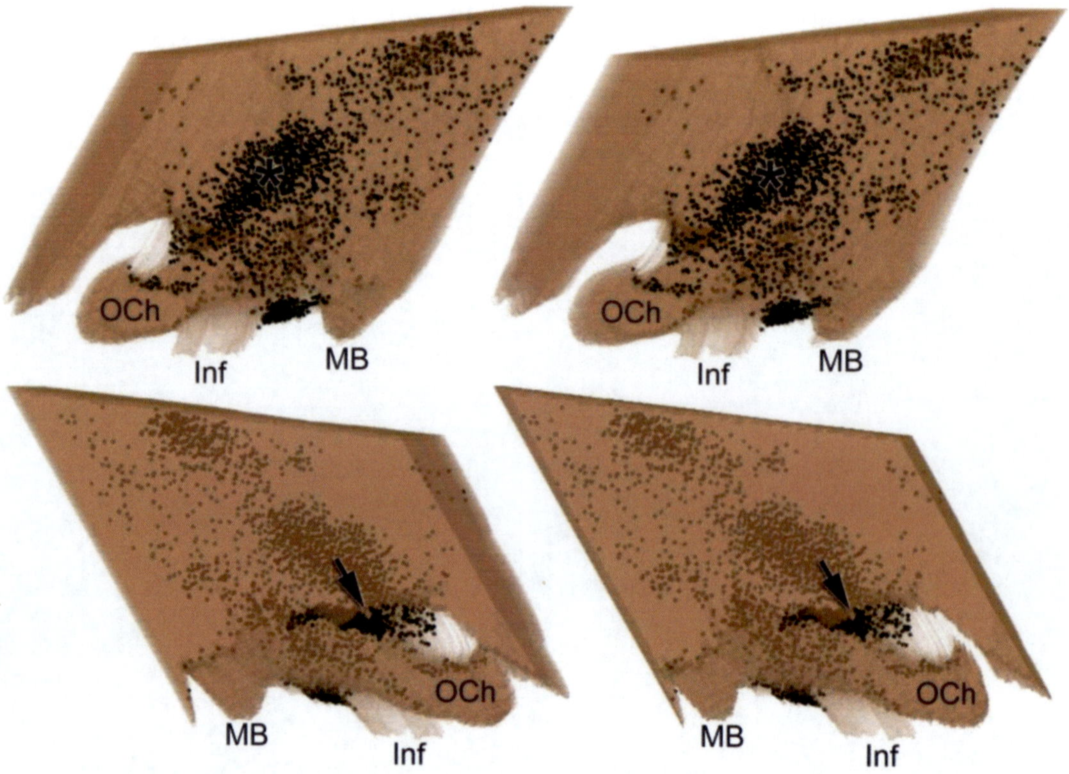

Figure 11. Distribution of catecholaminergic, tyrosine hydroxylase-immunoreactive (TH-IR) perikarya in the human hypothalamus from medial aspect (upper images) and lateral aspect (lower images). Since adrenergic and noradrenergic cell bodies can not be detected in the human hypothalamus, it is plausible that the hypothalamic TH-IR cell bodies are all dopaminergic. Stereoscopic images can be seen using U or parallel vision. The eyes are relaxed to look into the distance until the pair of the images fuse, and then refocused by the brain. With this technique a 3D hypothalamus can be seen on the figure, appearing to float in front of the paper, with the immunolabelled perikarya (marked by black dots) discernible at different depth. The optimal viewing distance is about 20 inches from the paper surface (average reading distance). If the separation is too great for the eyes (double vision), move the picture away and the required viewing angle will decrease. Abbreviations: Inf: infundibulum; MB, mammillary body; OCh, optic chiasm. Asterisks denote the paraventricular nucleus and arrows point to the supraoptic nucleus.

In the tuberal region, TH-IR perikarya are found in the basal part of the periventricular area (Figure 10A,C); a substantial number of perikarya can be observed in the median eminence, while the basal part of the infundibulum contains a relatively small number of TH-IR cells (Figure 11). The posterior hypothalamus contains relatively few neurons that are either periventricularly arranged or surround the mammillary body (Figure 11). Morphologically, the TH-IR neurons are typically fusiform, with thin cell bodies and two processes emanating from their opposite poles; multipolar neurons are located mainly in the PVN and SON (Figure 12). TH-IR axonal varicosities form a dense network primarily in the periventricular and infundibular areas and they appear primarily as relatively thick fiber varicosities (Figure 10A,C). Additionally, thin, TH-IR fibers were also detected primarily in the basal part of the periventricular and medial hypothalamic areas (Figure 10A,C), in the SON and in the medial zone of the lateral hypothalamus, although these were often obscured by the thicker fibers and the TH-IR perikarya. Labeled axon varicosities can be also observed in the lateral hypothalamus and in the septal area (Figure 11). Since DBH-IR and PNMT-IR neuronal elements are almost exclusively represented by thin fiber varicosities (Figures 8,10B,D), it is conceivable that the thick TH-IR fibers represent primarily dopaminergic axonal varicosities while the thin ones are mostly either noradrenergic or adrenergic.

In the PVN and SON, TH-IR axonal varicosities often form well-defined terminal fields around the contours of fusiform neurons that are apparently not TH-positive (Dudás et al., 2006; Dudás & Merchenthaler, 2001)(Figure 12A). Since PNMT-IR structures do not participate in the formation of such structures, instead they run straight, often parallel with the surface of the 3rd ventricle forming numerous varicosities along their course (Figure 8), it is conceivable that the detected TH-IR fiber baskets must be either noradrenergic or dopaminergic. Since previous studies revealed TH-IR fibers forming similar terminal fields around oxytocinergic (Semeniken et al., 2009) and vasopressinergic neurons (Dudás et al., 2006), it is likely that these fiber baskets represent the morphological substrate of norepinephrine- or dopamine-modulated oxytocin and vasopressin release.

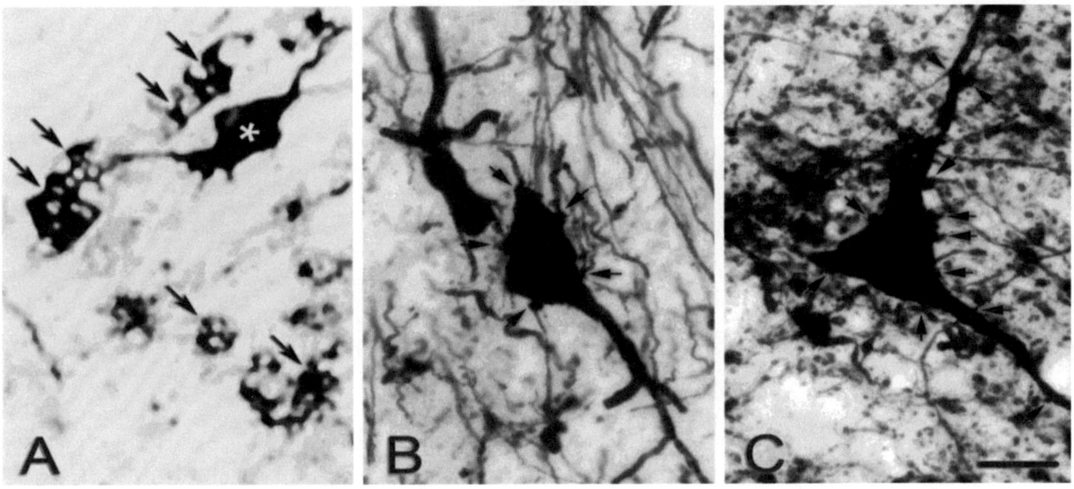

Figure 12. Tyrosine hydroxylase-immunoreactive (TH-IR) elements in the human hypothalamus. Catecholaminergic fiber baskets (arrows) formed by TH-IR axon varicosities emanating from TH-IR perikarya (asterisk) in the SON (A). TH-IR neurons receive abutting TH-IR axonal varicosities (arrowheads) in the PVN (B) and SON (C). Scale bar: 20 μm.

The source of the hypothalamic TH-IR axonal varicosities is not entirely clear in humans. Although previous studies described TH-IR fibers that also exhibited dopamine transporter (DAT)-immunoreactivity in humans (Ciliax et al., 1999), hypothalamic neurons appear to have no detectable DAT-immunoreactivity. These finding suggest that at least some of these dopaminergic, DAT-IR fibers may originate from mesencephalic areas and/or some hypothalamic neurons may have different mechanisms to regulate their extracellular dopamine levels (Ciliax et al., 1999).

Associations between the Catecholaminergic Elements

Double label immunohistochemistry visualizing first DBH-IR and then TH-IR neuronal elements in the hypothalamus revealed that DBH-IR fiber varicosities often surround TH-IR, but DBH-negative, dopaminergic perikarya in the PVN (Figure 13A), SON, infundibulum/infundibular nucleus (Figure 13B) and in the periventricular zone of the hypothalamus (Figure 13C).

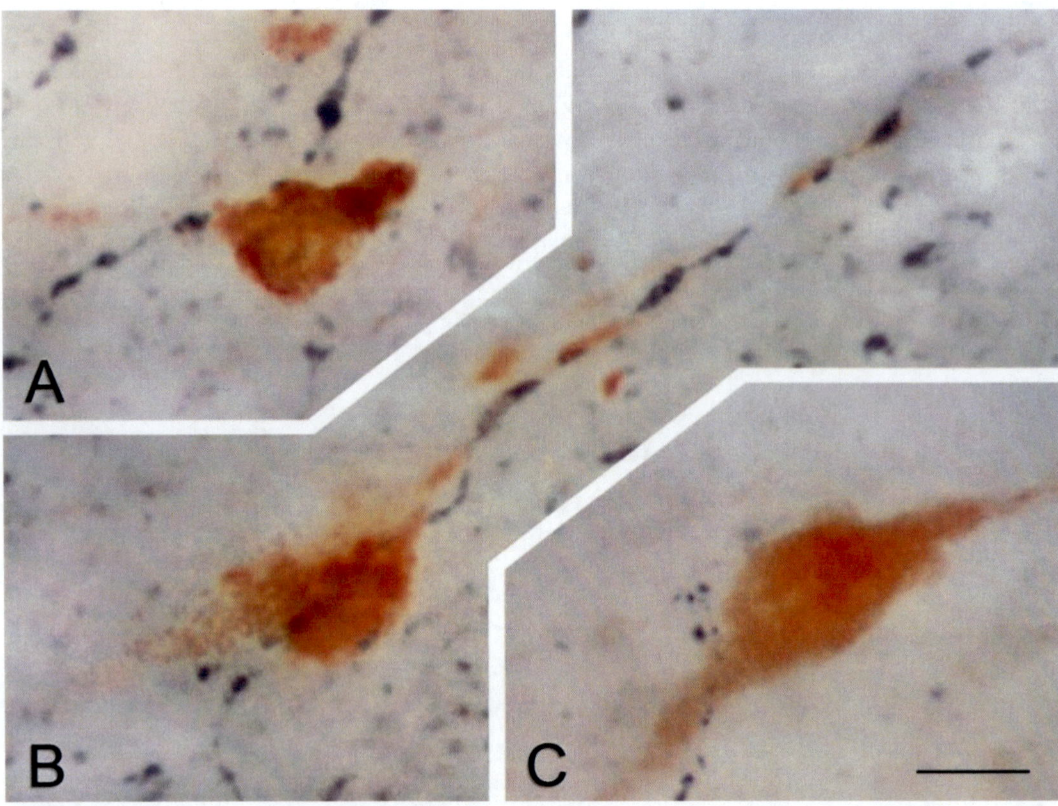

Figure 13. Double label immunohistochemistry revealed dopamine-beta hydroxylase (DBH)-immunoreactive (IR) fiber varicosities (black) surrounding dopaminergic perikarya (brown) in the PVN (A), infundibulum (B) and the SON (C). Since the first immunohistochemical signal, that was used to reveal the DBH-IR elements, was silver-intensified, the second immunohistochemical signal reveals those TH-IR elements only that do not contain DBH, thus being dopaminergic. Scale bar: 20 μm. Reprinted with permission from Elsevier (Dudás et al., 2010).

Despite the frequent close appositions, only few juxtapositions can be observed between the dopaminergic and the DBH-IR neurotransmitter systems, suggesting insignificant adrenergic/noradrenergic control on the dopaminergic system. In addition to these findings, no PNMT-IR fiber varicosities are located in the vicinity of DBH-IR or TH-IR neuronal elements (Dudás et al., 2010). In contrast, juxtapositions between TH-IR fibers and perikarya is relatively common in the tuberal region, PVN and SON (Figure 12B,C). Due to the small number of DBH-TH associations, the majority of these TH-TH contacts may represent dopaminergic autocontrol in humans. Since the density of DBH-IR neural elements is significantly less than that of the TH-IR structures, it is plausible that the far majority of the juxtapositions previously described between the TH-IR axonal varicosities and the GnRH- (Dudás & Merchenthaler, 2001), GHRH- (unpublished data) and NPY-IR perikarya (Ko et al., 2011) represent dopaminergic-peptidergic synapses.

Summary and Conclusion

- Since no DBH- and PNMT-IR cell bodies can be detected in the human hypothalamus, it is conceivable that all of the hypothalamic catecholaminergic perikarya represent dopaminergic neurons in humans.
- The density of the hypothalamic DBH- and PNMT-IR axon varicosities is significantly less than that of the TH-IR fibers, indicating that the majority of the catecholaminergic fibers are dopaminergic in the human hypothalamus.
- Due to the extremely small number of detectable PNMT-IR, adrenergic structures in the human hypothalamus, the DBH-IR fibers appear to represent almost exclusively noradrenergic neuronal processes.
- These findings suggest that the juxtapositions between the TH-IR and numerous peptidergic systems revealed by previous reports indicate primarily dopaminergic synapses.

References

Amaral, D. G. & Sinnamon, H. M. (1977). The locus coeruleus: neurobiology of a central noradrenergic nucleus. *Prog.Neurobiol., 9,* 147-196.

Armstrong, D. M., Ross, C. A., Pickel, V. M., Joh, T. H., & Reis, D. J. (1982). Distribution of dopamine-, noradrenaline-, and adrenaline-containing cell bodies in the rat medulla oblongata: demonstrated by the immunocytochemical localization of catecholamine biosynthetic enzymes. *J Comp Neurol, 212,* 173-187.

Astier, B., Kitahama, K., Denoroy, L., Jouvet, M., & Renaud, B. (1987). Immunohistochemical evidence for the adrenergic medullary longitudinal bundle as a major ascending pathway to the hypothalamus. *Neurosci.Lett., 78,* 241-246.

Axelsson, S., Bjorklund, A., Falck, B., Lindvall, O., & Svensson, L. A. (1973). Glyoxylic acid condensation: a new fluorescence method for the histochemical demonstration of biogenic monoamines. *Acta Physiol Scand., 87,* 57-62.

Bernstein-Goral, H. & Bohn, M. C. (1989) Phenylethanolamine N-methyltransferase-immunoreactive terminals synapse on adrenal preganglionic neurons in rat spinal cord. *Neuroscience, 32,* 521-538.

Bjorklund, A., Lindvall, O., & Nobin, A. (1975). Evidence of an incerto-hypothalamic dopamine neurone system in the rat. *Brain Res., 89,* 29-42.

Bjorklund, A. & Nobin, A. (1973). Fluorescence histochemical and microspectrofluorometric mapping of dopamine and noradrenaline cell groups in the rat diencephalon. *Brain Res., 51,* 193-205.

Bjorklund, A. & Skagerberg, G. (1979). Evidence for a major spinal cord projection from the diencephalic A11 dopamine cell group in the rat using transmitter-specific fluorescent retrograde tracing. *Brain Res., 177,* 170-175.

Bohn, M. C., Goldstein, M., & Black, I. B. (1986a). Expression and development of phenylethanolamine N-methyltransferase (PNMT) in rat brain stem: studies with glucocorticoids. *Dev.Biol., 114,* 180-193.

Ciliax, B. J., Drash, G. W., Staley, J. K., Haber, S., Mobley, C. J., Miller, G. W. et al. (1999). Immunocytochemical localization of the dopamine transporter in human brain. *J.Comp Neurol., 409,* 38-56.

Cunningham, E. T., Jr., Bohn, M. C., & Sawchenko, P. E. (1990). Organization of adrenergic inputs to the paraventricular and supraoptic nuclei of the hypothalamus in the rat. *J.Comp Neurol., 292,* 651-667.

Dahlstrom, A. & Fuxe, K. (1964). Localization of monoamines in the lower brain stem. *Experientia, 20,* 398-399.

Dudás, B., Baker, M., Rotoli, G., Grignol, G., Bohn, M. C., & Merchenthaler, I. (2010). Distribution and morphology of the catecholaminergic neural elements in the human hypothalamus. *Neuroscience, 171,* 187-195.

Dudás, B. & Merchenthaler, I. (2001). Catecholaminergic axons innervate LH-releasing hormone immunoreactive neurons of the human diencephalon. *J.Clin.Endocrinol.Metab, 86,* 5620-5626.

Dudás, B. & Merchenthaler, I. (2006). Three-dimensional representation of the neurotransmitter systems of the human hypothalamus: inputs of the gonadotrophin hormone-releasing hormone neuronal system. *J.Neuroendocrinol., 18,* 79-95.

Dudás, B., Semeniken, K. R., & Merchenthaler, I. (2006). Morphological substrate of the catecholaminergic input of the vasopressin neuronal system in humans. *J.Neuroendocrinol., 18,* 895-901.

Ericson, H., Blomqvist, A., & Kohler, C. (1989). Brainstem afferents to the tuberomammillary nucleus in the rat brain with special reference to monoaminergic innervation. *J.Comp Neurol., 281,* 169-192.

Fallon, J. H., Koziell, D. A., & Moore, R. Y. (1978). Catecholamine innervation of the basal forebrain. II. Amygdala, suprarhinal cortex and entorhinal cortex. *J Comp Neurol, 180,* 509-532.

Fallon, J. H. & Moore, R. Y. (1978a). Catecholamine innervation of the basal forebrain. III. Olfactory bulb, anterior olfactory nuclei, olfactory tubercle and piriform cortex. *J Comp Neurol, 180,* 533-544.

Fallon, J. H. & Moore, R. Y. (1978b). Catecholamine innervation of the basal forebrain. IV. Topography of the dopamine projection to the basal forebrain and neostriatum. *J Comp Neurol, 180,* 545-580.

Felten, D. L. (1976). Catecholamine neurons in the squirrel monkey hypothalamus. *J.Neural Transm., 39,* 269-280.

Felten, D. L., Laties, A. M., & Carpenter, M. B. (1974). Monoamine-containing cell bodies in the squirrel monkey brain. *Am.J.Anat., 139,* 153-165.

Felten, D. L. & Sladek, J. R., Jr. (1983). Monoamine distribution in primate brain V. Monoaminergic nuclei: anatomy, pathways and local organization. *Brain Res.Bull., 10,* 171-284.

Foster, G. A., Hokfelt, T., Coyle, J. T., & Goldstein, M. (1985a). Immunohistochemical evidence for phenylethanolamine-N-methyltransferase-positive/tyrosine hydroxylase-negative neurones in the retina and the posterior hypothalamus of the rat. *Brain Res, 330,* 183-188.

Foster, G. A., Schultzberg, M., Goldstein, M., & Hokfelt, T. (1985b). Ontogeny of phenylethanolamine N-methyltransferase- and tyrosine hydroxylase-like immunoreactivity in presumptive adrenaline neurones of the foetal rat central nervous system. *J.Comp Neurol., 236,* 348-381.

Hokfelt, T., Fuxe, K., Goldstein, M., & Johansson, O. (1973). Evidence for adrenaline neurons in the rat brain. *Acta Physiol Scand., 89,* 286-288.

Hokfelt, T., Johansson, O., Fuxe, K., Goldstein, M., & Park, D. (1976). Immunohistochemical studies on the localization and distribution of monoamine neuron systems in the rat brain. I. Tyrosine hydroxylase in the mes- and diencephalon. *Med.Biol., 54,* 427-453.

Hokfelt, T., Phillipson, O., & Goldstein, M. (1979). Evidence for a dopaminergic pathway in the rat descending from the A11 cell group to the spinal cord. *Acta Physiol Scand., 107,* 393-395.

Howe, P. R., Costa, M., Furness, J. B., & Chalmers, J. P. (1980). Simultaneous demonstration of phenylethanolamine N-methyltransferase immunofluorescent and catecholamine fluorescent nerve cell bodies in the rat medulla oblongata. *Neuroscience, 5,* 2229-2238.

Jaeger, C. B., Ruggiero, D. A., Albert, V. R., Park, D. H., Joh, T. H., & Reis, D. J. (1984). Aromatic L-amino acid decarboxylase in the rat brain: immunocytochemical localization in neurons of the brain stem. *Neuroscience, 11,* 691-713.

Jansen, A. S., Schmidt, E. D., Voorn, P., & Tilders, F. J. (2003). Substance induced plasticity in noradrenergic innervation of the paraventricular hypothalamic nucleus. *Eur.J.Neurosci., 17,* 298-306.

Kitahama, K., Denoroy, L., Berod, A., & Jouvet, M. (1986). Distribution of PNMT-immunoreactive neurons in the cat medulla oblongata. *Brain Res Bull., 17,* 197-208.

Kitahama, K., Denoroy, L., Goldstein, M., Jouvet, M., & Pearson, J. (1988). Immunohistochemistry of tyrosine hydroxylase and phenylethanolamine N-methyltransferase in the human brain stem: description of adrenergic perikarya and characterization of longitudinal catecholaminergic pathways. *Neuroscience, 25,* 97-111.

Kitahama, K., Luppi, P. H., Berod, A., Goldstein, M., & Jouvet, M. (1987). Localization of tyrosine hydroxylase-immunoreactive neurons in the cat hypothalamus, with special reference to fluorescence histochemistry. *J.Comp Neurol., 262,* 578-593.

Kitahama, K., Pearson, J., Denoroy, L., Kopp, N., Ulrich, J., Maeda, T. et al. (1985). Adrenergic neurons in human brain demonstrated by immunohistochemistry with antibodies to phenylethanolamine-N-methyltransferase (PNMT): discovery of a new group in the nucleus tractus solitarius. *Neurosci.Lett., 53,* 303-308.

Ko, L., Rotoli, G., Grignol, G., Hu, W., Merchenthaler, I., & Dudás, B. A putative morphological substrate of the catecholamine-influenced NPY release in the human hypothalamus. *Neuropeptides,* (in press).

Kopp, N., Denoroy, L., Renaud, B., Pujol, J. F., Tabib, A., & Tommasi, M. (1979). Distribution of adrenaline-synthesizing enzyme activity in the human brain. *J.Neurol.Sci., 41,* 397-409.

Leshin, L. S., Kraeling, R. R., Kineman, R. D., Barb, C. R., & Rampacek, G. B. (1996). Immunocytochemical distribution of catecholamine-synthesizing neurons in the hypothalamus and pituitary gland of pigs: tyrosine hydroxylase and dopamine-beta-hydroxylase. *J.Comp Neurol., 364,* 151-168.

Lew, J. Y., Matsumoto, Y., Pearson, J., Goldstein, M., Hokfelt, T., & Fuxe, K. (1977). Localization and characterization of phenylethanolamine N-methyl transferase in the brain of various mammalian species. *Brain Res, 119,* 199-210.

Li, Y. W., Halliday, G. M., Joh, T. H., Geffen, L. B., & Blessing, W. W. (1988). Tyrosine hydroxylase-containing neurons in the supraoptic and paraventricular nuclei of the adult human. *Brain Res, 461,* 75-86.

Lindvall, O. & Bjorklund, A. (1974). The organization of the ascending catecholamine neuron systems in the rat brain as revealed by the glyoxylic acid fluorescence method. *Acta Physiol Scand.Suppl, 412,* 1-48.

Lindvall, O., Bjorklund, A., & Skagerberg, G. (1983). Dopamine-containing neurons in the spinal cord: anatomy and some functional aspects. *Ann.Neurol, 14,* 255-260.

Lindvall, O., Bjorklund, A., & Skagerberg, G. (1984). Selective histochemical demonstration of dopamine terminal systems in rat di- and telencephalon: new evidence for dopaminergic innervation of hypothalamic neurosecretory nuclei. *Brain Res., 306,* 19-30.

Lindvall, O. & Stenevi, U. (1978). Dopamine and noradrenaline neurons projecting to the septal area in the rat. *Cell Tissue Res., 190,* 383-407.

Mefford, I. N. (1988). Epinephrine in mammalian brain. *Prog. Neuropsychopharmacol. Biol.Psychiatry, 12,* 365-388.

Mezey, E. (1989). Phenylethanolamine N-methyltransferase-containing neurons in the limbic system of the young rat. *Proc.Natl.Acad.Sci.U.S.A, 86,* 347-351.

Miachon, S., Berod, A., Leger, L., Chat, M., Hartman, B., & Pujol, J. F. (1984). Identification of catecholamine cell bodies in the pons and pons-mesencephalon junction of the cat brain, using tyrosine hydroxylase and dopamine-beta-hydroxylase immunohistochemistry. *Brain Res., 305,* 369-374.

Moore, R. Y. (1978). Catecholamin innervation of the basal forebrain. I. The septal area. *J Comp Neurol, 177,* 665-684.

Moore, R. Y. & Bloom, F. E. (1978). Central catecholamine neuron systems: anatomy and physiology of the dopamine systems. *Annu.Rev.Neurosci., 1,* 129-169.

Moreno, M. L., Villanua, M. A., & Esquifino, A. I. (1992). Serum prolactin and luteinizing hormone levels and the activities of hypothalamic monoamine oxidase A and B and phenylethanolamine-N-methyl transferase are changed during sexual maturation in male rats treated neonatally with melatonin. *J.Pineal Res, 13,* 167-173.

Nagatsu, T., Kato, T., Numata, Y., Ikuta, K., & Sano, M. (1977). Phenylethanolamine N-methyltransferase and other enzymes of catecholamine metabolism in human brain. *Clin.Chim.Acta, 75,* 221-232.

Nieuwenhuys, R. (1985). *Chemoarchitecture of the brain.* Berlin Heidelberg: Springer-Verlag.

Nobin, A. & Bjorklund, A. (1973). Topography of the monoamine neuron systems in the human brain as revealed in fetuses. *Acta Physiol Scand.Suppl, 388,* 1-40.

Ochi, J. & Shimizu, K. (1978). Occurrence of dopamine-containing neurons in the midbrain raphe nuclei of the rat. *Neurosci.Lett., 8,* 317-320.

Olson, L., Boreus, L. O., & Seiger, A. (1973a). Histochemical demonstration and mapping of 5-hydroxytryptamine- and catecholamine-containing neuron systems in the human fetal brain. *Z.Anat.Entwicklungsgesch., 139,* 259-282.

Olson, L., Nystrom, B., & Seiger, A. (1973b). Monoamine fluorescence histochemistry of human post mortem brain. *Brain Res., 63,* 231-247.

Palkovits, M., Mezey, E., Skirboll, L. R., & Hokfelt, T. (1992). Adrenergic projections from the lower brainstem to the hypothalamic paraventricular nucleus, the lateral hypothalamic area and the central nucleus of the amygdala in rats. *J.Chem.Neuroanat., 5,* 407-415.

Panayotacopoulou, M. T., Guntern, R., Bouras, C., Issidorides, M. R., & Constantinidis, J. (1991). Tyrosine hydroxylase-immunoreactive neurons in paraventricular and supraoptic nuclei of the human brain demonstrated by a method adapted to prolonged formalin fixation. *J.Neurosci.Methods, 39,* 39-44.

Panayotacopoulou, M. T., Malidelis, Y., van, H. J., Unmehopa, U., & Swaab, D. (2005). Individual differences in the expression of tyrosine hydroxylase mRNA in neurosecretory neurons of the human paraventricular and supraoptic nuclei: positive correlation with vasopressin mRNA. *Neuroendocrinology, 81,* 329-338.

Ruggiero, D. A., Ross, C. A., Anwar, M., Park, D. H., Joh, T. H., & Reis, D. J. (1985). Distribution of neurons containing phenylethanolamine N-methyltransferase in medulla and hypothalamus of rat. *J.Comp Neurol., 239,* 127-154.

Sawchenko, P. E. & Bohn, M. C. (1989). Glucocorticoid receptor-immunoreactivity in C1, C2, and C3 adrenergic neurons that project to the hypothalamus or to the spinal cord in the rat. *J.Comp Neurol., 285,* 107-116.

Semeniken, K., Merchenthaler, I., Hu, W., & Dudás, B. (2009). Catecholaminergic input to the oxytocin neurosecretory system in the human hypothalamus. *J.Chem.Neuroanat., 37,* 229-233.

Skagerberg, G., Bjorklund, A., Lindvall, O., & Schmidt, R. H. (1982). Origin and termination of the diencephalo-spinal dopamine system in the rat. *Brain Res.Bull., 9,* 237-244.

Skagerberg, G., Lindvall, O., & Bjorklund, A. (1984). Origin, course and termination of the mesohabenular dopamine pathway in the rat. *Brain Res., 307,* 99-108.

Swanson, L. W. (1982). The projections of the ventral tegmental area and adjacent regions: a combined fluorescent retrograde tracer and immunofluorescence study in the rat. *Brain Res.Bull., 9,* 321-353.

Swanson, L. W. & Hartman, B. K. (1975). The central adrenergic system. An immunofluorescence study of the location of cell bodies and their efferent connections in the rat utilizing dopamine-beta-hydroxylase as a marker. *J.Comp Neurol., 163,* 467-505.

Ungerstedt, U. (1971). Stereotaxic mapping of the monoamine pathways in the rat brain. *Acta Physiol Scand.Suppl, 367,* 1-48.

Zoli, M., Agnati, L. F., Tinner, B., Steinbusch, H. W., & Fuxe, K. (1993). Distribution of dopamine-immunoreactive neurons and their relationships to transmitter and hypothalamic hormone-immunoreactive neuronal systems in the rat mediobasal hypothalamus. A morphometric and microdensitometric analysis. *J.Chem.Neuroanat., 6,* 293-310.

In: The Central Catecholaminergic System
Editor: Bertalan Dudás

ISBN: 978-1-63117-937-2

Chapter 2

Biochemistry of Catecholamines

Thomas D. Corso and Bertalan Dudás

Synthesis

Catecholamines are widely distributed molecules in the central nervous system with a number of pivotal functions, and they are a class of monoamines that contain a catechol and an amine (Figure 1). The catechols consist of an aromatic ring with an *ortho* pair of phenolic hydroxyl groups (Morrison & Boyd, 1973).

Catechol 3,4-dihydroxy benzylamine

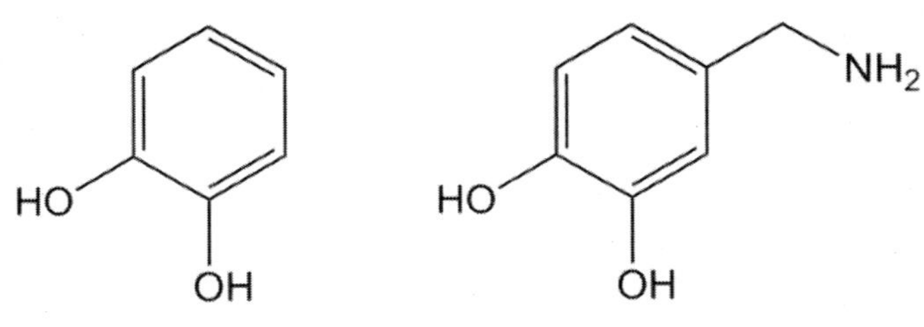

Figure 1. Depiction of the molecule catechol and an example of a catecholamine known as 3,4-dihydroxy benzylamine (DHBA). DHBA is a non-biologically occurring molecule used as a common internal standard in HPLC analysis of the catecholamines.

The most biologically relevant catecholamines are dopamine, noradrenaline (also known as norepinephrine), and adrenaline (also known as epinephrine). For consistency with the other chapters in this book, the terms noradrenaline and adrenaline will be used. These catecholamines are derived from the essential amino acid phenylalanine or the non-essential amino acid tyrosine (Nelson & Cox, 2013). The synthesis of the three most important catecholamines from the amino acid phenylalanine is depicted in Figure 2.

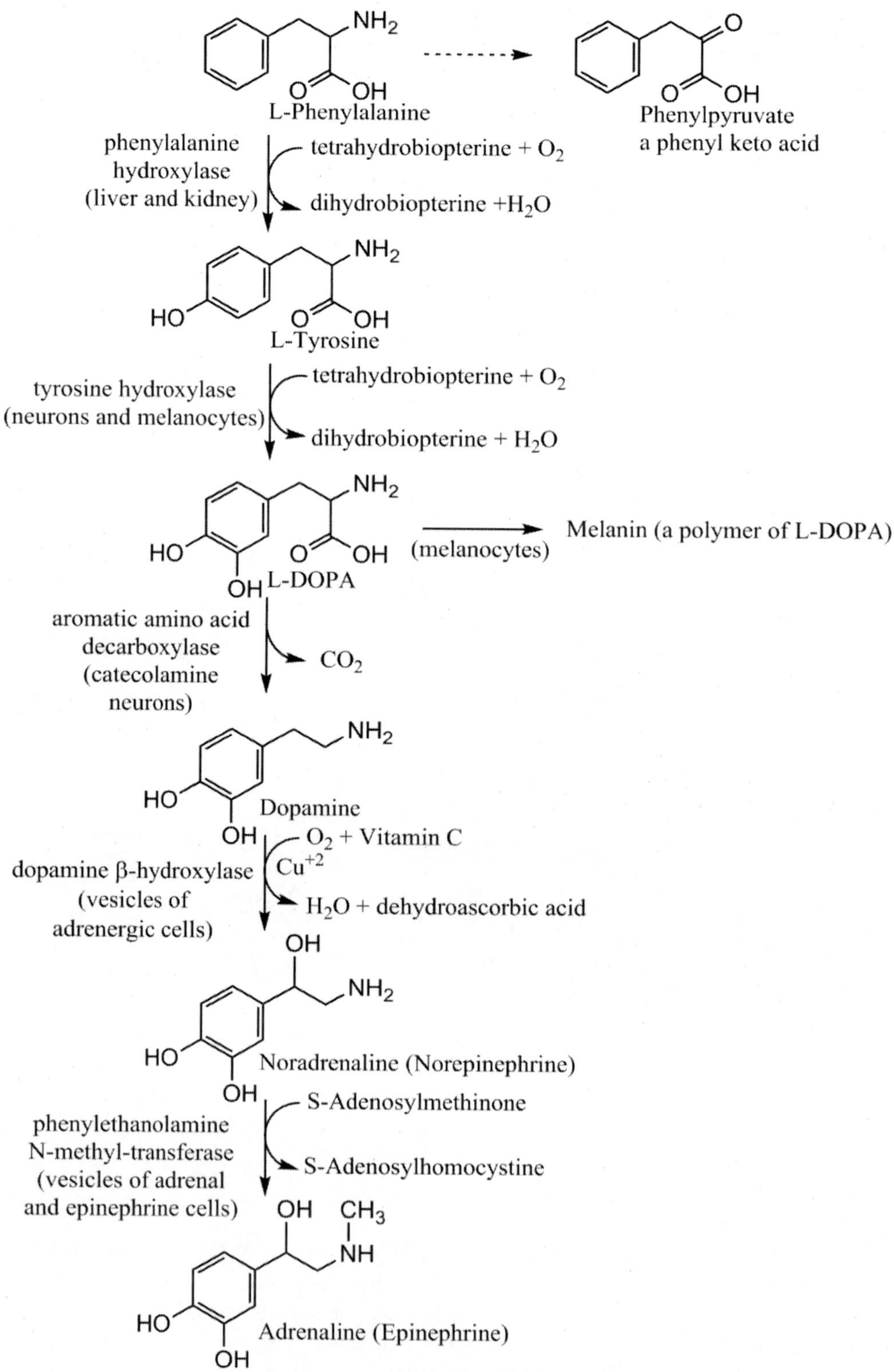

Figure 2. Synthesis of the catecholamines from amino acids. Additional pathways leading to phenylketonuria (PKU) and melanin synthesis are also depicted (horizontal arrows).

Phenylalanine, commonly abbreviated to Phe or the single letter F, is an essential amino acid that can be hydroxylated by the tetrahydrobiopterin-dependent mixed function oxidase enzyme, phenylalanine hydroxylase (PH), to the conditionally non-essential amino acid tyrosine (Nelson & Cox, 2013). Tyrosine, commonly abbreviated to Tyr or the single letter Y, is also hydroxylated by a tetrahydrobiopterin dependent enzyme, tyrosine hydroxylase (TH) to L-3,4-dihydroxy phenylalanine (L-DOPA). Tyrosine hydroxylase is the rate-limiting step for the biosynthesis of the catecholamines (Siegle et al., 1999) and a common immunological target for identifying the histological location of catecholamine neurons. The locations of these TH-immunopositive cells are mapped out in Chapter 1, Figures 2, 3 and 4 of this book. L-DOPA is decarboxylated to dopamine by a pyridoxal phosphate dependent enzyme originally called DOPA decarboxylase, but now renamed as aromatic amino acid decarboxylase, because it is also used to synthesize serotonin from 5-hydroxytrytophan (Siegle et al., 1999). Immunostaining for this enzyme would tag both catecholamine and indolamine cells. For dopamine cells, this is the end of the pathway.

In adrenergic and noradrenergic cells an additional enzyme called dopamine beta-hydroxylase (DBH) is found in the synaptic vesicles (Cooper et al., 2003). This enzyme hydroxylates dopamine to noradrenaline. Immunostaining for this enzyme labels both adrenergic and noradrenergic cells (for the distribution see Figures 3 and 4 in Chapter 1). Adrenergic cells contain one more enzyme not found in the dopaminergic or noradrenergic cells called phenylethanolamine N-methyltransferase (PNMT). Antibodies to this enzyme would target adrenergic cells only without labeling noradrenergic cells (Figure 4 in Chapter 1).

Additional Pathways

The beginning of this overall pathway is also associated with the genetic disorder phenylketonuria (PKU), which is caused by a defect of the enzyme phenylalanine hydroxylase. If this enzyme is defective, then phenylalanine becomes a substrate for an aminotransferase enzyme (horizontal dashed arrow in Figure 2) that removes the amine and replaces it with a ketone creating phenylpyruvate. Elevated concentrations of this highly acidic phenyl ketone molecule results in phenylketonuria. Prolonged exposure to this phenyl ketoacidosis will result in decreased IQ scores, motor abnormality, tremors and seizures (Lieberman & Marks, 2013). A similar syndrome called dihydrobiopterin reductase deficiency also causes a phenylketonuria. Dihydrobiopterin reductase is a NAD(P)H-dependent enzyme that regenerates tetrahydrobiopterin from dihydrobiopternin (Lieberman & Marks, 2013).

An additional pathway linked to the catecholamine pathway is the synthesis of melanin from L-DOPA in melanocytes and other pigmented cells (Figures 2,3). Eumelanin is polymerized from L-leucoDOPAchrome and L-DOPAchrome that are the derivatives of L-DOPA (Figure 3). This polymerization takes place primarily in melanocytes, but melanin can also be found in catecholaminergic cells, most notably the dopaminergic substantia nigra pars compacta and the noradrenergic locus coeruleus (Figure 4).

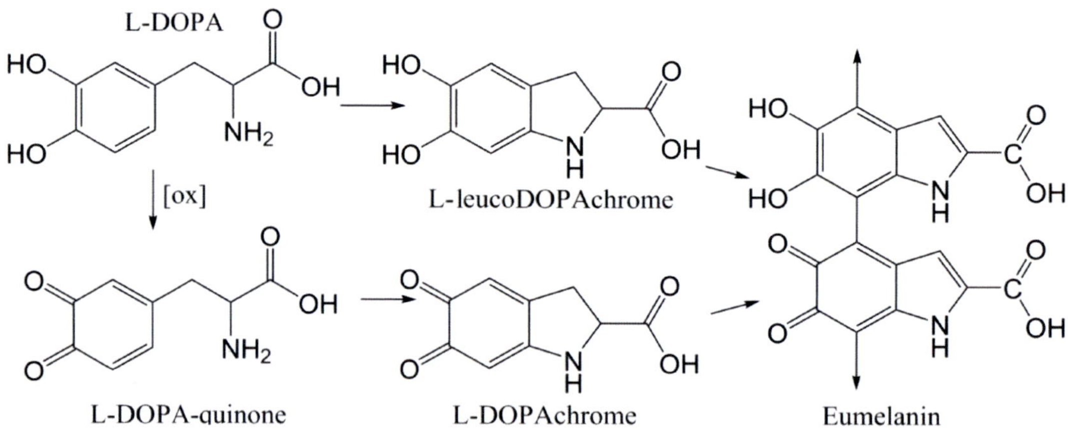

Figure 3. Oxidation and cyclic products of L-DOPA and a portion of eumelanin, the polymerization product of L-Leucodopachrome and L-DOPAchrome.

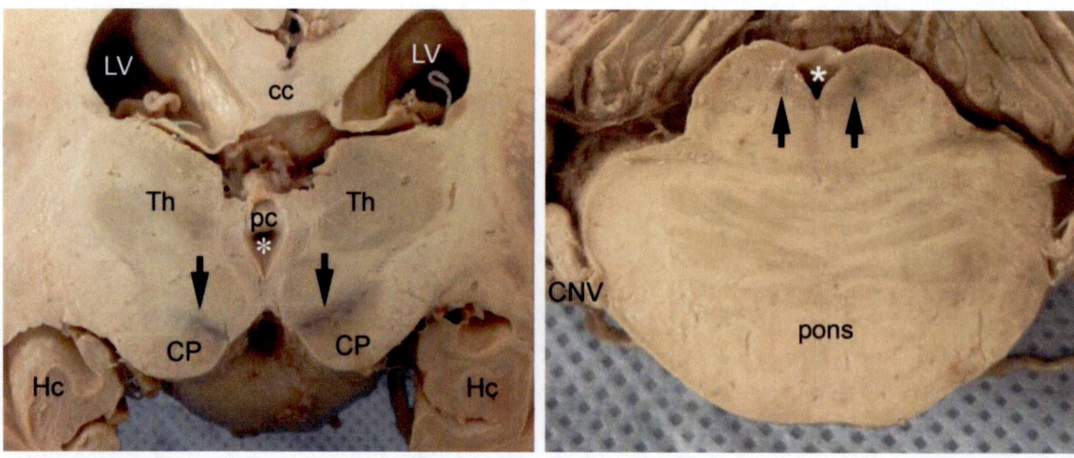

Figure 4. Substantia nigra (left insert, arrows) and locus coeruleus (right insert, arrows) contain pigmented neurons. The human brain was fixed in formalin. Abbreviations: cc, corpus callosum; CNV, trigeminal nerve; CP, cerebral peduncle; Hc, hippocampus; LV, lateral ventricle; pc, posterior commissure, Th, thalamus. Six-pointed asterisk under the posterior commissure marks the posterior part of the 3rd ventricle, while five pointed asterisk denotes the 4th ventricle.

Catabolism

Because of this inherent instability of the catecholamines, the ultimate catabolic products of catecholamines are methylated to retard the quinone formation and the consequent polymerization products (1st column, Figure 5). Catechol stabilization via methylation serves a protective function in these pathways (Siegle et al., 1999; Cooper et al., 2003).

The center of the catabolic pathway is L-DOPA and its decarboxylation product dopamine (2nd column, Figure 5). Dopamine can be oxidized by monoamine oxidase (MAO) to 3,4-dihydroxyphenylacetaldehyde (DOPAL). DOPAL is a very short-lived molecule and found in very low concentrations.

DOPAL can be either oxidized by aldehyde dehydrogenase (ALDH) or reduced by aldehyde reductase (AldR). The reduction product is generally the minor pathway which produces 3,4-dihydroxyphenylethanol (DOPET). DOPET can be oxidized by alcohol dehydrogenase (AlcD) back to DOPAL or sulfated (to be discussed in shortly). DOPAL is preferentially oxidized by ALDH to 3,4-dihydroxyphenylacetic acid (DOPAC). DOPAL, being an aldehyde is more unstable than all of the other dopamine metabolites and it is generally found in the lowest concentration of all these intermediates. MAO and ALDH form a complex on the outer surface of the mitochondria and participate in substrate channeling, where the MAO creates DOPAL, but ALDH quickly oxidizes DOPAL to DOPAC before much of it has a chance to escape into the cytosol.

Due to the fact that the catechols are chemically unstable and are prone to oxidation and polymerization, the enzyme catechol-O-methyl transferase transfers a methyl group from S-adenosyl-methionine (SAM) to the number 3 hydroxyl of the catechol. All of the methylated metabolites are shown in the first column of Figure 5. These methylated catechols are significantly less able to be oxidized and form polymers, which would make them more biologically suitable elimination products.

All of molecules depicted in the 3rd column of Figure 5 have a hydroxyl group in the beta position and they are metabolites of noradrenaline and adrenaline. Molecules illustrated in the 4th column of Figure 5 are the corresponding methylated catechols for each of those same intermediates in the 3rd column. Unlike dopamine, the catabolism of the noradrenergic and adrenergic metabolites favors the production of the reduced glycol (MOPEG) rather than the carboxylic acid (VMA). The MOPEG is then sulfated by the liver and eliminated as the sulfate conjugate.

The importance of methylation can be seen by simply comparing the unbuffered shelf-life of dopamine metabolites that are commonly used as standards for HPLC analysis. In addition to the enzymatic formation of melanin, L-DOPA and the other non-methylated catecholamines can spontaneously oxidize in the presence of oxygen to form dark precipitates. If the solutions are not used quickly or not stored in a buffered antioxidant containing solution, they darken and form a precipitate and do so more quickly when exposed to light (Figure 6).

In addition to methylation, the metabolites discussed in Figure 5 can also be sulfated or conjugated with other small molecules both in the brain and liver (Lemke et al., 2013). The sulfation takes place on the phenolic hydroxyl groups and would affect all the structures shown in Figure 5. Sulfation products of the dopamine, noradrenaline and adrenaline are common both in the blood and urine. The reduced noradrenergic and adrenergic metabolites also appear as sulfated elimination products.

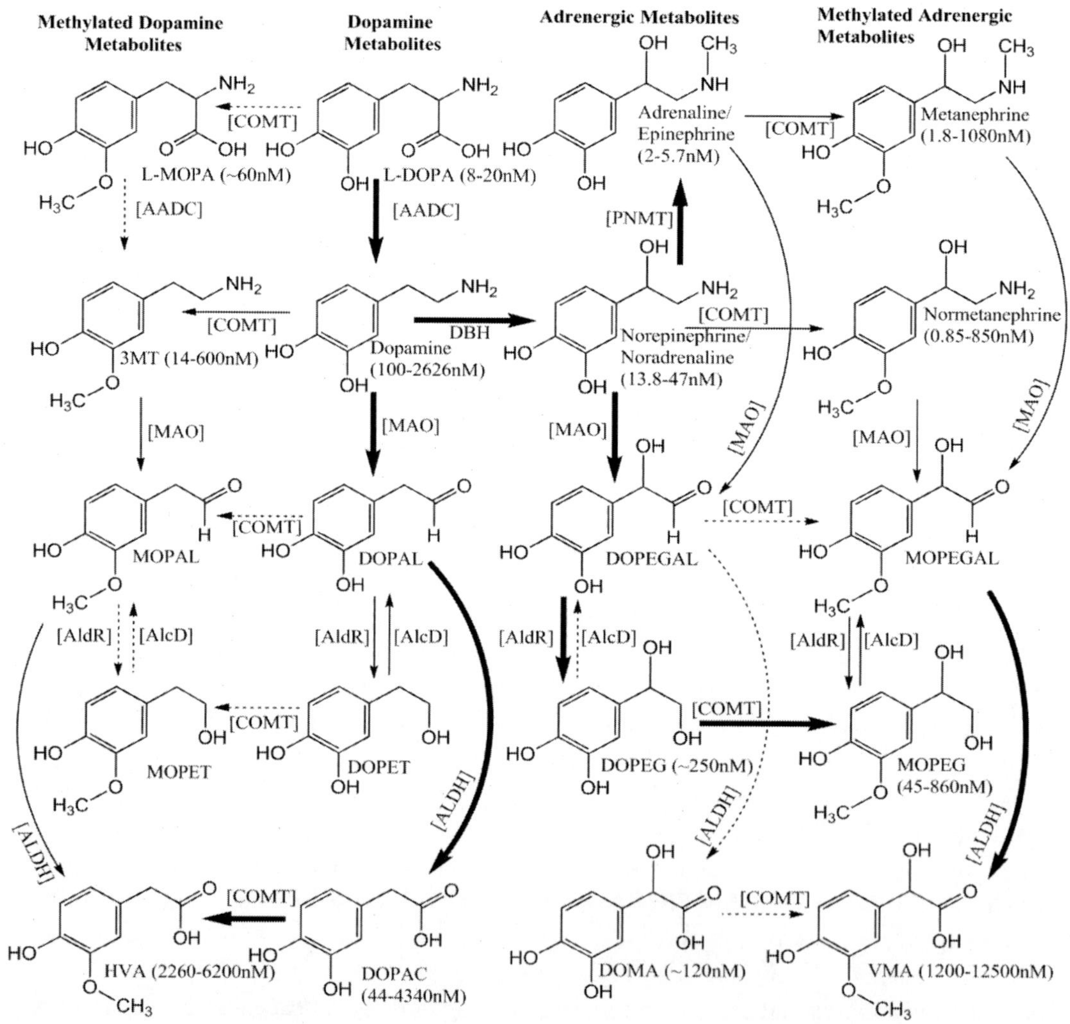

Figure 5. Catabolites of the catechols. The approximate urine concentrations of each of these metabolites are listed under each structure as taken from the Human Metabolome Database, http://www.serummetabolome.ca/ (Psychogios N. et al., 2014). These numbers put some perspective on the ultimate concentration of each of these metabolites. The metabolites with no numbers are presumably and most likely found in very low concentrations. The heavy arrows are the major pathways, the dotted arrows are minor pathways and the thin arrows are the other significant pathways. Chemical abbreviations: L-MOPA (L-4-methoxy-3-hydroxy-phenylalanine), L-DOPA (L-3,4-dihydroxyl-phenylalanine), 3-MT (3-methoxy-tyramine), MOPAL (3-methoxy-4-hydroxy-phenyl-acetaldehyde), DOPAL (3,4-dihydroxy-phenyl-acetaldehyde), DOPEGAL (3,4-dihydroxy-phenyl-glycol-aldehyde), MOPEGAL (3-methoxy-4-hydroxy-phenyl-glycol-aldehyde), MOPET (3-methoxy-4-hydroxy-phenyl-ethanol), DOPET (3,4-dihydroxy-phenyl-ethanol), DOPEG (3,4-dihydroxy-phenyl-glycol), MOPEG (3-methoxy-4-hydroxy-phenyl-glycol), HVA (homovanillic acid), DOPAC (3,4-dihydroxy-phenyl-acetic acid), DOMA (3,4-dihydroxy-mandelic acid), VMA (vanillyl-mandelic acid). Enzyme Abbreviations: AADC (aromatic amino acid decarboxylase, aka dopa decarboxylase), MAO (monoamine oxidase), ALDH (aldehyde dehydrogenase), AldR (aldehyde reductase, aka AR), AlcD (alcohol dehydrogenase), COMT (catechol-O-methyl transferase), DBA (dopamine beta hydroxylase), PNMT (phenylethylamine-N-methyl transferase).

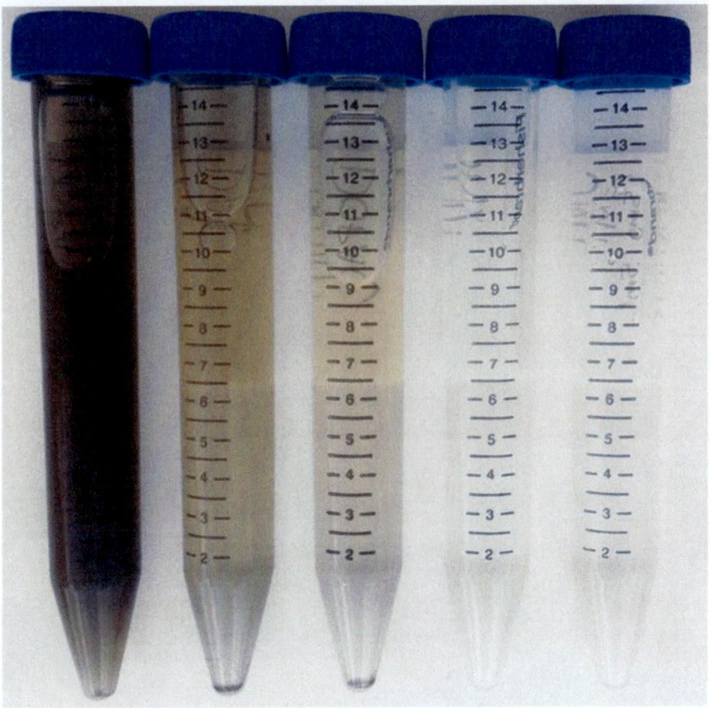

L-DOPA DA DOPAC HVA 3-MT

Figure 6. Photograph of 1 mg/ml dopamine metabolites in deionized water exposed to light for six months at room temperature. Notice that the methylated metabolites of HVA (homovanillic acid) and 3-MT (3-methoxytyramine) stayed clear and the non-methylated metabolites have discolored, especially L-DOPA and DA (dopamine).

Transporter Systems

It is well established that neurons are polarized due to the action of the sodium/potassium ATPase pump, which uses ATP and pumps out 3 sodium ions for each 2 potassium ions that are pumped in (Nelson & Cox, 2013). This is called primary active transport since it is directly coupled to the use of ATP. This transporter is also called an antiporter since it pumps out molecules or ions while pumping in other different molecules or ions. In this case 3 sodium ions are pumped out and 2 potassium ions are pumped in. The asymmetry of pumping out 3 positive charges and 2 back in results in losing net positive charges that makes the inside of the cell negatively charged relative to the outside (Nelson & Cox, 2013).

Both dopamine and noradrenaline, following release from the presynaptic axon can be recycled via either sodium dependent dopamine transporter (DAT) or the sodium dependent noradrenaline transporter (NET), respectively (Cooper et al., 2003)(Figure 7). Both of these transporters utilize a sodium gradient across the membrane that was created by the sodium/potassium ATPase pump, to provide the energy to pump these neurotransmitters back into the presynaptic cell. Most of this neurotransmitter is then taken up into the vesicles using the VMAT-2.

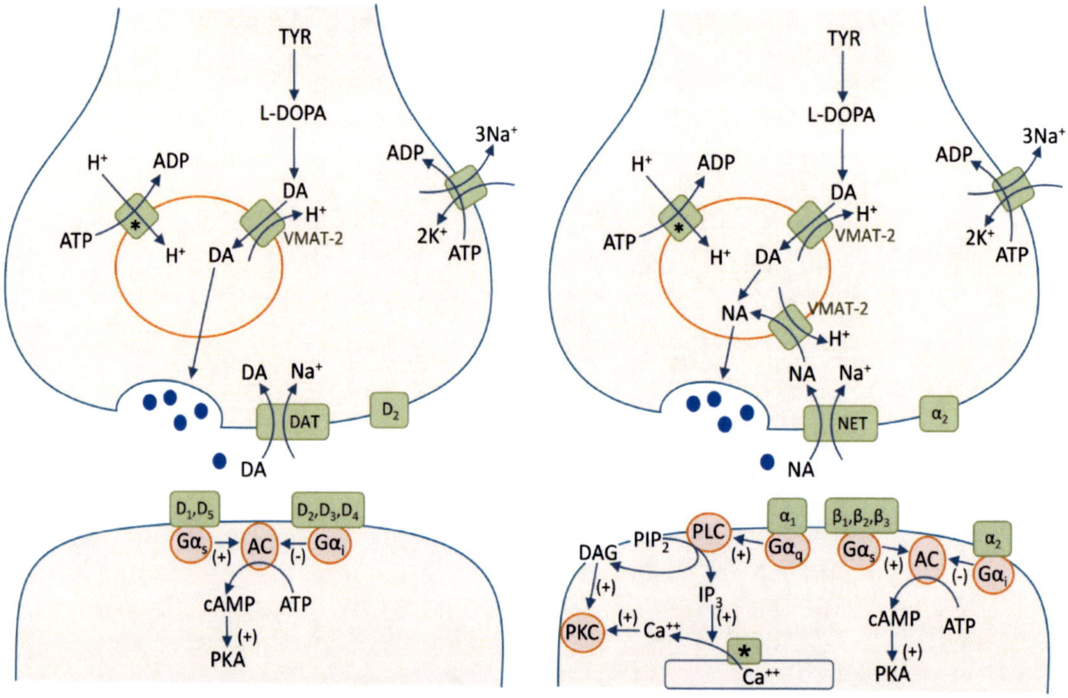

Figure 7. Depiction of pre- and postsynaptic elements of the dopaminergic (left insert) and noradrenergic synapses (NA; right insert). The Na+/K+ ATPase pumps that create membrane potential of all cells are illustrated at the right side of the presynaptic elements. The synaptic vesicles are depicted by the orange open circles. The V-type ATPase proton pumps (indicated by the 6 point asterisk) make the interior of the vesicle more acidic than the cytoplasm by using ATP to pump protons in and create the proton gradient. This proton gradient also drives the vesicle monoamine transporters (VMAT-2) which is a secondary active transport pump that drives dopamine (DA) and/or noradrenaline (NA) in as the protons are permitted back out. In dopaminergic cells, VMAT-2 pumps in both newly synthesized DA and recycled DA from the reuptake system. In the noradrenergic cells, the VMAT-2 pumps in newly synthesized DA as well as recycled NA from its reuptake system, and the *de novo* synthesis of NA takes place in the vesicle where DA is hydroxylated to NA by dopamine beta-hydroxylase (DBH). The reuptake transporters are the dopamine transporter (DAT) for dopaminergic neurons and norepinephrine transporter (NET) for noradrenergic cells. Both transporters are neurotransmitter/Na^+ antiporters and use the Na^+ gradient created by the Na+/K^+ ATPase pump. There are 3 classes of receptors for these catecholamine systems, two excitatory and one inhibitory, and all of them are linked to trimeric G-protein signaling. The α_1 receptors activate the G_q class of G-proteins. When activated, the alpha subunit of this trimeric system ($G\alpha_q$) stimulates phospholipase C (PLC). PLC converts the membrane lipid phosphatidyl inositol bisphosphate (PIP_2) into diacylglycerol (DAG) and inositol trisphosphate (IP_3). IP_3 acts on ligand gated calcium channels (indicated by the 5 point asterisk) to release calcium (Ca^{++}) stored in the endoplasmic reticulum to the cytoplasm. The combination of DAG and Ca^{++} activate protein kinase C to phosphorylate its target proteins. The D_1, D_5 and all 3 types of the β receptors are linked to the G_s timeric system. The alpha subunit ($G\alpha_s$) activates adenylate cyclase (AC) to convert adenosine triphosphate (ATP) into cyclic adenosine monophosphate (cAMP), which then activates protein kinase A (PKA) to phosphorylate its target proteins. The D_2, D_3, D_4 and α_2 receptors are inhibitory by activating the G_i class of trimeric G-proteins. The $G\alpha_i$ inhibits AC and this reduces the concentration of cAMP and thus the activity of PKA. A type of D_2 and α_2 receptors can also be found presynaptically and serve as inhibitory autoreceptors.

Vesicle Uptake

The storage of the neurotransmitters, prior to synaptic release, takes place inside membranous vesicles pinched off from the Golgi apparatus (Figure 7). These synaptic vesicles contain V-type ATPase proton pumps that use peripheral (cytoplasmic) ATP to pump protons into vacuolar structures including these synaptic vesicles of neurons. These transporters are also found on analogous vesicles in endocrine cells, as well as lysosomes, endosomes and Golgi cisternae (Nelson & Cox, 2013). The acidification of these vesicles also decreases the spontaneous non-enzymatic oxidation rate of the catecholamines. These acidified vesicles contain proton-neurotransmitter antiporters (secondary active transport) that pump catecholamines into the vesicle as protons escape back out to the cytoplasm. These vesicular monoamine transporters are termed VMAT's. VMAT-1 is found in the adrenal medulla and VMAT-2 is found in catecholamine and serotonin cells (Cooper et al., 2003).

VMAT-2 takes up and concentrates all catecholamines (Cooper et al., 2003; Siegle et al., 1999). In dopaminergic neurons, recycled dopamine as well as newly created dopamine synthesized in the cytoplasm are taken up by VMAT-2 (Figure 7). In noradrenergic cells, the dopamine synthesized in the cytoplasm is taken up into the vesicle via the VMAT-2 and then encounters the enzyme, dopamine beta-hydroxylase (DHB) inside the vesicle. Therefore, the actual synthesis of noradrenaline from dopamine takes place in the vesicle and not in the cytoplasm. However, noradrenaline that is taken back up into the cytoplasm via the reuptake system is also transported into the vesicle by the same VMAT-2 (Figure 7).

Adrenergic cells contain both DBH and the enzyme PNMT. In these neurons, dopamine is synthesized in the cytoplasm, taken up into the vesicles, and then converted first to noradrenaline, and then to adrenaline.

Catecholaminergic Receptors

Anatomical Overview of the Catecholaminergic System

The anatomy of the catecholamine systems is discussed in detail in Chapter 1, therefore, we include only a brief overview necessary to understand the correlation between the distribution of the catecholaminergic elements and the adrenergic and dopaminergic receptors. In summary, the largest and longest dopaminergic pathways include the nigrostriatal pathway originating in the pigmented (neuromelanin containing) substantia nigra pars compacta cells in the midbrain (Figure 4) and projecting to the caudate and putamen cells, also known collectively as the striatum due to its striated appearance caused by the projecting fibers into this region (Felten & Sladek, Jr., 1983; Moore & Bloom, 1978; Nieuwenhuys, 1985). The mesolimbic pathway originates primarily from neurons in the vental tegmental area, which are midline cells adjacent to the substantia nigra. These cells have a significant projection, as the name of the pathway implies, to the limbic areas, including the cingulate gyrus, hippocampus, nucleus accumbens and also to the medial orbital region of the frontal cortex (Blumenfeld, 2002; Felten & Sladek, Jr., 1983; Moore & Bloom, 1978; Nieuwenhuys, 1985). The mesocortical pathway includes fibers from both the substantia nigra pars compacta and the vental tegmental area to the prefrontal cortex

(Blumenfeld, 2002; Felten & Sladek, Jr., 1983; Moore & Bloom, 1978; Nieuwenhuys, 1985). An additional significant dopaminergic fiber system originates primarily in the hypothalamus with projections to the septum, pituitary and spinal cord (Bjorklund & Nobin, 1973; Dudás et al., 2010; Ungerstedt, 1971).

Within the central nervous system, the lightly pigmented region called the locus coeruleus (Figure 4) in the rostral pons and the lateral tegmental area (a diffuse area in the pons and medulla) are the primary source of noradrenergic projections in the central nervous system, including projections to the entire forebrain (Camps et al., 1989; Cortes et al., 1989b; Dahlstrom & Fuxe, 1964; Hall et al., 1994; Nieuwenhuys, 1985; Nobin & Bjorklund, 1973; Olson et al., 1973b; Olson et al., 1973a). The noradrenergic cells of the lateral pons and medulla are involved in sympathetic function. A small number of adrenergic neurons in the brain stem are the source of the adrenergic fibers in the central nervous system (Astier et al., 1987; Cunningham, Jr. et al., 1990; Dahlstrom & Fuxe, 1964; Kitahama et al., 1985; Kitahama et al., 1986; Kitahama et al., 1988; Sawchenko & Bohn, 1989).

Adrenergic Receptors

The adrenergic receptors include the alpha (α) and the beta (β) receptors. The alpha-adrenergic receptors can be subdivided into the α_1 and α_2 subtypes. The α_1 subtypes can be further subdivided into types A, B, C and D. All of the α_1 subtypes are transmembrane proteins that contain 7 helixes and are commonly referred to as heptahelical receptors but also known as serpentine receptors because they "snake" their way through the membrane (Cooper et al., 2003; Siegle et al., 1999; Nelson & Cox, 2013; Lieberman & Marks, 2013). Following binding with either adrenaline or noradrenaline, these receptors interact with a trimeric G-protein (Figure 7). The specific trimeric G-protein activated by the α_1 subtypes contains an alpha subunit called the Gα_q protein. All G-proteins are called G-proteins because they bind GTP or GDP. The alpha subunit of the inactive G-proteins binds GDP. Upon activation, G-proteins dislodge the GDP and bind GTP, which activate the alpha subunit and also causes it to disassociate from the beta and gamma subunits. The dissociated and active Gα_q interacts with another membrane protein, phospholipase C (PLC). The Gα_q protein continues to activate PLC as long as GTP is bound. The Gα proteins have a GTPase activity and eventually hydrolyse the GTP to GDP. At that point the Gα subunit inactivates and eventually reassociates with another beta and gamma subunits. Therefore, the duration of action of these G-proteins is self-limiting due to the GTPase activity.

The activated PLC cleaves the membrane lipid phosphatidyl inositol bisphophate (PIP_2) to the second messengers diacylglycerol (DAG) and the water soluble inositol trisphosphate (IP_3). IP_3 binds to intracellular calcium receptors on the endoplasmic reticulum and induces the release of sequestered calcium into the cytoplasm of the post-synaptic cell (Figure 7). The combination of DAG and calcium activates protein kinase C (PKC) that phosphorylates selected proteins. This phosphorylation causes activation of some proteins and inactivation others that usually counter the activity of the activated proteins. These α_1 adrenergic receptors are therefore considered to be excitatory metabotropic receptors and have a stimulatory effect on the target cells. The α_1 adrenergic receptors have a higher affinity for noradrenaline than for adrenaline, but they do respond to both transmitters.

The α_1 adrenergic receptors are widely distributed in the brain; the highest concentration of α_1 mRNA has been observed in the cerebral cortex, amygdala, thalamus, brain stem and spinal motor nuclei (Pieribone et al., 1994). High concentration of $\alpha_{1A/D}$ receptor mRNA has been also described in the inferior olivary nucleus, hippocampus, olfactory bulb, while α_{1B} mRNA is abundant in the intermediolateral cell column of the spinal cord (Pieribone et al., 1994).

The α_2 adrenergic receptors are inhibitory metabotropic receptors that respond to adrenaline more than noradrenaline. These receptors are found both on the post-synaptic and pre-synaptic membranes, and thus, they also serve as adrenergic autoreceptors (Figure 7). The α_2 receptors can also be subdivided pharmacologically into additional subtypes A, B and C. All of these receptor subtypes are heptahelical serpentine receptors that are coupled to a trimeric G-protein whose alpha subunit is called the $G\alpha_i$. These G-proteins, similarly to other G protein classes, dislodge their GDP and replace it with GTP, when activated; however, their action is inhibitory. They interact with a membrane protein called adenylate cyclase, which converts ATP to cAMP. The $G\alpha_i$ protein inhibits adenylate cyclase, thus decreasing the rate of cAMP formation. The function of cAMP is to activate protein kinase A (PKA), which phosphorylates proteins in a similar manner as PKC. Therefore, this cascade decreases the level of stimulation on a cell. A type of α_2 can also be found presynaptically and they serve as autoreceptors.

The α_2 receptors are widely distributed in the brain (Aoki et al., 1994; McCune et al., 1993; Nicholas et al., 1993a; Rosin et al., 1993; Scheinin et al., 1994; Tavares et al., 1996). The α_{2A}- and α_{2B}-subtypes has been observed in the cerebellum, brain stem, hypothalamus and various cortical areas (Tavares et al., 1996). The α_{2A} receptors are believed to play a pivotal role in maintaining vascular sympathetic tone. Indeed, α_{2A}-adrenergic receptor-like immunoreactivity has been described in most of noradrenergic and adrenergic cells of the brainstem (Rosin et al., 1993).

The beta-adrenergic receptors are subdivided into β_1, β_2, and β_3. These receptors are excitatory metabotropic receptors. Similarly to other catecholamine receptors, they are heptahelical serpentine receptors that, when activated, associate with a trimeric G-protein. This time the alpha subunit of the trimeric G-protein is the $G\alpha_s$. This class of G-proteins stimulates adenylate cyclase and thus increases the synthesis of cAMP, which activates PKA and its associated proteins. The β_1 receptors have a higher affinity for adrenaline than noradrenaline, the β_2 receptors have about the same affinity for adrenaline and noradrenaline and the β_3 receptors have a lower affinity for adrenaline than noradrenaline. The β_1 and β_2 receptors are widely distributed in the central nervous system and can be found in the thalamus, brain stem nuclei, spinal cord, substantia nigra, olfactory tubercle and various cortical areas, where highly laminar organization of the subtypes has been described (Nicholas et al., 1993b; Joyce et al., 1992; Rainbow et al., 1984). β_1 receptors are also located in high density in the hippocampus, while the molecular layer of cerebellum contains high levels of β_2 receptors (Joyce et al., 1992; Nicholas et al., 1993b; Rainbow et al., 1984). β_3 receptors are primarily localized in adipose tissue (Krief et al., 1993; Lonnqvist et al., 1993), however, the antidepressant effects of the selective β_3 agonist amibegron suggests that β_3 receptors are also present in the central nervous system (Overstreet et al., 2008).

Dopamine Receptors

The excitatory dopamine receptors are the also known as the D_1-type receptors. The D_1-type receptors can be pharmacologically subdivided into the D_1 and D_5 subtypes. These receptors are similar to the beta-adrenergic receptors in that they are coupled to $G\alpha_s$, cAMP and activation of PKA.

The inhibitory dopamine receptors are known as the D_2-type receptors. These D_2-type receptors can be subdivided into the subtypes: D_{2s}, D_{2L}, D_3 and D_4 (S and the L are for short and long forms and refers to different isoforms of the protein created by alternative splicing). These inhibitory receptors are similar to the α_2 receptors in that they are linked to $G\alpha_i$ and the inhibition of cAMP synthesis. The D_{2s} is found presynaptically as autoreceptor.

The distribution of the dopamine receptors in post mortem human brain tissue has been extensively studied [for review see (Beaulieu & Gainetdinov, 2011)]. The pattern of dopamine receptors in human and rat approximately corresponds to the distribution of the dopaminergic terminals in these species (Cortes et al., 1989b). In human, D_1 and D_2 binding sites are primarily located in the basal ganglia, including the substantia nigra, nucleus accumbens, caudate nucleus, putamen and globus pallidus (Camps et al., 1989; Cortes et al., 1989a; Cortes et al., 1989b; Hall et al., 1994; Beaulieu & Gainetdinov, 2011; Gerfen, 2000; Missale et al., 1998; Vallone et al., 2000). Significant density of D_1 and D_2 binding sites can also be observed in the amygdala and the hippocampus, while the diencephalon, cerebellum and brain stem contains lower level of D_1 binding sites (Cortes et al., 1989b). In the cerebral cortex, the density of D_1 receptors is higher than that of D_2 receptors (Camps et al., 1989; Cortes et al., 1989b; Hall et al., 1994). The distribution of D_3 receptor is associated with the mesolimbic pathway; highest densities can be found in the nucleus accumbens, olfactory tubercle and the islands of Calleja (Missale et al., 1998; Sokoloff et al., 1992; Sokoloff et al., 2006), but absent from the ventral tegmental area, where D_2 receptors can be detected (Gurevich & Joyce, 1999). The expression of D_4 receptors is limited in the brain and confined to the amygdala, hippocampus, hypothalamus, basal ganglia, frontal cortex and thalamus (Beaulieu & Gainetdinov, 2011; Missale et al., 1998; Rondou et al., 2010). D_5 receptors are restricted primarily to the substantia nigra, hypothalamus, hippocampus and multiple cortical areas (Beaulieu & Gainetdinov, 2011; Missale et al., 1998).

Conclusion

The synthesis of the most important catecholamines, dopamine, noradrenaline and adrenaline from the amino acid tyrosine involves 3 major key enzymes: tyrosine hydroxylase (TH), dopamine beta-hydroxylase (DBH), and phenylethanolamine N-methyltransferase (PNMT). Adrenergic neurons contain all of these three enzymes, noradrenergic cells contain DBH and TH, and dopaminergic cells TH only. The synthesis of melanin is closely linked to the catecholamine synthesis. Dopamine is eventually catabolyzed to homovanillic acid (HVA), while adrenaline and noradrenaline is catabolyzed to vanillylmandelic acid (VMA) and also the sulphate conjugates of the reduced glycol intermediates (DHPG and MHPG).

Catecholamines are synthesized in the cytoplasm of the neurons and they are transported into the synaptic vesicles by vesicle monoamine transporters (VMAT-2). Catecholamines released from the vesicles are either recycled to the presynaptic element by dopamine transporter (DAT) for dopaminergic neurons and norepinephrine transporter (NET) for noradrenergic cells or bind to the presynaptic and postsynaptic adrenergic and dopaminergic receptors. These receptors can be subdivided into 3 major classes, two excitatory and one inhibitory, and all of them are linked to trimeric G-protein signaling. The α_1 receptors activate the G_q class of G-proteins and exert their action by protein kinase C to phosphorylate target proteins. D_1, D_5 and all 3 types of the β receptors are linked to the G_s timeric system and act via the activation of protein kinase A (PKA). D_2, D_3, D_4 and α_2 receptors are inhibitory and activate G_i class of trimeric G-proteins that eventually cause activation of PKA. Adrenergic and dopaminergic receptors, with the exception of β_3 receptor, are widely distributed in the central nervous system.

References

Aoki, C., Go, C. G., Venkatesan, C., & Kurose, H. (1994). Perikaryal and synaptic localization of alpha 2A-adrenergic receptor-like immunoreactivity. *Brain Res., 650,* 181-204.

Astier, B., Kitahama, K., Denoroy, L., Jouvet, M., & Renaud, B. (1987). Immunohistochemical evidence for the adrenergic medullary longitudinal bundle as a major ascending pathway to the hypothalamus. *Neurosci.Lett., 78,* 241-246.

Beaulieu, J. M. & Gainetdinov, R. R. (2011). The physiology, signaling, and pharmacology of dopamine receptors. *Pharmacol.Rev., 63,* 182-217.

Bjorklund, A. & Nobin, A. (1973). Fluorescence histochemical and microspectrofluorometric mapping of dopamine and noradrenaline cell groups in the rat diencephalon. *Brain Res., 51,* 193-205.

Blumenfeld, H. (2002). *Neuroanatomy through Clinical Cases*. Sinauer.

Camps, M., Cortes, R., Gueye, B., Probst, A., & Palacios, J. M. (1989). Dopamine receptors in human brain: autoradiographic distribution of D2 sites. *Neuroscience, 28,* 275-290.

Cooper, J. R., Bloom, F. E., & Roth, R. H. (2003). *Biochemical Basis of Neuropharmacology*. (8th ed.) New York, NY: Oxford University Press.

Cortes, R., Camps, M., Gueye, B., Probst, A., & Palacios, J. M. (1989a). Dopamine receptors in human brain: autoradiographic distribution of D1 and D2 sites in Parkinson syndrome of different etiology. *Brain Res., 483,* 30-38.

Cortes, R., Gueye, B., Pazos, A., Probst, A., & Palacios, J. M. (1989b). Dopamine receptors in human brain: autoradiographic distribution of D1 sites. *Neuroscience, 28,* 263-273.

Cunningham, E. T., Jr., Bohn, M. C., & Sawchenko, P. E. (1990). Organization of adrenergic inputs to the paraventricular and supraoptic nuclei of the hypothalamus in the rat. *J.Comp Neurol., 292,* 651-667.

Dahlstrom, A. & Fuxe, K. (1964). Localization of monoamines in the lower brain stem. *Experientia, 20,* 398-399.

Dudás, B., Baker, M., Rotoli, G., Grignol, G., Bohn, M. C., & Merchenthaler, I. (2010). Distribution and morphology of the catecholaminergic neural elements in the human hypothalamus. *Neuroscience, 171,* 187-195.

Felten, D. L. & Sladek, J. R., Jr. (1983). Monoamine distribution in primate brain V. Monoaminergic nuclei: anatomy, pathways and local organization. *Brain Res.Bull., 10,* 171-284.

Gerfen, C. R. (2000). Molecular effects of dopamine on striatal-projection pathways. *Trends Neurosci., 23,* S64-S70.

Gurevich, E. V. & Joyce, J. N. (1999). Distribution of dopamine D3 receptor expressing neurons in the human forebrain: comparison with D2 receptor expressing neurons. *Neuropsychopharmacology, 20,* 60-80.

Hall, H., Sedvall, G., Magnusson, O., Kopp, J., Halldin, C., & Farde, L. (1994). Distribution of D1- and D2-dopamine receptors, and dopamine and its metabolites in the human brain. *Neuropsychopharmacology, 11,* 245-256.

Joyce, J. N., Lexow, N., Kim, S. J., Artymyshyn, R., Senzon, S., Lawrence, D. et al. (1992). Distribution of beta-adrenergic receptor subtypes in human post-mortem brain: alterations in limbic regions of schizophrenics. *Synapse, 10,* 228-246.

Kitahama, K., Denoroy, L., Berod, A., & Jouvet, M. (1986). Distribution of PNMT-immunoreactive neurons in the cat medulla oblongata. *Brain Res Bull., 17,* 197-208.

Kitahama, K., Denoroy, L., Goldstein, M., Jouvet, M., & Pearson, J. (1988). Immunohistochemistry of tyrosine hydroxylase and phenylethanolamine N-methyltransferase in the human brain stem: description of adrenergic perikarya and characterization of longitudinal catecholaminergic pathways. *Neuroscience, 25,* 97-111.

Kitahama, K., Pearson, J., Denoroy, L., Kopp, N., Ulrich, J., Maeda, T. et al. (1985). Adrenergic neurons in human brain demonstrated by immunohistochemistry with antibodies to phenylethanolamine-N-methyltransferase (PNMT): discovery of a new group in the nucleus tractus solitarius. *Neurosci.Lett., 53,* 303-308.

Krief, S., Lonnqvist, F., Raimbault, S., Baude, B., van, S. A., Arner, P. et al. (1993). Tissue distribution of beta 3-adrenergic receptor mRNA in man. *J Clin.Invest, 91,* 344-349.

Lemke, T. L., Williams, D. A., Roche, V. F., & Zito, S. W. (2013). *Foye's Princliples of Medicinal Chemistry.* (7th ed.) Lippencott Williams & Wilkins.

Lieberman, M. & Marks, A. D. (2013). *Marks' Basic Medical Biochemistry, A Clinical Approach.* (4th ed.) Lippincott Williams & Wilkins.

Lonnqvist, F., Krief, S., Strosberg, A. D., Nyberg, S., Emorine, L. J., & Arner, P. (1993). Evidence for a functional beta 3-adrenoceptor in man. *Br.J Pharmacol., 110,* 929-936.

McCune, S. K., Voigt, M. M., & Hill, J. M. (1993). Expression of multiple alpha adrenergic receptor subtype messenger RNAs in the adult rat brain. *Neuroscience, 57,* 143-151.

Missale, C., Nash, S. R., Robinson, S. W., Jaber, M., & Caron, M. G. (1998). Dopamine receptors: from structure to function. *Physiol Rev., 78,* 189-225.

Moore, R. Y. & Bloom, F. E. (1978). Central catecholamine neuron systems: anatomy and physiology of the dopamine systems. *Annu.Rev.Neurosci., 1,* 129-169.

Morrison, R. T. & Boyd, R. N. (1973). *Organic Chemistry.* (3rd ed.) Boston: Allyn and Bacon.

Nelson, D. L. & Cox, M. M. (2013). *Lehninger Principles of Biochemistry.* (6th ed.) New York, NY: Freeman and Company.

Nicholas, A. P., Pieribone, V., & Hokfelt, T. (1993a). Distributions of mRNAs for alpha-2 adrenergic receptor subtypes in rat brain: an in situ hybridization study. *J Comp Neurol, 328,* 575-594.

Nicholas, A. P., Pieribone, V. A., & Hokfelt, T. (1993b). Cellular localization of messenger RNA for beta-1 and beta-2 adrenergic receptors in rat brain: an in situ hybridization study. *Neuroscience, 56,* 1023-1039.

Nieuwenhuys, R. (1985). *Chemoarchitecture of the brain.* Berlin Heidelberg: Springer-Verlag.

Nobin, A. & Bjorklund, A. (1973). Topography of the monoamine neuron systems in the human brain as revealed in fetuses. *Acta Physiol Scand.Suppl, 388,* 1-40.

Olson, L., Boreus, L. O., & Seiger, A. (1973a). Histochemical demonstration and mapping of 5-hydroxytryptamine- and catecholamine-containing neuron systems in the human fetal brain. *Z.Anat.Entwicklungsgesch., 139,* 259-282.

Olson, L., Nystrom, B., & Seiger, A. (1973b). Monoamine fluorescence histochemistry of human post mortem brain. *Brain Res., 63,* 231-247.

Overstreet, D. H., Stemmelin, J., & Griebel, G. (2008). Confirmation of antidepressant potential of the selective beta3 adrenoceptor agonist amibegron in an animal model of depression. *Pharmacol.Biochem.Behav., 89,* 623-626.

Pieribone, V. A., Nicholas, A. P., Dagerlind, A., & Hokfelt, T. (1994). Distribution of alpha 1 adrenoceptors in rat brain revealed by in situ hybridization experiments utilizing subtype-specific probes. *J Neurosci., 14,* 4252-4268.

Psychogios N., Hau D.D, Peng J., Guo A.C., Mandal R., Bouatra S et al. (2014). The Human Serum Metabolome. *PLoS One, 6,* e16957.

Rainbow, T. C., Parsons, B., & Wolfe, B. B. (1984). Quantitative autoradiography of beta 1- and beta 2-adrenergic receptors in rat brain. *Proc.Natl.Acad.Sci.U.S.A, 81,* 1585-1589.

Rondou, P., Haegeman, G., & Van, C. K. (2010). The dopamine D4 receptor: biochemical and signalling properties. *Cell Mol.Life Sci., 67,* 1971-1986.

Rosin, D. L., Zeng, D., Stornetta, R. L., Norton, F. R., Riley, T., Okusa, M. D. et al. (1993). Immunohistochemical localization of alpha 2A-adrenergic receptors in catecholaminergic and other brainstem neurons in the rat. *Neuroscience, 56,* 139-155.

Sawchenko, P. E. & Bohn, M. C. (1989). Glucocorticoid receptor-immunoreactivity in C1, C2, and C3 adrenergic neurons that project to the hypothalamus or to the spinal cord in the rat. *J.Comp Neurol., 285,* 107-116.

Scheinin, M., Lomasney, J. W., Hayden-Hixson, D. M., Schambra, U. B., Caron, M. G., Lefkowitz, R. J. et al. (1994). Distribution of alpha 2-adrenergic receptor subtype gene expression in rat brain. *Brain Res.Mol.Brain Res., 21,* 133-149.

Siegle, G. J., Agranoff, B. W., Albers, R. W., Fisher, S. K., & Uhler, M. D. (1999). *Basic Neurochemistry, Molecular, Cellular and Medical Aspects.* (6th ed.) Philadelphia: Lippincott Williams & Wilkins.

Sokoloff, P., Diaz, J., Le, F. B., Guillin, O., Leriche, L., Bezard, E. et al. (2006). The dopamine D3 receptor: a therapeutic target for the treatment of neuropsychiatric disorders. *CNS.Neurol Disord.Drug Targets., 5,* 25-43.

Sokoloff, P., Giros, B., Martres, M. P., Andrieux, M., Besancon, R., Pilon, C. et al. (1992). Localization and function of the D3 dopamine receptor. *Arzneimittelforschung., 42,* 224-230.

Tavares, A., Handy, D. E., Bogdanova, N. N., Rosene, D. L., & Gavras, H. (1996). Localization of alpha 2A- and alpha 2B-adrenergic receptor subtypes in brain. *Hypertension, 27,* 449-455.

Ungerstedt, U. (1971). Stereotaxic mapping of the monoamine pathways in the rat brain. *Acta Physiol Scand.Suppl, 367,* 1-48.

Vallone, D., Picetti, R., & Borrelli, E. (2000). Structure and function of dopamine receptors. *Neurosci.Biobehav.Rev., 24,* 125-132.

In: The Central Catecholaminergic System
Editor: Bertalan Dudás
ISBN: 978-1-63117-937-2

Chapter 3

Catecholaminergic Regulation of the Hypothalamic Neuropeptide Y (NPY) and Galanin Systems

Bertalan Dudás and István Merchenthaler

Introduction

Neuropeptide Y (NPY) and galanin are neuropeptides widely distributed in the hypothalamus with broad range of cardiovascular, respiratory, immune and reproductive functions. It is a common consensus that both of these neuropeptides are controlled by the catecholaminergic system, and thus, they exert their regulatory role on numerous hypothalamic systems under catecholaminergic modulation. In this regard, galanin and NPY are considered to be key neurotransmitters/neuromodulators by which stress may regulate hypothalamic functions. Indeed, previous studies revealed that perikarya immunoreactive (IR) for gonadotropin-releasing hormone (GnRH, also called luteinizing hormone-releasing hormone: LHRH) and growth hormone-releasing hormone (GHRH) receive dense NPY-IR fiber varicosities that appear to be synapses (Deltondo et al., 2008; Dudás et al., 2000). In rodents, NPY-IR fibers from the arcuate nucleus (Toni et al., 1990) and from the brain stem (Wittmann et al., 2002) innervate thyrotropin-releasing hormone (TRH-IR) neurons in the paraventricular nucleus (PVN) and thus, modulate energy homeostasis. Similarly to TRH, corticotropin-releasing hormone (CRH)-IR neurons in the PVN are also innervated by NPY-IR fibres originating mostly from the brain stem and the arcuate nucleus (Fuzesi et al., 2007; Mihaly et al., 2002). NPY, acting via NPY Y1 receptors on CRH neurons (Dimitrov et al., 2007), may modulate the activity of the hypothalamo-hypophyseal-adrenal axis.

Similarly to the NPY, galanin has been shown to play important roles in the regulation of hypophyseal hormone secretion by acting directly on anterior hypophyseal cells whereby it functions as a hypophysiotropic peptide. In addition, galanin modulates the activity of several hypothalamic neuronal systems by acting as a neuromodulator/neurotransmitter. Some of these galanin-innervated neurons are hypophysiotropic (GnRH, GHRH, growth hormone release-inhibiting hormone [SRIF], TRH, and CRH) and release their products into the hypophysial portal circulation, while others are interneurons participating in different neuronal circuits in the brain (Merchenthaler, 2010). Thus, stress, conveyed by, at least partially, the catecholaminergic system may have a profound impact on a number of vital hypothalamic functions via the NPY and galaninergic neurons.

NPY and Stress

Neuropeptide Y (NPY) is a 36 amino acid peptide with complex biological functions (Chronwall & Zukowska, 2004). A large body of evidence indicates that NPY is fundamentally involved in stress responses, and thus, it can be considered a stress molecule (Carrasco & Van de Kar, 2003; Kakui & Kitamura, 2007; Morris et al., 1987; Rudehill et al., 1987; Zukowska-Grojec et al., 1988; Zukowska-Grojec & Vaz, 1988; Zukowska-Grojec et al., 1996). Plasma NPY levels are raised by various physical and emotional stressors in several species. In rats, electric shock and prolonged immobilization (Castagne et al., 1987; Zukowska-Grojec et al., 1988), cold water exposure (Zukowska-Grojec et al., 1988), handling (Castagne et al., 1987), and transfer to a new environment (Zukowska-Grojec et al., 1988) increase plasma NPY levels. Moreover, hemorrhagic stress in rats (Morris et al., 1987) and pigs (Rudehill et al., 1987) as well as academic stress in humans have been shown to significantly increase NPY levels in the plasma (Al-Ayadhi, 2005). Although stress-induced NPY secretion appears to be independent from the activation of the hypothalamic-hypophyseal-adrenal (HPA) axis in rats (Castagne et al., 1987) and the NPY detected in the peripheral blood is originated primarily from the adrenal medulla and from postganglionic sympathetic nerves (Allen et al., 1984; Bernet et al., 1998; Fuzesi et al., 2007; Lundberg et al., 1983) there is a growing body of evidence that stress also regulates NPY release centrally, in the hypothalamus.

Catecholamines are believed to play a major role in NPY-mediated stress response. NPY has been shown to co-localize with noradrenaline in sympathetic nerves (Lundberg et al., 1982; Lundberg et al., 1983) and with noradrenaline and adrenaline in the chromaffin cells of adrenal medulla (Allen et al., 1984). When released from the adrenal medulla, NPY stimulates catecholamine release in a paracrine fashion (Cavadas et al., 2001; Cavadas et al., 2006; Nussdorfer, 1996) through the activation of NPY Y_1 and Y_3 receptors. The observation that the stress response can be blocked by NPY Y_1 receptor antagonists (Zhang et al., 1997; Zukowska-Grojec & Vaz, 1988; Zukowska-Grojec et al., 1996) indicates the pivotal role of NPY Y_1 receptor in mediating the stress response. Thus, during stress, catecholamine release is modulated by, among others, neuropeptides, including NPY.

A large body of evidence suggests that NPY plays a crucial role on feeding. Feeding-related hormones including insulin, ghrelin and leptin, appear to wield their central effects via NPY-synthesizing neurons of the hypothalamic arcuate nucleus (Gruninger et al., 2007; Meister, 2007). It is also well established that stress has a fundamental impact on feeding behaviour (Gruninger et al., 2007; Meister, 2007; Thorsell, 2008). These results suggest that stressors, at least partially, may trigger stress-related food intake changes via the hypothalamic NPY system.

Catecholamines and NPY

The majority of the peripheral noradrenergic axons have been shown to contain NPY (Domeij et al., 1991; Schalling et al., 1991). Moreover, catecholamines co-localize with NPY in neurons of the human (Hokfelt et al., 1983a) and rat (Domeij et al., 1991; Hokfelt et al., 1983b; Sawchenko et al., 1985; Schalling et al., 1991) brain stem. Although this co-localization may contribute to the amplification of NPY and/or catecholamine secretion, the relased NPY can further stimulate the release of catecholamines in a paracrine fashion (Rosmaninho-Salgado et al., 2007). In addition to the co-localization, it is conceivable that direct catecholaminergic-NPY synapses may also play a crucial role in the catecholamine-induced NPY-release during stress. Catecholamines, in addition to interacting with NPY in the brainstem (Fuxe et al., 1987; Fuzesi et al., 2007; Harfstrand, 1987; Sawchenko et al., 1985), can modulate NPY neuronal activity in the hypothalamus and thus, regulate indirectly the hypothalamo-hypophyseal-gonadal, -thyroid, -adrenal and growth hormone systems (Collu et al., 1979; Collu et al., 1984; Dieguez et al., 1988; Dorn & Chrousos, 1993; Sapolsky & Krey, 1988; Stratakis et al., 1995) via the NPY system.

The morphology and distribution of the NPY-IR neuronal elements in the human hypothalamus have been previously described (Dudás et al., 2000; Dudás & Merchenthaler, 2006). NPY-IR neurons are distributed throughout the human hypothalamus and their number decrease mediolaterally (Figure 1). NPY-IR perikarya are detected periventricularly in the septal region, in the medial preoptic area and in the infundibular region. In the posterior hypothalamus, NPY-IR cell bodies are scattered around the mamillary body. NPY-IR perikarya are typically fusiform or multipolar. NPY-IR fibers with axonal varicosities form dense networks in the periventricular zone of the medial preoptic area and infundibulum as well as along the diagonal band of Broca. Numerous well-defined NPY-IR terminal fields can be observed in the lateral preoptic area.

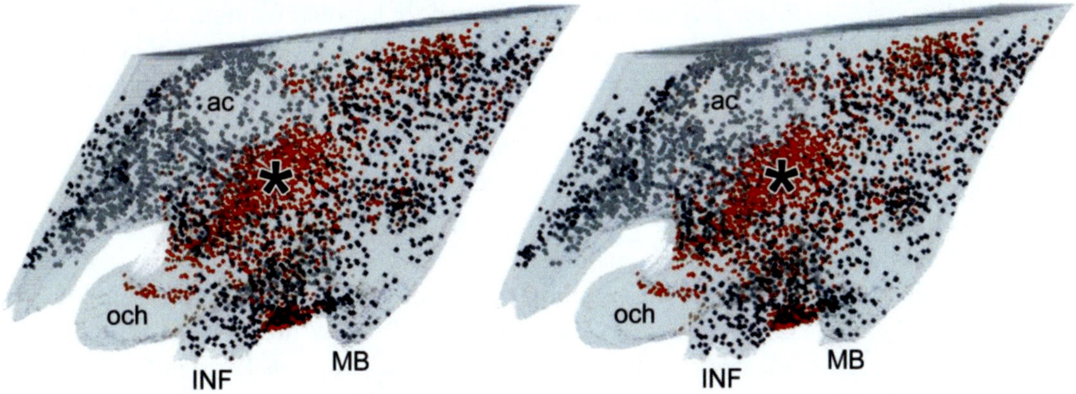

Figure 1. Stereoscopic images of the human diencephalon illustrating TH-IR perikarya (red dots) and NPY-IR perikarya (blue dots). The overlapping sites between these systems are primarily located in the infundibular nucleus/median eminence and in the periventricular zone of the tuberal region and preoptic area. Stereoscopic images can be seen using U or parallel vision. The eyes are relaxed to look into the distance until the pair of the images fuse, and then refocused by the brain. The optimal viewing distance is about 20 inches from the paper surface. Asterisk denotes the paraventricular nucleus. Abbreviations: INF, infundibulum; MB, mamillary body; och, optic chiasm; ac, anterior commissure. Reprinted with permission from Elsevier (Ko et al., 2011).

The distribution of catecholaminergic and NPY-IR neural elements overlap primarily in the infundibular nucleus/median eminence and in the periventricular zone of the preoptic area and the tuberal region (Figure 1). In these areas, catecholaminergic fibers can be found in the close proximity of the NPY neurons (Figure 2) often abutting on the surface of NPY-IR perikarya, typically forming multiple synapse-like contacts in *en passant* fashion while passing by. From these overlapping sites between the catecholaminergic and NPY systems, the majority of these juxtapositions between the catecholaminergic, TH-IR fiber varicosities and NPY-IR perikarya can be observed in the periventricular zone of the tuberal region (Figure 2A-C) where approximately half of the observed NPY-IR perikarya receive more than three contacting catecholaminergic fibre varicosities (Figure 2A-C); the rest of the NPY-IR cell bodies form juxtapositions with 1-3 catecholaminergic fibres or do not receive any apparent catecholaminergic innervation. Although surrounded by catecholaminergic fibers, the subpopulation of NPY-IR neurons located in the infundibular nucleus/median eminence (Figure 2D) generally receive less dense networks of abutting catecholaminergic fibre varicosities comparing to the periventricularly located subpopulation. Here, the majority of the NPY-IR perikarya does not form juxtapositions with catecholaminergic elements; only few of them receive light (1-3 contacts per cell) catecholaminergic innervation. In the PVN and SON as well as in the lateral and posterior zones of the hypothalamus, the number of catecholaminergic-NPY juxtapositions is negligible. Close examination of the hypothalamic sections with oil immersion revealed no gaps between the contacting elements, supporting the concept that these juxtapositions are indeed functional synapses.

In general, juxtapositions between the DBH-IR and NPY-IR elements are less abundant than the TH-NPY associations, indicating that the majority of the observed TH-NPY juxtapositions, at least in the periventricular zone of the basal infundibular area, may represent dopaminergic synapses. Similarly to the pattern of the TH-NPY contacts, the majority of the DBH-NPY juxtapositions are found periventricularly in the basal part of the infundibulum. Here, some of the NPY-IR perikarya receive dense network of abutting DBH-IR axonal varicosities in *en passant* fashion (Figure 2E). Although thin DBH-IR fibre varicosities generally surround some of the NPY-IR perikarya in the infundibular nucleus, DBH-NPY juxtapositions are uncommon here; although few fibers appear to abut NPY-IR cell bodies, due to the thinness of these DBH-IR fibres the verification of the actual contacts is difficult with light microscopy. Since the quantity of the PNMT-IR fibres is rather limited in the human hypothalamus, it is conceivable that the vast majority of the DBH-IR fibre varicosities represent noradrenergic structures. Consequently, the negligible amount of adrenergic, PNMT-IR fibres in the human hypothalamus virtually rules out any significant impact of the hypothalamic adrenergic system on the NPY system.

The adrenergic, PNMT-IR system is represented only by few fibers in the infundibular region of the human hypothalamus; however, these PNMT-IR axonal varicosities are not located in the close proximity of the NPY-IR perikarya, indicating that adrenergic system does not play a role in the direct influence of hypothalamic NPY release. These findings in human are in contrast to rodent data, where all three adrenergic cell groups in the medulla (C1-3) are shown to innervate hypothalamic nuclei (Cunningham, Jr. et al., 1990), suggesting significant species differences in the morphology of the central catecholaminergic system. Indeed, the distribution of dopaminergic, noradrenergic and adrenergic elements in the human hypothalamus appear to exhibit significant differences when compared to that of rodents (Cunningham, Jr. & Sawchenko, 1988; Cunningham, Jr. et al., 1990; Sawchenko et al., 1985).

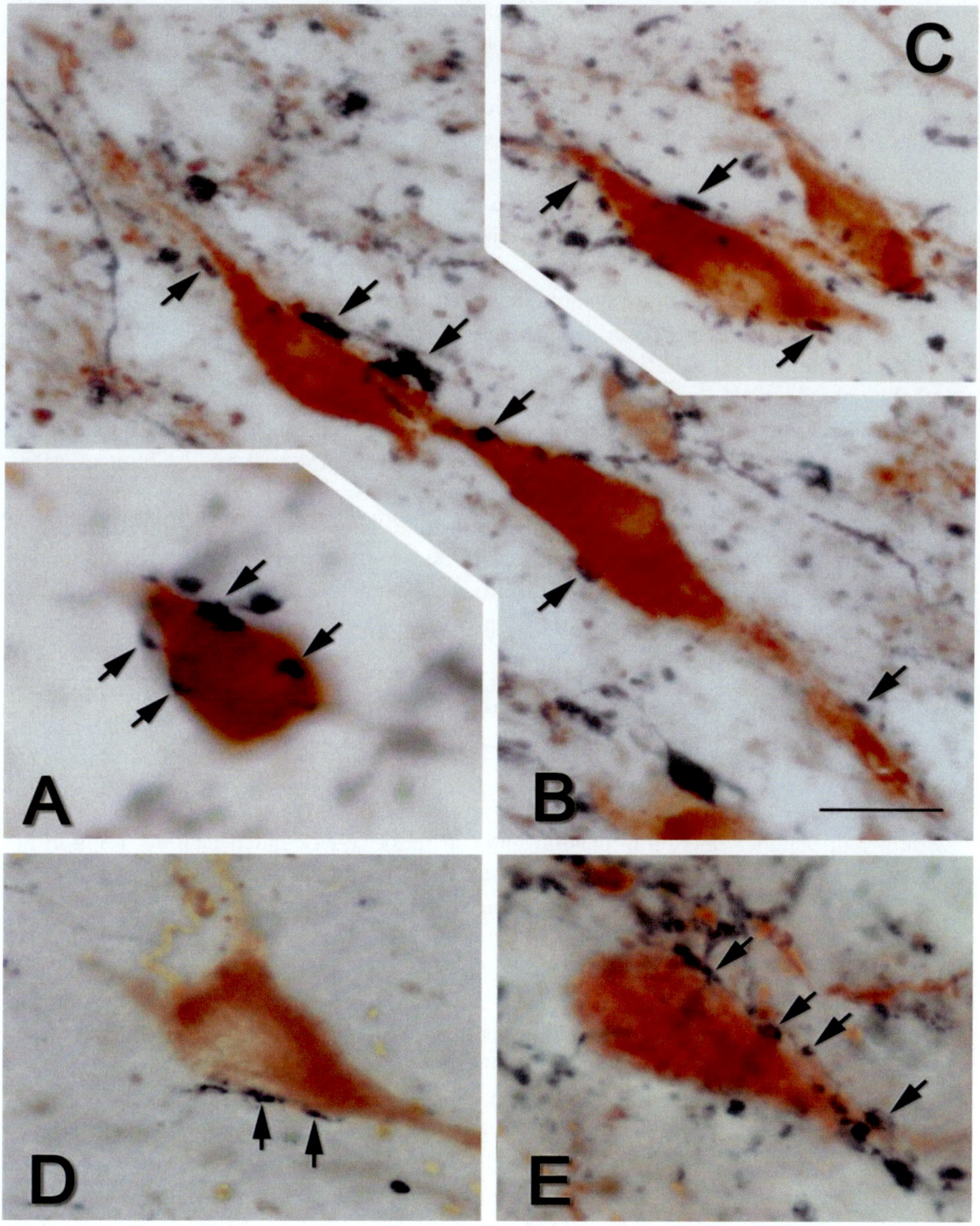

Figure 2. Double-label immunohistochemistry illustrates black, NiDAB labelled, TH-IR, catecholaminergic fibre varicosities abutting brown, DAB labelled, NPY-immunoreactive perikarya primarily in the medial zone of the infundibulum of the human hypothalamus (A-C), while in the infundibular nucleus, the TH-NPY juxtapositions were less numerous (D). Few juxtapositions between the DBH-IR fibre varicosities and the NPY-IR perikarya were also observed in the periventricular zone of the infundibulum (E). The catecholaminergic fibre varicosities often form numerous en passant type contacts with NPY-IR perikarya (arrowheads). Scale bar: 10 μm. Reprinted with permission from Elsevier (Ko et al., 2011).

The morphology and the abundance of the juxtapositions between the catecholaminergic and NPY-IR elements indicate that these contacts may be functional synapses, and may represent the morphological substrate of the catecholamine-induced NPY release. Moreover, the distinct difference between the densities of catecholaminergic axonal varicosities associated with NPY-IR perikarya in the periventricular area of the infundibular region and in the infundibular nucleus/median eminence indicate that the periventricular NPY-IR neuronal subpopulations may play a unique role in the stress response. In addition to the peripheral elevation of catecholamines and NPY derived from the adrenal medulla and postganglionic nerve endings under stress conditions, catecholamines in the hypothalamus may also influence NPY secretion via direct synaptic mechanisms.

It has previously been described that NPY-IR axonal varicosities form intimate associations with GnRH, GHRH, CRH and TRH neurotransmitter systems in the human diencephalons (Deltondo et al., 2008; Dudás et al., 2000; Mihaly et al., 2000; Mihaly et al., 2002). The function of these systems is also known to be suppressed by various stressors in humans (Collu et al., 1979; Collu et al., 1984; Dieguez et al., 1988; Dorn & Chrousos, 1993; Sapolsky & Krey, 1988; Stratakis et al., 1995). Since NPY release has been demonstrated to be induced by stress, the juxtapositions between the catecholaminergic and NPY-IR neuronal elements may also represent a crucial factor in the suppression of reproductive functions, growth, and metabolism in stressful conditions, via the human GnRH, GHRH, CRH and TRH systems.

The Morphology and Function of Galaninergic System

Galanin, a 29 (30 in human) amino acid neuropeptide (Tatemoto et al., 1983) is a member of a family of peptides, including galanin, galanin message-associated peptide (Lang et al., 2007; Rokaeus & Brownstein, 1986), galanin-like peptide (Ohtaki et al., 1999; Santic et al., 2007), and alarin (Santic et al., 2007). Galanin is broadly distributed in the central nervous system and the hypothalamus is particularly rich in galanin-synthesizing neurons and nerve processes (Merchenthaler et al., 1993). Depending on the target, galanin may function as a neuromodulator/neurotransmitter when innervating other neurons or as a hypophysiotropic messenger when it is released into the hypothalamo-hypophysial portal circulation and reaches the anterior hypophysis. Although galanin seems to play a modulatory function at both locations, this does not diminish the importance of its function (Merchenthaler, 2010). Numerous neuropeptides, catecholamines, indolamines and hormones regulate the activity of galanin-IR neurons acting via their corresponding membrane or nuclear receptors (see Merchenthaler, 2010 for a review). When released from nerve terminals, galanin acts via its receptors including Gal_1, Gal_2 and Gal_3. Gal_1 and Gal_3 primarily activate Gi/o types of G-proteins mediating inhibition via adenylate cyclase. In contrast, the Gal_2 subtype transmits either stimulatory effects of galanin, for example, on neurotransmitter release acting via Gq/11 types of G-proteins, or inhibits neurotransmission via Gi/o subtypes. The discovery of galanin receptors and galanin receptor antagonists [see (Branchek et al., 2000; Lang et al., 2007; Santic et al., 2007)] have advanced our understanding on how this neuropeptide functions in the brain, including the hypothalamus. However, much of our knowledge on galanin's distribution, connectivity, and function is based on studies performed in rodents.

Although the confirmation of the connectivity of galanin-immunoreactive (galanin-IR) neurons in the human hypothalamus is important because such observations provide a foundation for existing or future physiological and pharmacological studies and may result in the discovery of species differences, only a few studies has been conducted in primates, including humans (Beal et al., 1988; Bonnefond et al., 1990; Dudás & Merchenthaler, 2004; Garcia-Falgueras et al., 2011; Gentleman et al., 1989; Kordower & Mufson, 1990; Merchenthaler et al., 2010; Michener et al., 1990),

Previous studies revealed that galaninergic perikarya are concentrated mostly at the infundibular nucleus in humans (Dudás & Merchenthaler, 2004). A significant number of galanin-IR perikarya are also detected in the periventricular zone of the preoptic and tuberal regions, the basal perifornical area, the dorsomedial and ventrolateral subdivisions of the ventromedial nucleus, and in the paraventricular nucleus. In the posterior hypothalamus, galanin-IR neurons are found in the periventricular area and around the mammillary nuclei. Dense network of galaninergic axonal varicosities can be observed in the periventricular zone of the entire hypothalamus as well as in the infundibulum/median eminence; smaller amount of galanin-IR fibers reside in the lamina terminalis, along the diagonal band of Broca, and in the tuberomammillary nucleus. Only few galaninergic fiber varicosities are located in the lateral hypothalamus.

Catecholaminergic Control of Hypothalamic Functions via Galanin

Since stress has an impact on numerous hypothalamic functions via the catecholaminergic system, it is conceivable that in addition to the direct catecholaminergic influence, hypothalamic functions may be regulated by catecholamines via the galaninergic neurons. This regulation postulates direct interactions between the catecholaminergic and galaninergic neurons. Indeed, hypothalamic catecholaminergic and galaninergic systems overlap in the infundibular nucleus/median eminence and in the periventricular zone (Figure 3). Here, juxtapositions between the catecholaminergic, TH-IR and galanin-IR neural elements can be found (Merchenthaler et al., 2013). The vast majority of the detected juxtapositions are located in the basal part of the periventricular region of the infundibular area (Figure 4A-F). Here, galaninergic perikarya are surrounded by dense network of TH-IR axonal varicosities that often formed multiple contacts with the cell bodies while abutting, in *en passant* fashion. Many of these close associations are located directly beneath the ependymal layer of the 3rd ventricle. The vast majority of the periventricular galaninergic neurons appear to be heavily innervated by TH-IR fibers, often receiving 3-5 contacts/cell (Figure 4A-F). An additional subpopulation of galanin-IR neurons receive contacting TH-IR axon varicosities in the infundibular nucleus (Figure 4G-I). These juxtapositions are generally more delicate, the abutting TH-IR fiber varicosities are thinner and the TH-galanin contacts are less numerous, averaging 2-4 contacts/cell.

Occasionally, galaninergic axonal varicosities form contacts with the catecholaminergic, TH-IR neurons while abutting on the surface of the perikarya in the infundibular nucleus (Merchenthaler et al., 2013). These contacts are generally more delicate due to the thinness of the galaninergic fiber varicosities and much less frequent than those observed between the TH-IR fiber varicosities and the galaninergic perikarya.

Intimate associations between the DBH-IR and galaninergic elements are far less abundant than TH-galanin associations. Occasional contacts between the DBH-IR axonal varicosities and the galanin-IR perikarya are observed in the periventricular area of the tuberal region and in the infundibular nucleus (Fig 4K). As typical to the catecholaminergic fibers, these juxtapositions are usually *en passant* associations, where the DBH-IR fibers make contacts with the galanin IR cell bodies while passing by. PNMT-IR fiber varicosities are not observed in the close vicinity of the galaninergic perikarya (Figure 4J).

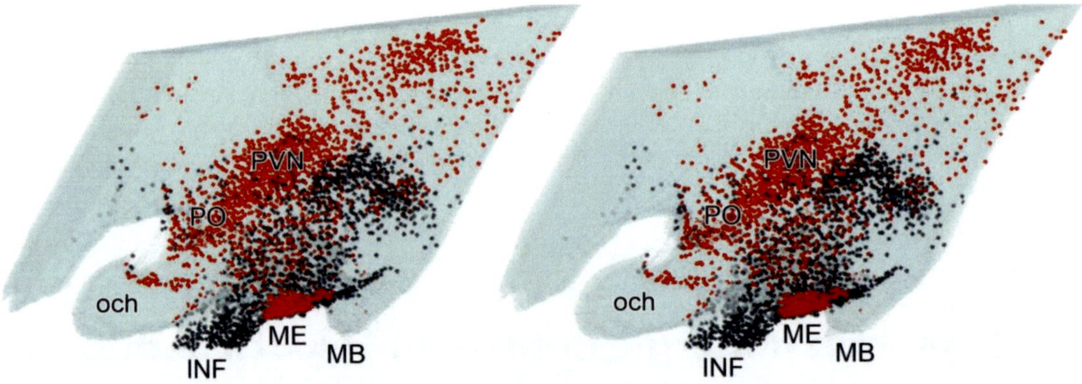

Figure 3. Stereoscopic images of the human diencephalon illustrating TH-IR perikarya (red dots) and galaninergic perikarya (black dots). The overlapping sites between these systems are primarily located in the infundibular nucleus/median eminence and in the periventricular zone of the tuberal region and preoptic area. Stereoscopic images can be seen using U or parallel vision. The eyes are relaxed to look into the distance until the pair of the images fuse, and then refocused by the brain. With this technique a 3D hypothalamus can be seen on the figure, appearing to float in front of the paper, with the immunolabeled perikarya (marked by blue and red dots) discernible at different depth. The optimal viewing distance is about 20 inches from the paper surface (average reading distance). If the separation is too great for the eyes (double vision), move the picture away and the required viewing angle will decrease. Asterisk denotes the paraventricular nucleus. Abbreviations: INF, infundibulum; MB, mamillary body; och, optic chiasm; ac, anterior commissure. Reprinted with permission from Elsevier (Merchenthaler et al., 2013).

Since the density and number of juxtapositions between the DBH-IR and galaninergic elements are far less than those between the TH-IR and galaninergic structures, the contacting TH-IR axonal varicosities on the surface of galaninergic perikarya may represent mainly dopaminergic-galaninergic juxtapositions. Similarly, since no PNMT-IR structures can be found in the close vicinity of the galaninergic structures, it is plausible that the detected juxtapositions between the DBH-IR neural elements and the galaninergic perikarya represent exclusively noradrenergic-galaninergic and not adrenergic-galaninergic associations. These findings are in general agreement with previous studies reporting significantly smaller adrenaline content in the human hypothalamus comparing to that of other species (Mefford, 1988).

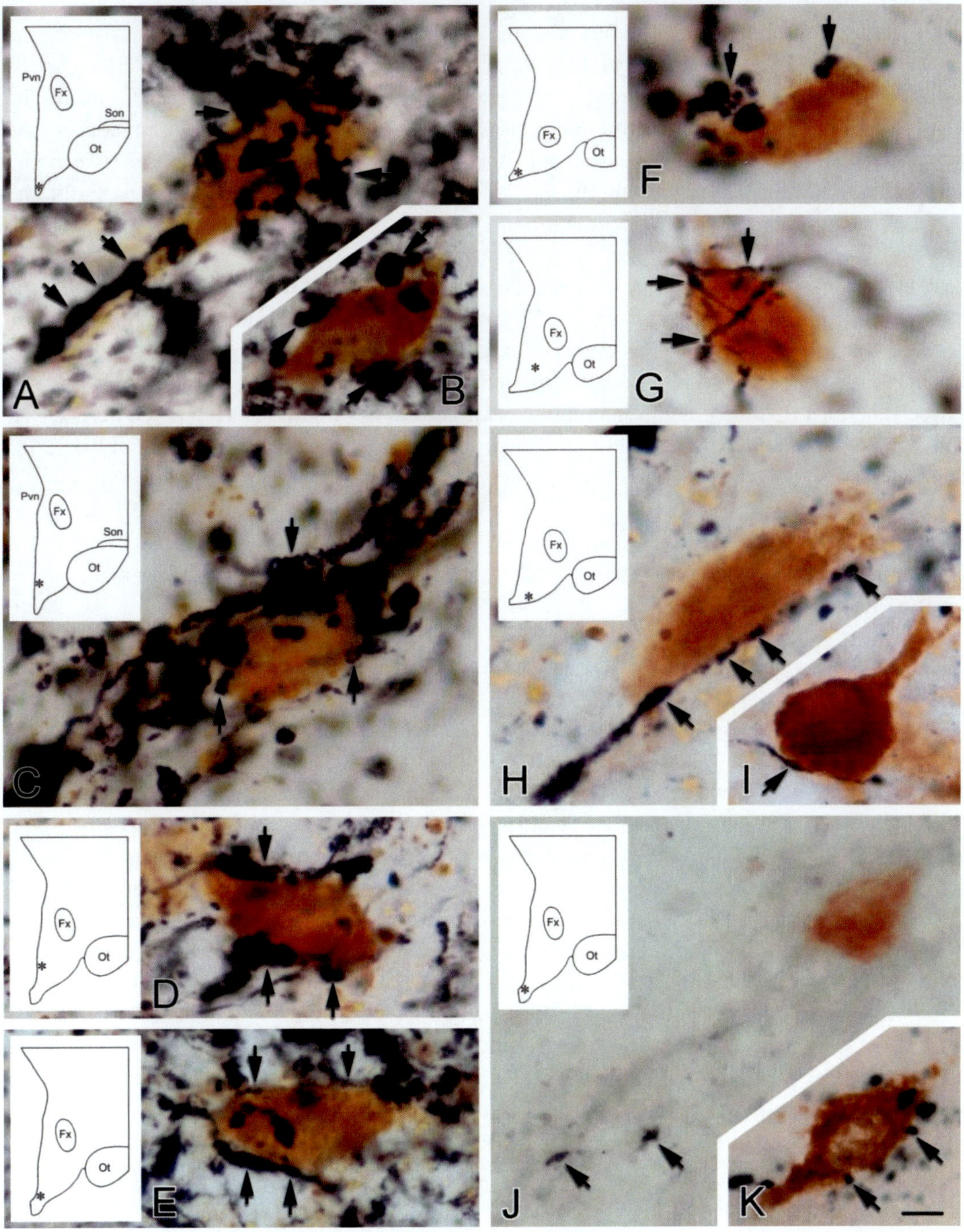

Figure 4. Double-label immunohistochemistry illustrates black, NiDAB labeled, catecholaminergic fiber varicosities forming numerous *en passant* type contacts with DAB labeled, galaninergic perikarya (arrowheads). These juxtapositions are located primarily at the basal part of the periventricular region of the infundibular area (A-F), and in the infundibular nucleus (G-I). Occasional DBH-galaninergic juxtapositions can be observed in the basal part of the infundibulum (K), while PNMT axonal varicosities are not located in the close vicinity of the galaninergic neurons (J). The positions of the illustrated neurons are depicted by asterisks on the coronal hypothalamic sections shown in the inserts. Scale bar: 10 μm. Reprinted with permission from Elsevier (Merchenthaler et al., 2013).

Although adrenergic cell bodies are present in the posterior hypothalamus of the rat (Foster et al., 1985; Ruggiero et al., 1985), no apparent hypothalamic perikarya can be detected in the human hypothalamus, suggesting discernible species differences regarding the distribution of the adrenergic structures. However, the paucity of PNMT elements in the human hypothalamus and the consequent lack of the apparent juxtapositions between the adrenergic, PNMT-IR elements and the galaninergic perikarya might be, at least partially, the result of the rapid *post-mortem* degradation of PNMT.

Due to the inability to utilize anterograde and retrograde tracing techniques in human there is no unequivocal evidence that the same galaninergic neurons that innervate specific hypophysiotropic neurons are innervated by catecholaminergic axon terminals. However, the density and morphology of the catecholaminergic-galaninergic associations indicate that catecholamines may indeed regulate hypothalamic functions via the galaninergic system. These functions involve galanin interacting with neurons synthesizing GnRH, GHRH, CRH, somatostatin and dopamine as most of the data on the action of galanin is well-established for these messengers.

Catecholamines-Galanin-GnRH and the Hypothalamic-Hypophyseal-Gonadal (HPG) Axis

In rodents, galanin is involved in the regulation of reproduction and reproductive behavior [see (Sahu et al., 1994) for a review]. The direct action of galanin on GnRH release is supported by the observations that in humans, galanin directly communicates with GnRH neurons via putative synaptic contacts (Dudás & Merchenthaler, 2004; Dudás & Merchenthaler, 2006) and by the presence of GAL_1 receptors reported in GnRH neurons (Mitchell et al., 1999). By expressing gonadal steroid hormone receptors, galanin-IR neurons, among others, may mediate the feedback action of sex steroids to GnRH neurons (Herbison, 1998; Horvath et al., 1995; Merchenthaler, 2010). Galaninergic neurons also receive TH- and DBH-IR but not PNMT-IR nerve terminals and they appear innervate GnRH neurons (Dudás & Merchenthaler, 2004) and therefore, they can mediate catecholaminergic action on GnRH neurons. However, noradrenaline, one of the most potent stimulators of GnRH neuronal activity, also has a direct action on GnRH neurons [(Dudás & Merchenthaler, 2001), for a review see (Herbison, 1997)]. These observations suggest that catecholamines modulate the activity of target neurons, including GnRH neurons both directly and indirectly, via other neurotransmitter sytems.

Catecholamines-Galanin-CRH and the Hypothalamic-Hypophyseal-Adrenal HPA Axis

Although galanin and its receptors are expressed in all anatomical components of the HPA axis; i.e, the hypothalamus (PVN), anterior hypohysis, and adrenal cortex, the exact role of galanin in the physiology and pathophysiology of the HPA axis has not been entirely understood. The expression of galanin in the PVN is modulated by a variety of physiological stimuli and the activity of galaninergic neurons is also regulated by noradrenergic inputs (Vacher et al., 2002). In contrast to vasopressin and oxytocin, the two neuropeptides co-localized with galanin in the magnocellular compartment of the PVN, the effects of galanin on CRH biosynthesis and release have not been thoroughly elucidated. It has been demonstrated however, that CRH secretion from perifused fetal rat hypothalamic neurons is augmented by galanin (Bergonzelli et al., 2001). Under *in vivo* conditions, galaninergic fibers targeting CRH-IR neurons in the PVN and consequently affecting CRH release may arise from the infundibulum (medial basal hypothalamus, including the arcuate nucleus in rodents) (Gundlach et al., 2001) or from local neurons in the magnocellular subdivisions of the PVN (Levin & Sawchenko, 1993; Palkovits, 2000). Thus catecholamines, primarily dopamine and noradrenaline, stimulate the activity of vasopressinergic, oxytocinergic and CRH-IR neurons directly, but at the same time, they also stimulate galaninergic neurons which in turn, inhibit the activity of vasopressinergic, oxytocinergic and CRH-IR neurons. These observations support the hypothesis that catecholamines may have dual actions: they stimulate the activity of a target circuit but at the same time, they protect from overstimulation by increasing the activity of an inhibitory circuit that operates, among other neurotransmitters, with galanin.

Catecholamines-Galanin-GHRH/somatostatin in the Neuroendocrine Regulation of Growth Hormone (GH) Secretion

Growth hormone secretion is controlled by two antagonistic hypophysiotrophic systems: somatostatin and GHRH. The neuronal network involved in the central control of GH also includes intrahypothalamic neurons such as those expressing galanin and extrahypothalamic neurons of the noradrenergic and cholinergic systems. These hypothalamic and extrahypothalamic systems participate in concert with other components not discussed in this chapter to regulate somatostatin and GHRH neuronal activity. Indeed, previous studies revealed that a dense network of catecholaminergic elements abut on the surface of GHRH neurons in the human hypothalamus, suggesting that stress, among other factors, modulates GH secretion via the hypothalamic GHRH neurons (Rotoli et al., 2011).

The stimulatory action of galanin on GH secretion, in addition to activating the GHRH neuronal system (Hohmann et al., 1998) may also be mediated via the inhibition of the somatostatinergic system. Indeed, it has been shown in rats that somatostatinergic neurons are innervated by galanin nerve terminals in the median eminence (Liposits et al., 1993) and that somatostatinergic neurons express galanin receptors (Chan et al., 1996). Selective blockade of the hypothalamic adrenergic and/or noradrenergic systems, blocks the stimulatory effect of galanin on GH secretion indicating that the actions of galanin on GHRH neuronal activity are mediated, at least partially, via the catecholaminergic system projecting from the brainstem or the infundibulum [for reviews on the regulation of GH secretion see (Bluet-Pajot et al., 1998; Hohmann et al., 1998; Merchenthaler et al., 1993)].

Catecholamines-Galanin Interaction and the Effect on Prolactin Secretion

Similarly to GH, the regulation of PRL is under the dual control. Prolactin secretion is stimulated by yet unidentified prolactin release-stimulating factor(s) (PRFs) and is inhibited by prolactin release-inhibiting factor (dopamine). The hypothalamus exerts a predominant inhibitory control on prolactin release via the tuberoinfundibular dopaminergic (TIDA) neurons. It is generally accepted that prolactin release is induced by exogenous galanin and the action of galanin is mediated via TIDA neurons. Galanin reduces the inhibitory tone provided by dopamine and thus stimulates prolactin secretion. Indeed, it has been reported that galaninergic axonal varicosities form contacts with catecholaminergic, TH-IR neurons in the infundibulum (Merchenthaler et al., 2013). Catecholamines may stimulate the activity of galanin neurons, which in turn, inhibit the activity of TIDA neurons, resulting in elevated prolactin secretion. However, several data indicate that galanin also regulates prolactin secretion by modulating the activity of the PRF system. Among the potential PRFs, the role of vasoactive intestinal polypeptide (VIP), opioid peptides, and catecholamines seems to be compelling [for a review see (Merchenthaler et al., 1993)].

Catecholaminergic Control of Hypothalamic Functions via NPY-Modulated Galanin Secretion

As we have demonstrated, both the galaninergic and NPY system is under catecholaminergic regulation in the hypothalamus. These systems, in turn, modulate vital hypothalamic functions by influencing numerous peptidergic systems, conveying indirect catecholaminergic influence on these functions. The central role of NPY and galanin in this indirect regulatory pathway suggests direct synaptic communication between these systems. Indeed, NPY and galanin appears to be functionally connected in the hypothalamus. Both NPY and galanin play roles in the neuronal circuitry regulating the pulsatile secretion of GnRH and subsequently, the pulsatile secretion of LH (Merchenthaler, 1991; Merchenthaler et al., 1993). Although NPYIR and galaninergic neurons are organized into distinct neuroanatomical pathways in the rat (Chronwall, 1988; Everitt & Hokfelt, 1989; Melander et al., 1986; Merchenthaler et al., 1993) and human hypothalamus (Figure 5) they have a remarkably similar effect on the hypothalamo-pituitary-gonadal axis.

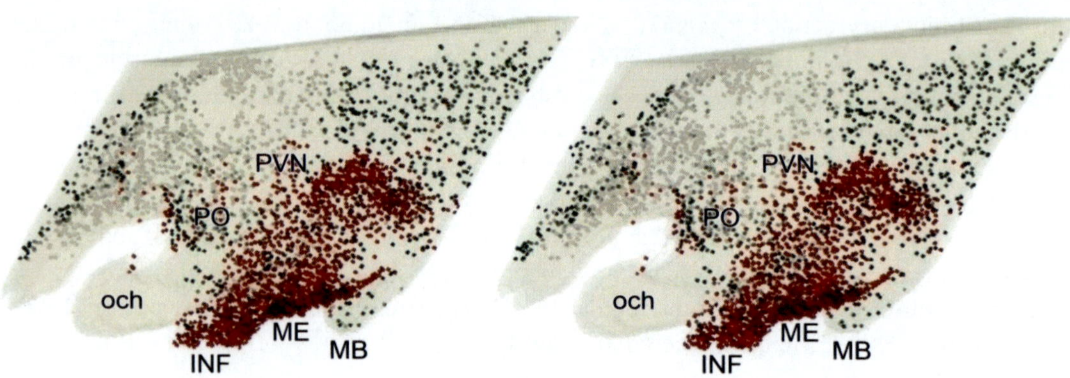

Figure 5. Stereoscopic images of the human diencephalon denoting galaninergic perikarya (red dots) and NPY-IR perikarya (blue dots). The overlapping sites between these systems are primarily located in the basal part of the infundibulum. Abbreviations: INF, infundibulum; MB, mamillary body; ME, median eminence; och, optic chiasm; PO, preoptic area; PVN, paraventricular nucleus. Reprinted with permission from Elsevier (Merchenthaler et al., 2010).

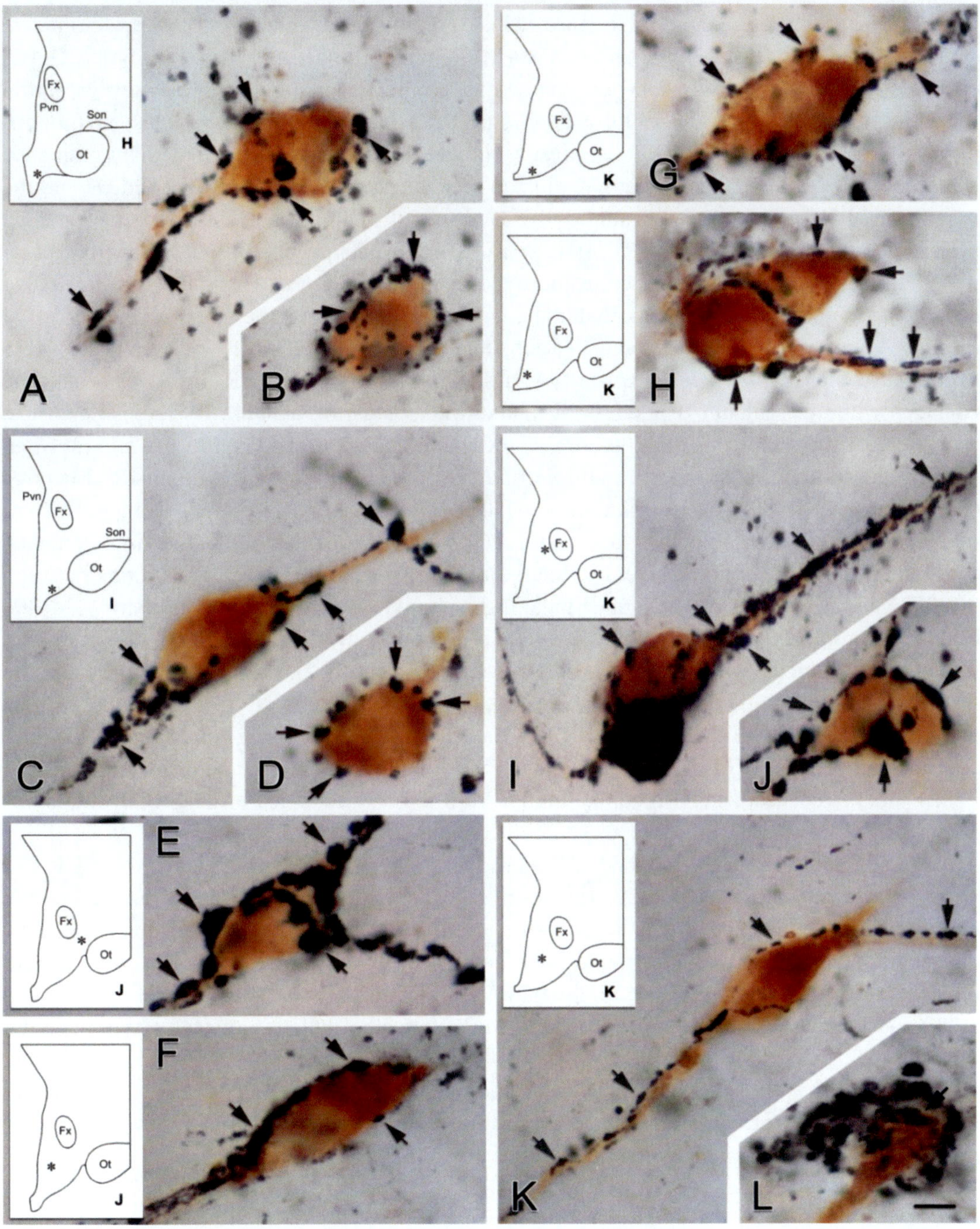

Figure 6. Juxtapositions between the NPY-IR fibers (black) and galanin-IR perikarya (brown) in the human hypothalamus illustrated by double-label immunohistochemistry. The positions of the demonstrated galanin-IR neurons are marked by asterisks on the hypothalamic coronal sections in the corners of the micrographs. NPY-IR axonal varicosities often covered a significant surface area of the galaninergic neurons forming numerous *en passant* type contacts. The thickness of the sections is 30 μm. Arrowheads point to some of the juxtapositions between the NPY-IR and galanin-IR elements. Scale bar: 15 μm. Abbreviations: fx, fornix; pvn, paraventricular nucleus; ot, optic tract; son, supraoptic nucleus. Reprinted with permission from Elsevier (Merchenthaler et al., 2010).

Both peptides augment LH release when administered centrally to ovariectomized, steroid-primed rats (Kalra & Crowley, 1984; Rajendren, 2002), and they can evoke GnRH efflux *in vitro* from the arcuate-nucleus/median eminence preparation (Crowley & Kalra, 1987; Lopez & Negro-Vilar, 1990; Rajendren, 2002). The finding that, at least in rodents, primarily galanin and not NPY is present in nerve terminals of the median eminence (Merchenthaler, 2008) suggest that galanin can mediate the actions of NPY on GnRH and the subsequent LH release. Indeed, studies by Horvath et al. (Horvath et al., 1996) revealed synaptic connections between NPY axon terminals and galanin neurons in the medial basal hypothalamus and the preoptic area of the hypothalamus of the rat. These findings have also been confirmed in the human hypothalamus, where the majority of the galaninergic perikarya receive abutting NPY-IR axonal varicosities (Merchenthaler et al., 2010). These juxtapositions are typically *en passant* type associations where NPY-IR fibers form multiple contacts with the galanin-IR cell bodies and the emanating galanin-IR axons/dendrites, characteristically following the contours of the galanin-IR neurons (Figure 6A-L) and often forming dense fiber network with multiple fiber varicosities around the galanin-IR structures (Figure 6B,E-H,J,L). Close examination of these juxtapositions with high magnification utilizing oil immersion objectives does not reveal any gaps between the contacting elements, suggesting that these contacts may be functional synapses. These close associations between the NPY-IR fiber varicosities and galanin-IR perikarya are located primarily in the infundibulum/median eminence of the human hypothalamus (Figure 6A-D,G-H). In the infundibular nucleus, where galanin-IR neurons are densely packed, the majority of the detected galaninergic perikarya appear to be heavily innervated by NPY-IR fiber varicosities that often cover a significant surface area of the galaninergic neuron forming more than five contacts/cell (Figure 6G,H). A significant number of the galaninergic neurons appear to be lightly innervated, receiving 1-5 contacting NPY-IR axon varicosities while only few galanin-IR perikarya does not have any apparent contacts with NPY fibers.

The attenuation of NPY-induced LH release with the galanin receptor antagonist, GLN *in vivo*, utilizing ovariectomized rats (Horvath et al., 1996) and *in vitro*, utilizing arcuate nucleus/median eminence preparations (Rajendren, 2002) supports the concept that NPY-dependent anterior pituitary hormone secretion is mediated, at least in part, by galanin released in response to NPY. The NPY-galanin communication shown in rats (Horvath et al., 1996) and humans (Figure 6) may provide a more delicate regulation of many hypothalamic functions than those elicited directly by NPY. This dual (direct via NPY and indirect via galanin) control appears to be a general phenomenon as it is present in many mammalian species, and may provide an alternative avenue via which catecholamines exert their regulatory role on numerous hypothalamic functions.

Conclusion

Catecholamines, either directly, or indirectly, modulate many hypothalamic neurons associated with the regulation of autonomic functions, including reproduction, stress, thermoregulation, metabolism and ingestive behavior, water and salt balance, etc., all organized by hypothalamic neuronal circuitries [reviewed in (Merchenthaler, 2010)]. In the present chapter, we have discussed the possibility that catecholamines regulate vital hypothalamic functions not only directly, by affecting hypophysiotropic neurons, but also indirectly, via the NPY and the galaninergic system.

Catecholaminergic fibers establishing contacts with NPY and galaninergic perikarya may represent the morphological substrate of interaction between these systems. Since the amount and density of juxtapositions observed between the DBH/PNMT-IR and NPY/galanin-IR neurons is much less that the number of intimate associations between the TH-IR and NPY/galanin-IR structures, in is conceivable that catecholaminergic system directly influences hypothalamic NPY and galanin release primarily via the dopaminergic system. According to these findings, various stressors may regulate hypothalamic functions via the central NPY and galaninergic system in the human diencephalon. The relative abundance of these catecholaminergic-NPY/galanin juxtapositions in the infundibular region of the hypothalamus suggests that this region may have a pivotal role in the stress response via the NPY and galaninergic system.

Adrenergic and noradrenergic fibers arise from perikarya in the brainstem and reach the hypothalamus via the medial forebrain bundle. Dopaminergic fibers may arise from the brainstem but also from the infundibular and other dopaminergic (TH-IR, but not DBH-IR and PNMT-IR) neurons. Galanin and NPY, innervated by these afferents, can be released into the hypopysial portal circulation and regulate directly anterior hypophyseal function or they can participate in synaptic transmissions innervating hypothalamic (hypophysiotropic and non-hypophysiotropic) neurons and regulate indirectly anterior hypophyseal or hypothalamic functions, respectively.

References

Al-Ayadhi, L. Y. (2005). Neurohormonal changes in medical students during academic stress. *Ann.Saudi.Med., 25,* 36-40.

Allen, J. M., Bircham, P. M., Bloom, S. R., & Edwards, A. V. (1984). Release of neuropeptide Y in response to splanchnic nerve stimulation in the conscious calf. *J.Physiol, 357,* 401-408.

Beal, M. F., Gabriel, S. M., Swartz, K. J., & MacGarvey, U. M. (1988). Distribution of galanin-like immunoreactivity in baboon brain. *Peptides, 9,* 847-851.

Bergonzelli, G. E., Pralong, F. P., Glauser, M., Cavadas, C., Grouzmann, E., & Gaillard, R. C. (2001). Interplay between galanin and leptin in the hypothalamic control of feeding via corticotropin-releasing hormone and neuropeptide Y. *Diabetes, 50,* 2666-2672.

Bernet, F., Dedieu, J. F., Laborie, C., Montel, V., & Dupouy, J. P. (1998). Circulating neuropeptide Y (NPY) and catecholamines in rat under resting and stress conditions. Arguments for extra-adrenal origin of NPY, adrenal and extra-adrenal sources of catecholamines. *Neurosci.Lett., 250,* 45-48.

Bluet-Pajot, M. T., Epelbaum, J., Gourdji, D., Hammond, C., & Kordon, C. (1998). Hypothalamic and hypophyseal regulation of growth hormone secretion. *Cell Mol.Neurobiol., 18,* 101-123.

Bonnefond, C., Palacios, J. M., Probst, A., & Mengod, G. (1990). Distribution of Galanin mRNA Containing Cells and Galanin Receptor Binding Sites in Human and Rat Hypothalamus. *Eur.J.Neurosci., 2,* 629-637.

Branchek, T. A., Smith, K. E., Gerald, C., & Walker, M. W. (2000). Galanin receptor subtypes. *Trends Pharmacol.Sci., 21,* 109-117.

Carrasco, G. A. & Van de Kar, L. D. (2003). Neuroendocrine pharmacology of stress. *Eur.J.Pharmacol., 463,* 235-272.

Castagne, V., Corder, R., Gaillard, R., & Mormede, P. (1987). Stress-induced changes of circulating neuropeptide Y in the rat: comparison with catecholamines. *Regul.Pept., 19,* 55-63.

Cavadas, C., Cefai, D., Rosmaninho-Salgado, J., Vieira-Coelho, M. A., Moura, E., Busso, N. et al. (2006). Deletion of the neuropeptide Y (NPY) Y1 receptor gene reveals a regulatory role of NPY on catecholamine synthesis and secretion. *Proc.Natl.Acad.Sci.U.S.A, 103,* 10497-10502.

Cavadas, C., Silva, A. P., Mosimann, F., Cotrim, M. D., Ribeiro, C. A., Brunner, H. R. et al. (2001). NPY regulates catecholamine secretion from human adrenal chromaffin cells. *J.Clin.Endocrinol.Metab, 86,* 5956-5963.

Chan, Y. Y., Grafstein-Dunn, E., Delemarre-van de Waal HA, Burton, K. A., Clifton, D. K., & Steiner, R. A. (1996). The role of galanin and its receptor in the feedback regulation of growth hormone secretion. *Endocrinology, 137,* 5303-5310.

Chronwall, B. B. (1988). Anatomical distribution of NPY and NPY messenger RNA in rat brain. In V.Mutt, K. Fuxe, T. Hokfelt, & J. Lundberg (Eds.), *Neuropeptide Y* (pp. 51-60). New York: Raven Press.

Chronwall, B. M. & Zukowska, Z. (2004). Neuropeptide Y, ubiquitous and elusive. *Peptides, 25,* 359-363.

Collu, R., Gibb, W., & Ducharme, J. R. (1984). Effects of stress on the gonadal function. *J.Endocrinol.Invest, 7,* 529-537.

Collu, R., Tache, Y., & Ducharme, J. R. (1979). Hormonal modifications induced by chronic stress in rats. *J.Steroid Biochem., 11,* 989-1000.

Crowley, W. R. & Kalra, S. P. (1987). Neuropeptide Y stimulates the release of luteinizing hormone-releasing hormone from medial basal hypothalamus in vitro: modulation by ovarian hormones. *Neuroendocrinology, 46,* 97-103.

Cunningham, E. T., Jr., Bohn, M. C., & Sawchenko, P. E. (1990). Organization of adrenergic inputs to the paraventricular and supraoptic nuclei of the hypothalamus in the rat. *J.Comp Neurol., 292,* 651-667.

Cunningham, E. T., Jr. & Sawchenko, P. E. (1988). Anatomical specificity of noradrenergic inputs to the paraventricular and supraoptic nuclei of the rat hypothalamus. *J.Comp Neurol., 274,* 60-76.

Deltondo, J., Por, I., Hu, W., Merchenthaler, I., Semeniken, K., Jojart, J. et al. (2008). Associations between the human growth hormone-releasing hormone- and neuropeptide-Y-immunoreactive systems in the human diencephalon: a possible morphological substrate of the impact of stress on growth. *Neuroscience, 153,* 1146-1152.

Dieguez, C., Page, M. D., & Scanlon, M. F. (1988). Growth hormone neuroregulation and its alterations in disease states. *Clin.Endocrinol.(Oxf), 28,* 109-143.

Dimitrov, E. L., DeJoseph, M. R., Brownfield, M. S., & Urban, J. H. (2007). Involvement of neuropeptide Y Y1 receptors in the regulation of neuroendocrine corticotropin-releasing hormone neuronal activity. *Endocrinology, 148,* 3666-3673.

Domeij, S., Dahlqvist, A., & Forsgren, S. (1991). Studies on colocalization of neuropeptide Y, vasoactive intestinal polypeptide, catecholamine-synthesizing enzymes and acetylcholinesterase in the larynx of the rat. *Cell Tissue Res., 263,* 495-505.

Dorn, L. D. & Chrousos, G. P. (1993). The endocrinology of stress and stress system disorders in adolescence. *Endocrinol.Metab Clin.North Am., 22,* 685-700.

Dudás, B. & Merchenthaler, I. (2001). Catecholaminergic axons innervate LH-releasing hormone immunoreactive neurons of the human diencephalon. *J.Clin.Endocrinol.Metab, 86,* 5620-5626.

Dudás, B. & Merchenthaler, I. (2004). Bi-directional associations between galanin and luteinizing hormone-releasing hormone neuronal systems in the human diencephalon. *Neuroscience, 127,* 695-707.

Dudás, B. & Merchenthaler, I. (2006). Three-dimensional representation of the neurotransmitter systems of the human hypothalamus: inputs of the gonadotrophin hormone-releasing hormone neuronal system. *J Neuroendocrinol., 18,* 79-95.

Dudás, B., Mihaly, A., & Merchenthaler, I. (2000). Topography and associations of luteinizing hormone-releasing hormone and neuropeptide Y-immunoreactive neuronal systems in the human diencephalon. *J Comp Neurol., 427,* 593-603.

Everitt, B. J. & Hokfelt, T. (1989). The coexistence of neuropeptide Y with other peptides and amines in the central nervous system. In V.Mutt, K. Fuxe, T. Hokfelt, & J. Lundberg (Eds.), *Neuropeptide Y* (pp. 61-72). New York: Raven Press.

Foster, G. A., Hokfelt, T., Coyle, J. T., & Goldstein, M. (1985). Immunohistochemical evidence for phenylethanolamine-N-methyltransferase-positive/tyrosine hydroxylase-negative neurones in the retina and the posterior hypothalamus of the rat. *Brain Res, 330,* 183-188.

Fuxe, K., Harfstrand, A., Agnati, L. F., Kalia, M., Fredholm, B., Svensson, T. et al. (1987). Central catecholamine-neuropeptide Y interactions at the pre- and postsynaptic level in cardiovascular centers. *J.Cardiovasc.Pharmacol., 10 Suppl 12,* S1-13.

Fuzesi, T., Wittmann, G., Liposits, Z., Lechan, R. M., & Fekete, C. (2007). Contribution of noradrenergic and adrenergic cell groups of the brainstem and agouti-related protein-synthesizing neurons of the arcuate nucleus to neuropeptide-y innervation of corticotropin-releasing hormone neurons in hypothalamic paraventricular nucleus of the rat. *Endocrinology, 148,* 5442-5450.

Garcia-Falgueras, A., Ligtenberg, L., Kruijver, F. P., & Swaab, D. F. (2011). Galanin neurons in the intermediate nucleus (InM) of the human hypothalamus in relation to sex, age, and gender identity. *J.Comp Neurol., 519,* 3061-3084.

Gentleman, S. M., Falkai, P., Bogerts, B., Herrero, M. T., Polak, J. M., & Roberts, G. W. (1989). Distribution of galanin-like immunoreactivity in the human brain. *Brain Res., 505,* 311-315.

Gruninger, T. R., LeBoeuf, B., Liu, Y., & Garcia, L. R. (2007). Molecular signaling involved in regulating feeding and other motivated behaviors. *Mol.Neurobiol., 35,* 1-20.

Gundlach, A. L., Burazin, T. C., & Larm, J. A. (2001). Distribution, regulation and role of hypothalamic galanin systems: renewed interest in a pleiotropic peptide family. *Clin.Exp.Pharmacol.Physiol, 28,* 100-105.

Harfstrand, A. (1987). Brain neuropeptide Y mechanisms. Basic aspects and involvement in cardiovascular and neuroendocrine regulation. *Acta Physiol Scand.Suppl, 565,* 1-83.

Herbison, A. E. (1997). Noradrenergic regulation of cyclic GnRH secretion. *Rev.Reprod., 2,* 1-6.

Herbison, A. E. (1998). Multimodal influence of estrogen upon gonadotropin-releasing hormone neurons. *Endocr.Rev., 19,* 302-330.

Hohmann, J. G., Clifton, D. K., & Steiner, R. A. (1998). Galanin: analysis of its coexpression in gonadotropin-releasing hormone and growth hormone-releasing hormone neurons. *Ann.N.Y.Acad.Sci., 863,* 221-235.

Hokfelt, T., Lundberg, J. M., Lagercrantz, H., Tatemoto, K., Mutt, V., Lindberg, J. et al. (1983a). Occurrence of neuropeptide Y (NPY)-like immunoreactivity in catecholamine neurons in the human medulla oblongata. *Neurosci.Lett., 36,* 217-222.

Hokfelt, T., Lundberg, J. M., Tatemoto, K., Mutt, V., Terenius, L., Polak, J. et al. (1983b). Neuropeptide Y (NPY)- and FMRFamide neuropeptide-like immunoreactivities in catecholamine neurons of the rat medulla oblongata. *Acta Physiol Scand., 117,* 315-318.

Horvath, T. L., Leranth, C., Kalra, S. P., & Naftolin, F. (1995). Galanin neurons exhibit estrogen receptor immunoreactivity in the female rat mediobasal hypothalamus. *Brain Res., 675,* 321-324.

Horvath, T. L., Naftolin, F., Leranth, C., Sahu, A., & Kalra, S. P. (1996). Morphological and pharmacological evidence for neuropeptide Y-galanin interaction in the rat hypothalamus. *Endocrinology, 137,* 3069-3078.

Kakui, N. & Kitamura, K. (2007). Direct evidence that stimulation of neuropeptide Y Y5 receptor activates hypothalamo-pituitary-adrenal axis in conscious rats via both corticotropin-releasing factor- and arginine vasopressin-dependent pathway. *Endocrinology, 148,* 2854-2862.

Kalra, S. P. & Crowley, W. R. (1984). Norepinephrine-like effects of neuropeptide Y on LH release in the rat. *Life Sci., 35,* 1173-1176.

Kordower, J. H. & Mufson, E. J. (1990). Galanin-like immunoreactivity within the primate basal forebrain: differential staining patterns between humans and monkeys. *J.Comp Neurol., 294,* 281-292.

Lang, R., Gundlach, A. L., & Kofler, B. (2007). The galanin peptide family: receptor pharmacology, pleiotropic biological actions, and implications in health and disease. *Pharmacol.Ther., 115,* 177-207.

Levin, M. C. & Sawchenko, P. E. (1993). Neuropeptide co-expression in the magnocellular neurosecretory system of the female rat: evidence for differential modulation by estrogen. *Neuroscience, 54,* 1001-1018.

Liposits, Z., Merchenthaler, I., Reid, J. J., & Negro-Vilar, A. (1993). Galanin-immunoreactive axons innervate somatostatin-synthesizing neurons in the anterior periventricular nucleus of the rat. *Endocrinology, 132,* 917-923.

Lopez, F. J. & Negro-Vilar, A. (1990). Galanin stimulates luteinizing hormone-releasing hormone secretion from arcuate nucleus-median eminence fragments in vitro: involvement of an alpha-adrenergic mechanism. *Endocrinology, 127,* 2431-2436.

Lundberg, J. M., Terenius, L., Hokfelt, T., & Goldstein, M. (1983). High levels of neuropeptide Y in peripheral noradrenergic neurons in various mammals including man. *Neurosci.Lett., 42,* 167-172.

Lundberg, J. M., Terenius, L., Hokfelt, T., Martling, C. R., Tatemoto, K., Mutt, V. et al. (1982). Neuropeptide Y (NPY)-like immunoreactivity in peripheral noradrenergic neurons and effects of NPY on sympathetic function. *Acta Physiol Scand., 116,* 477-480.

Mefford, I. N. (1988). Epinephrine in mammalian brain. *Prog. Neuropsychopharmacol. Biol. Psychiatry, 12,* 365-388.

Meister, B. (2007). Neurotransmitters in key neurons of the hypothalamus that regulate feeding behavior and body weight. *Physiol Behav., 92,* 263-271.

Melander, T., Hokfelt, T., & Rokaeus, A. (1986). Distribution of galaninlike immunoreactivity in the rat central nervous system. *J.Comp Neurol., 248,* 475-517.

Merchenthaler, I. (1991). The hypophysiotropic galanin system of the rat brain. *Neuroscience, 44,* 643-654.

Merchenthaler, I. (2008). Galanin and the neuroendocrine axis. *Cell.Mol.Life Sciences, 65,* 1826-1835.

Merchenthaler, I. (2010). Galanin and the neuroendocrine axes. *EXS, 102,* 71-85.

Merchenthaler, I., Lopez, F. J., & Negro-Vilar, A. (1993). Anatomy and physiology of central galanin-containing pathways. *Prog.Neurobiol., 40,* 711-769.

Merchenthaler, I., Rotoli, G., Grignol, G., & Dudás, B. (2010). Intimate associations between the neuropeptide Y system and the galanin-immunoreactive neurons in the human diencephalon. *Neuroscience, 170,* 839-845.

Merchenthaler, I., Rotoli, G., Peroski, M., Grignol, G., & Dudás, B. (2013). Catecholaminergic system innervates galanin-immunoreactive neurons in the human diencephalon. *Neuroscience, 238,* 327-334.

Michener, S. R., Aimone, L. D., Yaksh, T. L., & Go, V. L. (1990). Distribution of galanin-like immunoreactivity in the pig, rat and human central nervous system. *Peptides, 11,* 1217-1223.

Mihaly, E., Fekete, C., Lechan, R. M., & Liposits, Z. (2002). Corticotropin-releasing hormone-synthesizing neurons of the human hypothalamus receive neuropeptide Y-immunoreactive innervation from neurons residing primarily outside the infundibular nucleus. *J.Comp Neurol., 446,* 235-243.

Mihaly, E., Fekete, C., Tatro, J. B., Liposits, Z., Stopa, E. G., & Lechan, R. M. (2000). Hypophysiotropic thyrotropin-releasing hormone-synthesizing neurons in the human hypothalamus are innervated by neuropeptide Y, agouti-related protein, and alpha-melanocyte-stimulating hormone. *J.Clin.Endocrinol.Metab, 85,* 2596-2603.

Mitchell, V., Bouret, S., Prevot, V., Jennes, L., & Beauvillain, J. C. (1999). Evidence for expression of galanin receptor Gal-R1 mRNA in certain gonadotropin releasing hormone neurones of the rostral preoptic area. *J Neuroendocrinol., 11,* 805-812.

Morris, M., Kapoor, V., & Chalmers, J. (1987). Plasma neuropeptide Y concentration is increased after hemorrhage in conscious rats: relative contributions of sympathetic nerves and the adrenal medulla. *J.Cardiovasc.Pharmacol., 9,* 541-545.

Nussdorfer, G. G. (1996). Paracrine control of adrenal cortical function by medullary chromaffin cells. *Pharmacol.Rev., 48,* 495-530.

Ohtaki, T., Kumano, S., Ishibashi, Y., Ogi, K., Matsui, H., Harada, M. et al. (1999). Isolation and cDNA cloning of a novel galanin-like peptide (GALP) from porcine hypothalamus. *J Biol.Chem., 274,* 37041-37045.

Palkovits, M. (2000). Stress-induced expression of co-localized neuropeptides in hypothalamic and amygdaloid neurons. *Eur.J Pharmacol., 405,* 161-166.

Rajendren, G. (2002). Increased galanin synapses onto activated gonadotropin-releasing hormone neuronal cell bodies in normal female mice and in functional preoptic area grafts in hypogonadal mice. *J.Neuroendocrinol., 14,* 435-441.

Rokaeus, A. & Brownstein, M. J. (1986). Construction of a porcine adrenal medullary cDNA library and nucleotide sequence analysis of two clones encoding a galanin precursor. *Proc.Natl.Acad.Sci.U.S.A, 83,* 6287-6291.

Rosmaninho-Salgado, J., Alvaro, A. R., Grouzmann, E., Duarte, E. P., & Cavadas, C. (2007). Neuropeptide Y regulates catecholamine release evoked by interleukin-1beta in mouse chromaffin cells. *Peptides, 28,* 310-314.

Rotoli, G., Grignol, G., Hu, W., Merchenthaler, I., & Dudás, B. (2011). Catecholaminergic axonal varicosities appear to innervate growth hormone-releasing hormone-immunoreactive neurons in the human hypothalamus: the possible morphological substrate of the stress-suppressed growth. *J Clin.Endocrinol.Metab, 96,* E1606-E1611.

Rudehill, A., Olcen, M., Sollevi, A., Hamberger, B., & Lundberg, J. M. (1987). Release of neuropeptide Y upon haemorrhagic hypovolaemia in relation to vasoconstrictor effects in the pig. *Acta Physiol Scand., 131,* 517-523.

Ruggiero, D. A., Ross, C. A., Anwar, M., Park, D. H., Joh, T. H., & Reis, D. J. (1985). Distribution of neurons containing phenylethanolamine N-methyltransferase in medulla and hypothalamus of rat. *J.Comp Neurol., 239,* 127-154.

Sahu, A., Xu, B., & Kalra, S. P. (1994). Role of galanin in stimulation of pituitary luteinizing hormone secretion as revealed by a specific receptor antagonist, galantide. *Endocrinology, 134,* 529-536.

Santic, R., Schmidhuber, S. M., Lang, R., Rauch, I., Voglas, E., Eberhard, N. et al. (2007). Alarin is a vasoactive peptide. *Proc.Natl.Acad.Sci.U.S.A, 104,* 10217-10222.

Sapolsky, R. M. & Krey, L. C. (1988). Stress-induced suppression of luteinizing hormone concentrations in wild baboons: role of opiates. *J.Clin.Endocrinol.Metab, 66,* 722-726.

Sawchenko, P. E., Swanson, L. W., Grzanna, R., Howe, P. R., Bloom, S. R., & Polak, J. M. (1985). Colocalization of neuropeptide Y immunoreactivity in brainstem catecholaminergic neurons that project to the paraventricular nucleus of the hypothalamus. *J.Comp Neurol., 241,* 138-153.

Schalling, M., Dagerlind, A., Stieg, P., Lindquist, C., & Hokfelt, T. (1991). Colocalization of neurotransmitters analyzed by in situ hybridization. *Eur.Neuropsychopharmacol., 1,* 173-176.

Stratakis, C. A., Gold, P. W., & Chrousos, G. P. (1995). Neuroendocrinology of stress: implications for growth and development. *Horm.Res., 43,* 162-167.

Tatemoto, K., Rokaeus, A., Jornvall, H., McDonald, T. J., & Mutt, V. (1983). Galanin - a novel biologically active peptide from porcine intestine. *FEBS Lett., 164,* 124-128.

Thorsell, A. (2008). Central neuropeptide Y in anxiety- and stress-related behavior and in ethanol intake. *Ann.N.Y.Acad.Sci., 1148,* 136-140.

Toni, R., Jackson, I. M., & Lechan, R. M. (1990). Neuropeptide-Y-immunoreactive innervation of thyrotropin-releasing hormone-synthesizing neurons in the rat hypothalamic paraventricular nucleus. *Endocrinology, 126,* 2444-2453.

Wittmann, G., Liposits, Z., Lechan, R. M., & Fekete, C. (2002). Medullary adrenergic neurons contribute to the neuropeptide Y-ergic innervation of hypophysiotropic thyrotropin-releasing hormone-synthesizing neurons in the rat. *Neurosci.Lett., 324,* 69-73.

Zhang, W., Lundberg, J. M., & Thoren, P. (1997). Neuropeptide Y Y1 receptor antagonist (BIBP 3226) attenuates stress evoked tachycardia in conscious spontaneously hypertensive rats. *Cardiovasc.Drugs Ther., 11,* 801-806.

Zukowska-Grojec, Z., Dayao, E. K., Karwatowska-Prokopczuk, E., Hauser, G. J., & Doods, H. N. (1996). Stress-induced mesenteric vasoconstriction in rats is mediated by neuropeptide Y Y1 receptors. *Am.J.Physiol, 270,* H796-H800.

Zukowska-Grojec, Z., Konarska, M., & McCarty, R. (1988). Differential plasma catecholamine and neuropeptide Y responses to acute stress in rats. *Life Sci., 42,* 1615-1624.

Zukowska-Grojec, Z. & Vaz, A. C. (1988). Role of neuropeptide Y (NPY) in cardiovascular responses to stress. *Synapse, 2,* 293-298.

In: The Central Catecholaminergic System
Editor: Bertalan Dudás

ISBN: 978-1-63117-937-2

Chapter 4

Stress and Gonadal Functions: The Role of Catecholamines

Bertalan Dudás and István Merchenthaler

Introduction

It is a general consensus that stress plays a pivotal role in the regulation of gonadal functions in numerous mammalian species including humans. Acute and chronic stress as well as autonomic failure disrupt gonadal physiology (Collu et al., 1979; Collu et al., 1984; Sapolsky & Krey, 1988; Williams et al., 1989). Chronic stress appears to inhibit the amount of circulating LH in the human, baboon and rat (Collu et al., 1979; Collu et al., 1984; Sapolsky & Krey, 1988). Although numerous neurotransmitter systems are believed to be involved in the regulation of gonadal functions by stress, it is believed that stress impacts the hypothalamo-hypophysisal axis, at least partially, via the catecholaminergic system. Indeed, altered luteinizing hormone (LH) release is associated with central catecholaminergic deficiency in polycystic ovarian syndrome (Barnes et al., 1987; Paradisi et al., 1988; Shoupe & Lobo, 1984). Moreover, catecholamines are known to play a role in the preovulatory hormonal changes (Kalra & Kalra, 1983; Rance et al., 1981) and are essential for the initiation of ovulation (Barraclough et al., 1984; Coen & Coombs, 1983; Kalra & McCann, 1974).

Although the mechanisms involved in the gonadal regulation by catecholamines are not entirely understood, several studies indicate that they are based on the control of gonadotropin secretion by the hypothalamo-hypophyseal axis. Indeed, catecholamines have been implicated in the modulation of LH release; however, reports of their effects have been rather contradictory. Noradrenaline actively inhibits LH secretion and pulse frequency in the rat and ewe (Havern et al., 1991; Nagatani et al., 1996), as well as in isolated pig hypophyseal cells (Li, 1989). Moreover, dopamine and adrenaline administration present similar blocking effect in human, ewe and pig hypophyseal cell cultures (Havern et al., 1991; Li, 1989). In contrast to these findings, noradrenaline increases LH release in rats, possibly via the alpha-1 adrenergic receptors (Barraclough et al., 1984; Brann & Mahesh, 1991; Drouva & Gallo,

1976; Gitler & Barraclough, 1987; Martin et al., 1995; Rance et al., 1981; Rettori et al., 1981; Weiner et al., 1988). Indeed, α-1 but not α-2 antagonists block LH secretion and reduce Fos expression in gonadotropin-releasing hormone (GnRH, also called luteinizing hormone-releasing hormone: LHRH) neurons at the time of LH surge in the rat (Le et al., 1997). Administration of an alpha-adrenergic antagonist blocks LH secretion in ovarectomized rhesus monkeys (Pau et al., 1989). Electric stimulation of the locus ceruleus and medullary noradrenergic cell groups increases LH release in rats (Hartman et al., 1989). Moreover, the stimulatory and inhibitory effects of noradrenaline and dopamine appear to be altered during sexual maturation with inhibitory effects predominating in the prepubertal rat (Moguilevsky et al., 1990; Raum & Swerdloff, 1986).

The central regulation of gonadal functions by catecholamines has been suggested to take place at two distinct levels of the hypothalamo-hypophyseal axis. Although the presence of TH-IR elements in the hypophysis of several species (Leshin et al., 1996; Schussler et al., 1992) raise the possibility of direct catecholaminergic control of LH release, there is a general consensus that catecholamines influence LH secretion primarily through the hypothalamic GnRH system (Adler et al., 1983; Bukiia et al., 1986; Havern et al., 1991; Le et al., 1997; Pau et al., 1989; Rettori et al., 1981), either by direct morphological connection between catecholaminergic and GnRH-IR elements or via other neurotransmitter systems contacting the GnRH neurns.

The role of dopamine, epinephrine and norepinephrine in the control of GnRH neuronal activity is controversial and appears to be species-dependent (Herbison, 1997; Herbison, 1998). It seems that stimulatory or inhibitory roles of catecholamines in LH secretion depend on the endocrine milieu and may change during sexual maturation. On the basis of recent molecular and neuroanatomical data, it is proposed that estrogen influences noradrenergic neurons located in the brainstem, specifically within the nucleus tractus solitarius (A2), in order to facilitate synaptic transmission within the GnRH network. In this manner, norepinephrine is likely to play a role in increasing GnRH mRNA expression and secretion necessary for ovulation. In addition to conveying the effects of estrogen, the A2 norepinephrinergic system integrates several visceral and peripheral inputs, and therefore, it is well positioned to modulate the activity of GnRH and other neuropeptides/neurotransmitters interacting with GnRH neurons in response to homeostatic and environmental stimuli. Since adrenergic receptor antagonists block the actions of various neuropeptides/neurotransmitters on LH secretion (Kalra, 1993), norepinephrine is currently considered as a permissive factor promoting high output states of the GnRH neuronal network (Herbison, 1997). Although these findings were originally explained as a serial arrangement among the neuropeptides/neurotransmitters, norepinephrine and the GnRH neurones (Herbison, 1997; Herbison, 1998), it is now considered that there is a parallel relationship between the actions of neuropeptides/neurotransmitters and norepinephrine. With removal of the permissive effect of norepinephrine within the GnRH network, the effect of neuropeptides/neurotransmitters contacting GnRH neurons becomes silent (Herbison, 1997; Herbison, 1998). Thus, the demonstration of tyrosine-hydroxylase (TH)-IR fibers contacting GnRH-IR neurons in the human hypothalamus (Dudás & Merchenthaler, 2001) suggests an evolutionarily conserved role for the norepinephrine system.

Morphology of the GnRH System in Humans

The anatomical organization of the GnRH neuronal system in humans is quite different than that of rodents. In rats, the vast majority (over 90%) of GnRH-IR perikarya are located rostrally in the diagonal band of Broca, medial septum, and medial preoptic area. In contrast, GnRH-IR perikarya in humans occupy two major regions: about 50% of the neurons are located in the preoptic-septal region and the other 50% in the posterior region that involves the infundibulum and posterior hypothalamus (Bloch et al., 1992; Dudás & Merchenthaler, 2006; King et al., 1985; Rance et al., 1994; Silverman et al., 1994) (Figure 1). The majority of the labeled neurons are located in a 2-mm-wide periventricular zone of the hypothalamus, primarily in the periventricular zone of the preoptic region (Figure 1). The number of labeled cells gradually decreases in the mediolateral direction, and 16 mm laterally from the ventricular ependymal surface no GnRH-IR cell bodies are found. Similarly to this pattern, GnRH perikarya are located primarily in the anterior hypothalamus and septal regions, occupying areas along the diagonal band of Broca, in the preoptic and tuberal regions. Few GnRH-IR neurons are present in the paraventricular (PVN) and supraoptic nuclei (SON), as well as in the posterior hypothalamus distributed mainly around the mamillary body. The organum vasculosum of the lamina terminalis (OVLT) contains a significant population of GnRH-IR perikarya and fiber varicosities (Figure 2). Interestingly, *in situ* hybridization studies demonstrated a considerably larger number of cells expressing GnRH mRNA than GnRH neurons observed with immunohistochemistry (Abe et al., 1990; Barry, 1976; Barry, 1977; King & Anthony, 1984; King et al., 1985; Rance et al., 1994; Rance & Uswandi, 1996; Stopa et al., 1991).

Human and non-human primates express two chemical forms of GnRH (GnRH-I and GnRH-II). GnRH-II, like GnRH-I, is highly effective at stimulating gonadotropin release, both *in vitro* and *in vivo*, but the neurons that produce GnRH-II are completely distinct from those producing GnRH-I. The human GnRH neurons have three distinct morphological phenotypes: (1) small, heavily labeled, oval or fusiform, located primarily in the infundibulum, ventral preoptic area, and periventricular zone; (2) small, oval, weakly labeled neurons located in the septum and dorsal preoptic area; and (3) large, round neurons with medium staining density scattered within the magnocellular basal forebrain complex, extended amygdala, ventral pallium and putamen (Krajewski et al., 2003; Rance et al., 1994). GnRH-II expression in primates is concentrated to the PVN, SON, suprachiasmatic nucleus (SCN) and infundibulum and double labeling studies indicate that the two forms of GnRH are not co-expressed (Latimer et al., 2000).

Direct Associations between the Catecholaminergic and GnRH-IR Neurons in Humans

Catecholaminergic and GnRH systems are morphologically and functionally associated; they not only co-localize in certain brain areas (Ibata et al., 1979) but their perikarya comigrate during embryonic development (Verney et al., 1996). Earlier studies also revealed a close opposition between the GnRH cell bodies and catecholaminergic structures in rats

(Hoffman, 1985), mice (34) and humans (Dudás & Merchenthaler, 2001). The origin of these fibers is not entirely known. Most of noradrenergic terminals in the region of the GnRH perikarya in the rat medial septum/rostral preoptic area are believed to originate from ipsilateral neurons in areas A1 and A2 (Wright & Jennes, 1993). In contrast to these findings, dopaminergic neurotoxins administered in the rat preoptic area causes degeneration of the catecholamine terminals on GnRH neurons suggesting that the terminals do arise locally and are dopaminergic (Leranth et al., 1988).

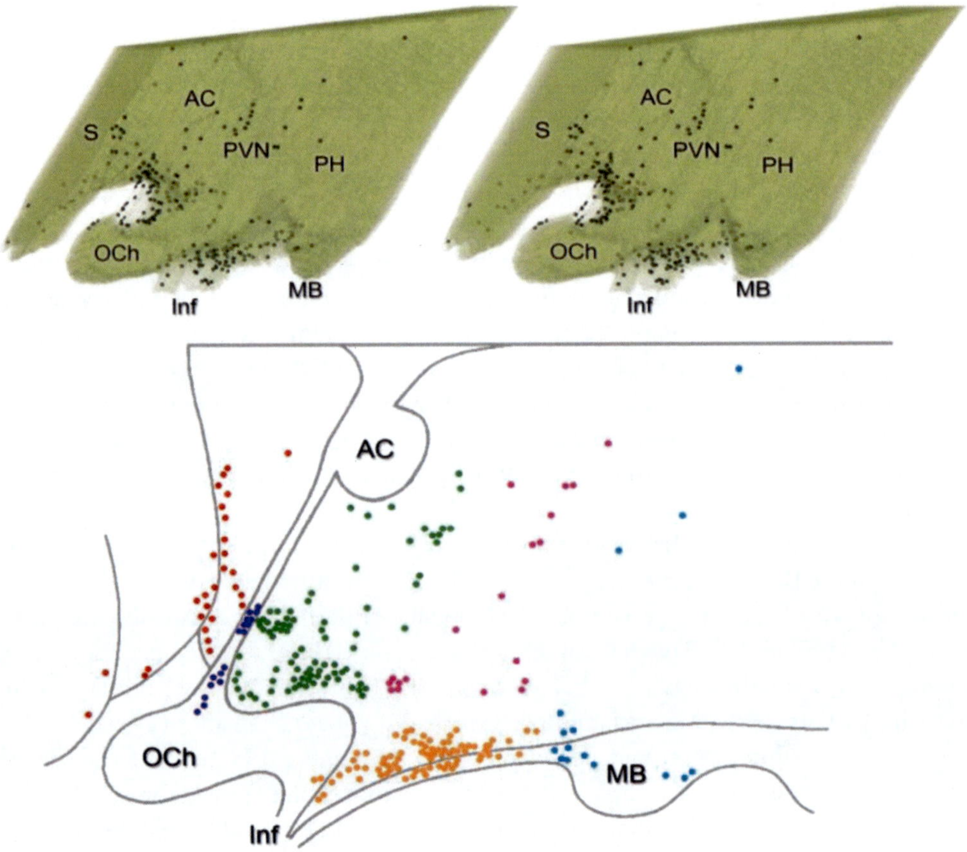

Figure 1. Stereoscopic images of the human hypothalamus illustrating the distribution of the GnRH perikarya denoted by dots (upper inserts). Stereoscopic images can be seen using parallel vision. The eyes are relaxed to look into the distance until the pair of the images fuse. Main subclasses of the GnRH-IR perikarya in the human diencephalon a (lower insert). Colored dots represent the cell bodies. The GnRH-IR cells appear to receive innervation from the NPY, SP, β-endorphin, leu-enkephalin, CRH, galanin, and TH (catecholaminergic) fiber varicosities, except the neurons in the septal area (red dots) that do not appear to form juxtapositions with any of these neurotransmitter systems. The most heavily innervated GnRH subclasses are located in the infundibulum and median eminence, followed by the preoptic area. GnRH-IR neurons in the posterior hypothalamus are only occasionally innervated. Color codes: red, septal area; blue, lamina terminalis; green, preoptic area; orange, infundibulum, median eminence; magenta, dorsal part of the tuberal region; cyan, posterior hypothalamus. Abbreviations: AC, anterior commissure; Inf, infundibulum; MB, mamillary body; OCh, optic chiasm; PH, posterior hypothalamus; PVN, paraventricular nucleus; S, septum. Reprinted with permission from Wiley (Dudás & Merchenthaler, 2006).

Superimposition of the maps of GnRH-IR and TH-IR elements reveals that these systems mainly overlap in the medial preoptic area and the median eminence. Partial overlap can be detected in the periventricular zone of the tuberal part of the hypothalamus, and in the PVN and SON. High magnification examination of the overlapping areas reveals black, TH-IR fibers abutting on brown GnRH-IR neurons forming multiple contacts with the cell bodies and the stem dendrites while passing by (Figure 2).

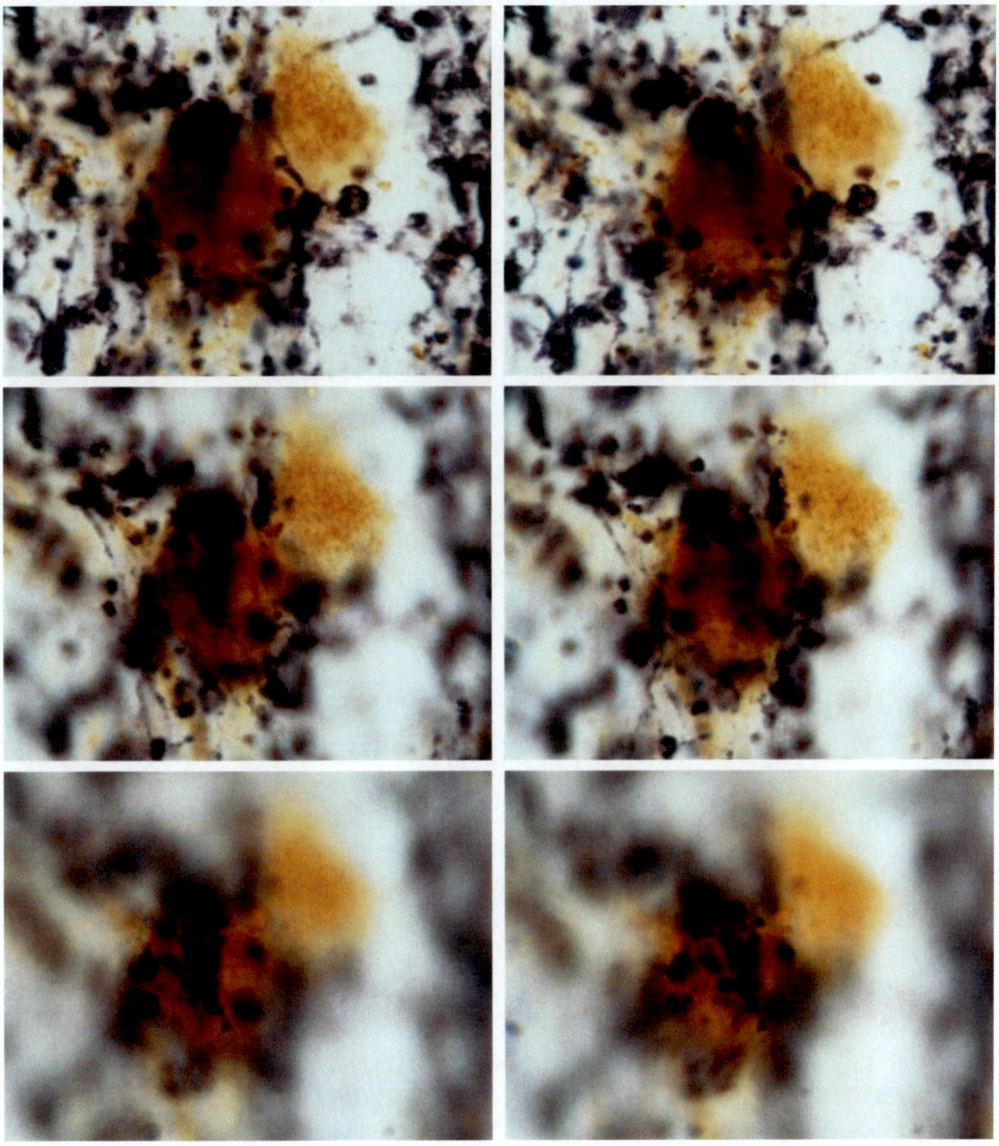

Figure 2. Stereoscopic images of catecholaminergic, TH-IR (black) axonal varicosities abutting on the surface of a GnRH-IR perikaryon (brown) and forming multiple contacts in the infundibular region of the human hypothalamus. Stereoscopic images can be seen using U or parallel vision. The eyes are relaxed to look into the distance until the pair of the images fuse, and then refocused as a 3D image by the brain. Stereoscopic magnifier is suggested to readers unfamiliar with U or parallel vision. Magnification: 400x.

The majority of juxtapositions between the GnRH-IR perikarya and TH-IR fibers (78%) are located in the infundibular region and median eminence. Here, most of the detected GnRH-IR cells are heavily (3-5 contacts) and lightly (1-3 contacts) innervated by TH-IR axon terminals, while one third of the cells do not appear to receive abutting TH-IR fibers. The medial preoptic area contains fewer juxtapositions, and in the majority of these cases the contacting TH varicosities lightly innervate the GnRH neurons with 1-3 contacts. Previous studies reported that the majority of the juxtapositions between GnRH-IR perikarya and TH-IR fibers are located in the medial preoptic area in rat (Hoffman, 1985). However, in humans, most of these GnRH-TH-IR associations are present in the infundibular region and median eminence, indicating significant species differences between the pattern of catecholaminergic innervation of GnRH system. Although few GnRH neurons are located in the PVN and SON, these cells do not appear to form juxtapositions with catecholaminergic fibers. Similar pattern of GnRH-TH associations can be found in human hypothalami irrespective of the sex or age (Dudás & Merchenthaler, 2001).

The infundibular nucleus contains only small numbers of TH-IR perikarya but a dense fiber network, while in the medial preoptic area TH cell bodies dominate. Earlier studies report that the cell bodies projecting to the medial preoptic area are located in areas A1 and A2 (Wright & Jennes, 1993) or the projecting fibers do arise locally (Leranth et al., 1988) in the preoptic area. The distribution of TH-IR perikarya and fibers suggests that TH-IR axon varicosities juxtaposing GnRH-IR perikarya in the medial preoptic area and in the median eminence may originate locally, whereas GnRH-IR cell bodies in the infundibular region may receive TH-IR fibers from distant hypothalamic or extrahypothalamic regions. The difference between the patterns of the TH-IR structures in these regions indicates that GnRH cell subpopulations may receive catecholaminergic innervation from different sources.

Catecholaminergic Influence on GnRH-IR Neurons via Neuropeptide Y

In addition to the direct associations between the catecholaminergic and GnRH-IR elements, catecholaminergic system is believed to regulate gonadal function via the hypothalamic NPY system. As it is described previously in Chapter 3, catecholaminergic fiber varicosities appear to innervate NPY-IR structures in the human diencephalon. Earlier morphological and pharmacological findings strongly suggested that, in turn, these steroid-responsive NPY neurons play a pivotal role in the regulation of LH secretion. In mammals, this regulation appears to occur at the level of the hypophysiotropic GnRH neurons where NPY stimulates GnRH release (Crowley & Kalra, 1988; Kasuya et al., 1998; Khorram et al., 1988; Pau et al., 1991; Pau et al., 1997; Sahu, 1998) and/or at the level of the gonadotroph cells of the hypophysis where NPY enhances LH release. Therefore, the stimulation of LH secretion by NPY can be direct (Chabot et al., 1988; Crowley & Kalra, 1988; McDonald et al., 1987) or indirect, via the potentiation of GnRH-induced LH release (Crowley et al., 1987; Crowley & Kalra, 1987; Crowley et al., 1990; Kalra et al., 2000; Leupen et al., 1997; Leupen & Levine, 1999; Sahu et al., 1995). These synergistic actions of NPY and GnRH on LH secretion are also confirmed in humans (Watanobe et al., 1994). In addition to a synergistic effect operating at the level of the anterior hypophysis, NPY neurons appear to modulate GnRH secretion directly, via direct NPY-GnRH associations.

A number of experimental data have emerged in support of the notion that the hypothalamic NPY-containing neuronal system may serve as a crucial factor in the regulation of the gonadal function (Kalra & Crowley, 1992). Exogenous NPY has been reported to have multiple effects on the reproductive function via the hypothalamo-hypophyseal-gonadal axis in rodents, rabbits and cattle (Evans, 1999; Gazal et al., 1998; Kaynard & Spies, 1991; Sahu et al., 1995; Sahu & Kalra, 1998). These effects include a sex hormone-dependent alteration of GnRH release from the hypophysiotropic neurons and an increased secretion of LH from the hypophyseal gonadotrophs (Kalra et al., 2000; Kasuya et al., 1998; Kaynard et al., 1990; Kaynard & Spies, 1991; Leupen et al., 1997; Leupen & Levine, 1999; Pau et al., 1995; Peng et al., 1993; Sahu & Kalra, 1998; Walsh & Kuenzel, 1997; Watanobe et al., 1994). Interestingly, the effect of centrally administered NPY on GnRH release appears to depend on the site of administration; for example, NPY stimulates GnRH secretion when it is administered into the median eminence, but inhibits GnRH release when injected into the third ventricle (Kaynard et al., 1990; Pau et al., 1995). These seemingly contradictory observations may be reconciled by presuming that NPY axonal varicosities may innervate hypothalamic GnRH neurons partly on their perikarya and dendrites (Li et al., 1999; Simonian et al., 1999; Tsuruo et al., 1990) and/or on their axon varicosities in the median eminence (Li et al., 1999; Pelletier et al., 1984; Silverman et al., 1977; Walter et al., 1990). It is also interesting that the effects of NPY on GnRH release in non-human primates is species-dependent (Kaynard et al., 1990; Pau et al., 1993; Pau et al., 1995), indicating the existence of several different action mechanisms, which may vary among the species.

A large body of evidence indicates that NPY plays a pivotal role in the regulation of the hypothalamic-hypophysial-gonadal axis by modulating LH release in a sex steroid-dependent manner. NPY gene expression has been shown to be enhanced before the onset of the LH surge in estrogen/progesterone-primed ovariectomized rats (Sahu et al., 1995). Concomitantly, an increase in NPY content can be observed in the infundibular nucleus and hypophyseal stalk preceding the LH surge (Sahu & Kalra, 1998). Similarly as in rodents and sheep, the effects of NPY on the LH surge may involve not only the hypophysis, but also an indirect, hypothalamic mechanism, via the hypophysiotropic GnRH neurons. Some *in vivo* (Khorram et al., 1987; Woller & Terasawa, 1991) and *in vitro* (Crowley & Kalra, 1987) experimental data have shown that NPY induces GnRH release in monkeys, rabbits and rats. This regulatory mechanism may involve synapses on GnRH-IR perikarya, dendrites or nerve terminals. The morphological basis of the hypothalamic action of NPY on the GnRH neurons in the preoptic area of rats (Danger et al., 1990; Li et al., 1999; Tsuruo et al., 1990) and sheep (Norgren, Jr. & Lehman, 1989) has already been confirmed.

Although the distribution of GnRH-IR neurons (Abe et al., 1990; Barry, 1976; Barry, 1977; King & Anthony, 1984; King et al., 1985; Stopa et al., 1991) and the neurons expressing GnRH mRNA (Rance et al., 1994; Rance & Uswandi, 1996) are not always identical, previous studies concerning the similar regional distributions of the GnRH-IR and NPY-IR neuronal structures suggest areas of possible communication between the two neurotransmitter systems in human. Indeed, the superimpositions of the maps of GnRH-IR and NPY-IR structures reveal a partial overlapping. The areas with the highest degree of overlap include the diagonal band of Broca, the periventricular areas at the preoptic region, and the infundibular nucleus, where NPY-IR varicose fibers are frequently observed to abut on GnRH-IR neurons. The individual GnRH-IR cells are often contacted at several sites by the axonal swellings of two or more NPY-IR fibers in *en passant* fashion. In some cases, NPY-IR fibers can be observed to twine around GnRH neurons (Figure 3). These juxtapositions are most numerous in the infundibular nucleus (Figure 3) where the majority of the GnRH-IR cells are in intimate contact with NPY-IR varicosities, while in the medial preoptic region 36%, in the anterior periventricular nucleus 25% of the identified GnRH-IR cells are found to be in contact with NPY-IR fibers. No NPY-GnRH contacts can be observed in the diagonal band of Broca. Although ultrastructural data regarding the membrane specializations between the NPY varicosities and the GnRH cell bodies are not available in humans, the morphology and the density of these associations indicate direct synaptic communication. However, a paracrine mechanism for the action of NPY on the GnRH system can not be ruled out. Several studies have reported the presence of NPY immunoreactivity around the capillaries of the median eminence in humans and rats (Abe et al., 1990; Barry, 1977; King & Anthony, 1984; King et al., 1985; Pelletier et al., 1984; Schwartzberg et al., 1990; Stopa et al., 1991) and thus, suggests a potential interaction between NPY and GnRH at this site. However, the presence of interneuronal connections (synapses, close contacts or paracrine mechanisms) between NPY-IR and GnRH-IR neuronal structures in the human brain described above indicate physiologically relevant interaction between these neuropeptides in the preoptic area and in the mediobasal hypothalamus in humans.

The origin of of NPY-IR fibers which may establish potential contacts with the GnRH neurons is not certain in humans. These fiber varicosities may arise from the infundibular nucleus, which exhibits the highest concentration of NPY in humans (Corder et al., 1990), from the septal and preoptic areas, from the scattered NPY perikarya in the medial hypothalamus, and also ftrom the catecholaminergic cell bodies in the brain stem, as indicated by rat data (Sawchenko et al., 1985). Since destruction of the neonatal infundibular nucleus by monosodium glutamate administration do not affect NPY immunostaining in rats, the NPY-containing fibers in the median eminence may originate from the lower brain stem (Meister et al., 1989). However, intrahypothalamic and septal origins are also probable.

Catecholaminergic Influence on the GnRH-IR Neurons via Galanin

Apart from the direct catecholaminergic-GnRH interaction, catecholaminergic system is also believed to regulate gonadal function via the hypothalamic galaninergic system. Catecholaminergic fiber varicosities appear to innervate galaninergic structures in the human diencephalon (Chapter 3). In turn, galaninergic neurons are believed to regulate gonadal functions via the hypothalamic GnRH neurons.

Galanin is a 29 amino acid peptide (Tatemoto et al., 1983) that is is widely distributed in the central and peripheral nervous systems. Galanin is a major cellular messenger within the central nervous system of rodents, regulating diverse physiological functions including cognition (Steiner et al., 2001), nociception (Liu et al., 2001; Wynick et al., 2001) and numerous aspects of neuroendocrine activity that are associated with feeding behavior and reproduction (Reimann et al., 1994; Xu et al., 2000; Yanagisawa et al., 1986).

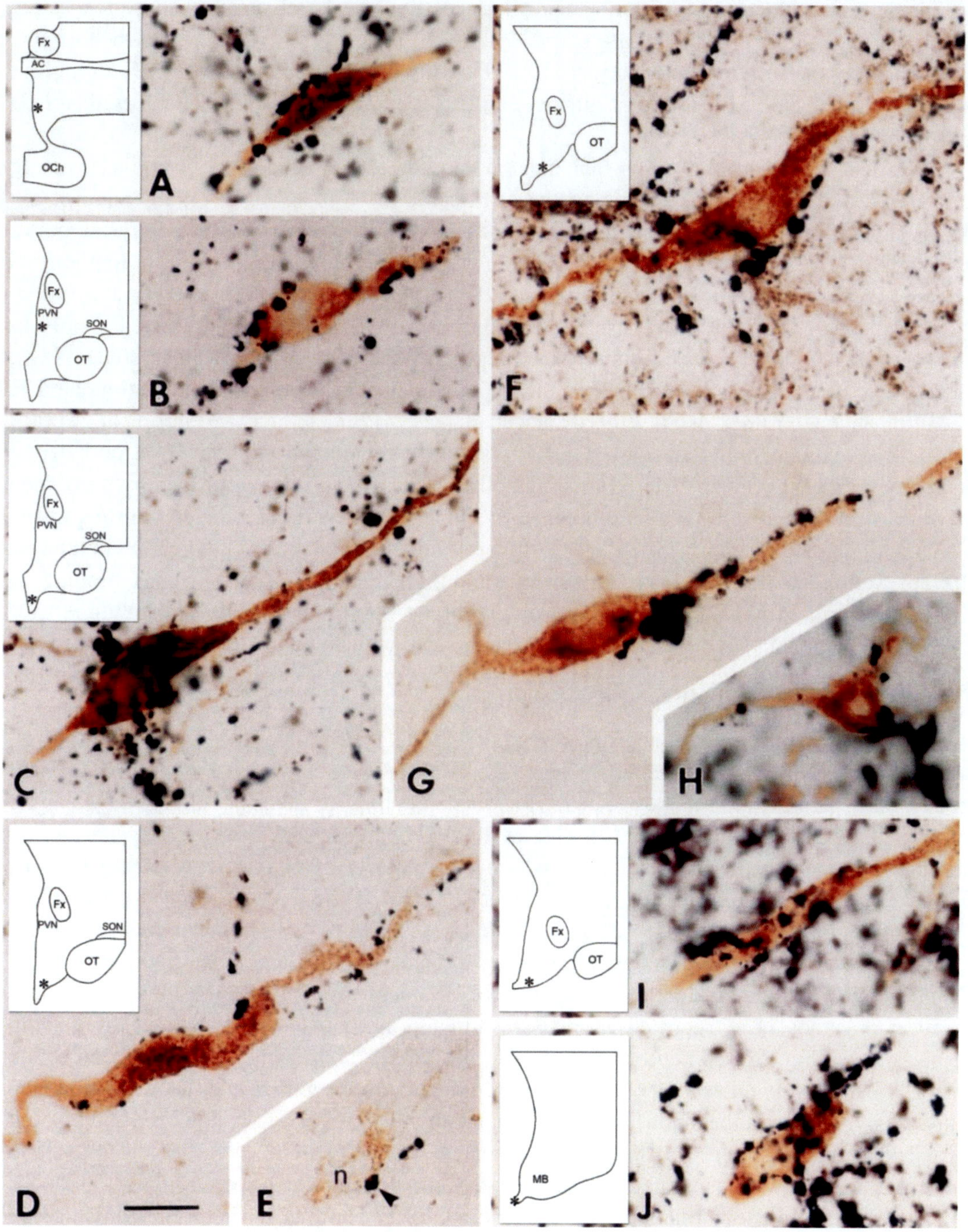

Figure 3. Simultaneous detection of NPY (black) and GnRH (brown) immunoreactive elements in the human hypothalamus. The position of the GnRH neurons is illustrated on schematic coronal sections of the human hypothalamus. Arrowheads point to the NPY-GnRH contacts. The thickness of the sections is 30 μm (A-D, F-J) and that of the plastic section is 1 μm (E). Abbreviations: AC, anterior commissure; Fx, fornix; MB, mammillary body; OCh, optic chiasm; OT, optic tract; PVN, paraventricular nucleus; SON, supraoptic nucleus. Scale bar, 20 μm. Reprinted with permission from Wiley (Dudás et al., 2000).

As a neuroendocrine regulator, galanin induces the release of prolactin (Grottoli et al., 1996; Koshiyama et al., 1990; Murakami et al., 1993; Ren et al., 1999), growth hormone (GH) and LH [see references (Carey et al., 1993; Crawley, 1995; Elsaesser, 2001; Hokfelt et al., 1998; Lopez et al., 1991; Merchenthaler et al., 1993; Sahu et al., 1994; Tanoh et al., 1993) for review].

There is a general consensus that galanin modulates LH release at two levels, acting directly at the hypophysis influencing the LH secretion (Kaplan et al., 1988; Sahu et al., 1994) and/or indirectly, via the regulation of GnRH release into the hypophysial portal circulation (Lopez et al., 1991). Indeed, galanin is synthesized in both the anterior hypophysis (Bennet et al., 1991; Kaplan et al., 1988) and the hypothalamus (Melander et al., 1986b; Merchenthaler et al., 1993; Skofitsch & Jacobowitz, 1985). Galanin, synthesized locally in the anterior hypophysis, has been shown to induce LH secretion in rats (Kaplan et al., 1988); in the same time, galanin synthesized in the hypothalamus has been observed to stimulate LH secretion in rats (Lopez et al., 1991; Sahu et al., 1994) and monkeys (Finn et al., 2000). Therefore, galanin, similarly to GnRH, is also considered to be a hypothalamic hypophysiotropic hormone. These functional observations have been confirmed by retrograde labeling studies from the median eminence in rats by demonstrating labeled neurons in the PVN and arcuate nucleus following peripheral injection of fluoro-gold (Merchenthaler, 1991b; Merchenthaler, 1991a). The observation that galanin enhances GnRH binding to GnRH receptors of hypophyseal gonadotrophs (Sahu et al., 1994) provide further support for galanin as a hypophysiotropic peptide in the human hypothalamus. A hypophyseal action of galanin is also supported by the intimate associations between galanin-IR fiber varicosities and the hypophyseal portal vessels in the infundibulum.

In the same time, galanin appears to regulate gonadal function at the hypothalamic level, via GnRH secretion. Indeed, galanin (Gai et al., 1990; Melander et al., 1986a; Merchenthaler et al., 1993; Skofitsch & Jacobowitz, 1985) and its receptors (Branchek et al., 2000; Melander et al., 1986a; Mitchell et al., 1999; Servin et al., 1987) are present in large concentration in the preoptic area of the hypothalamus, where the majority of GnRH synthesizing neurons reside (Dudás & Merchenthaler, 2006). In addition to being in a strategically important location of the hypothalamus, galanin is co-expressed with GnRH in neurons of the rat (Merchenthaler et al., 1990), mouse (Rajendren & Gibson, 1999) and ovine (Dufourny et al., 2003) medial preoptic area and diagonal band of Broca. However, the colocalization of these peptides has not been reported in primates, including humans. The pattern of galanin expression within GnRH neurons is sexually dimorphic in rodents (Merchenthaler et al., 1991; Rajendren & Gibson, 1999) but not in ovine (Dufourny et al., 2003) with more co-expressing neurons in the adult female than male animals. Interestingly, however, the amount of galanin in GnRH neurons is negatively regulated in mice (Rajendren & Gibson, 1999) and positively in rats (Merchenthaler, 1991b) by estrogen. Nevertheless, several lines of evidence suggest that galanin expression increases within GnRH neurons during their activation in proestrus or following administration of estrogen to ovariectomized rats [for review see (Gundlah et al., 2002; Herbison, 1998; Merchenthaler et al., 1993)]. Galanin, co-localized and co-released with GnRH (Merchenthaler et al., 1990), probably further enhances the pulsatile release of GnRH into the hypophyseal portal circulation (Pau & Spies, 1997; Zdrojewicz & Sowinska, 2000). Observations in rats, mice, and sheep suggest species differences not only in the presence of colocalization of galanin with GnRH but also in the mechanism of galanin-controlled GnRH release.

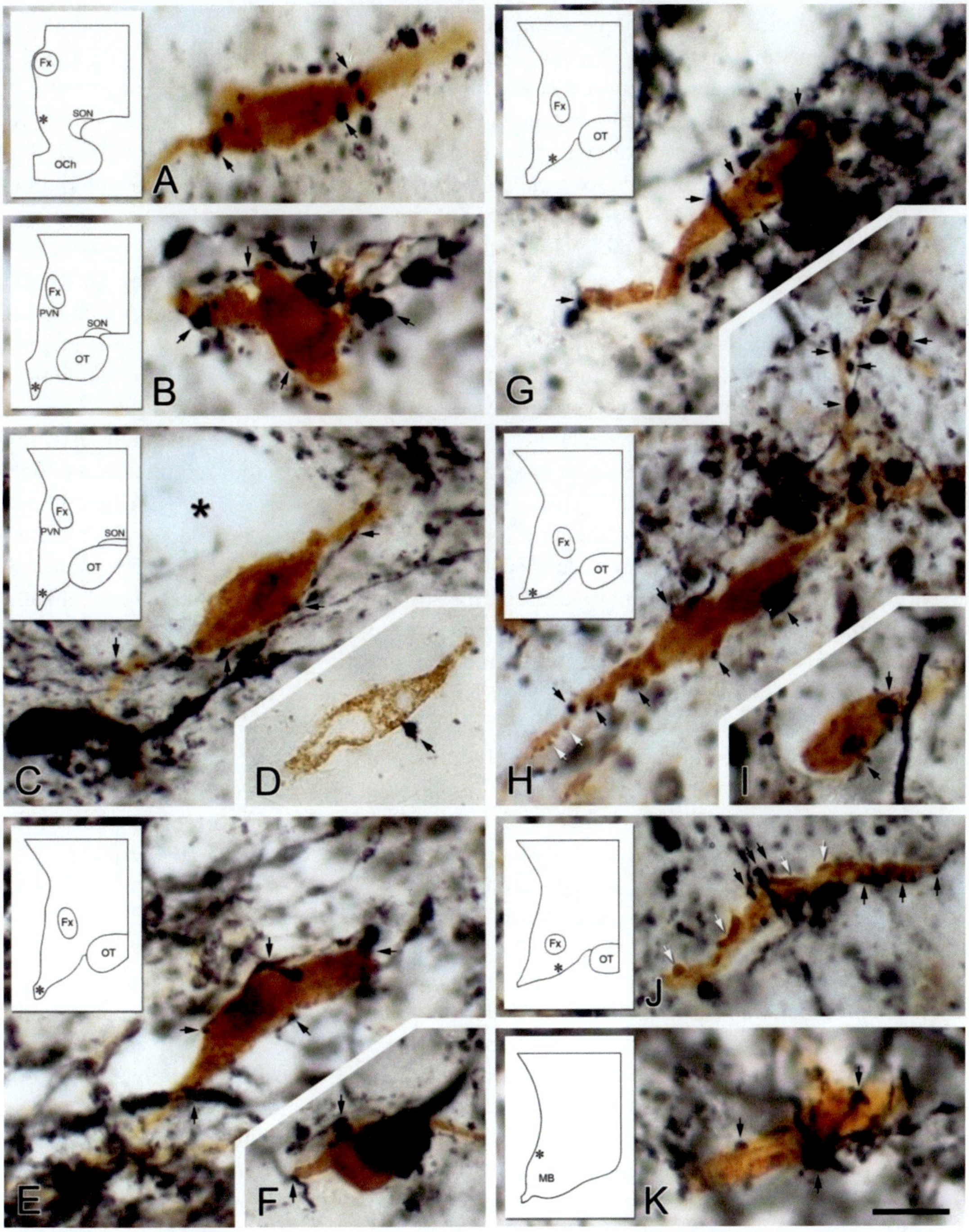

Figure 4. Galaninergic axonal varicosities (black) abut on GnRH-IR perikarya (brown) in the human hypothalamus forming contacts (black arrowheads). The location of the demonstrated GnRH neurons is marked by asterisks on the coronal sections at the upper corner of the micrographs. The thickness of the sections is 30 μm (A-C, E-K) and that of the plastic section is 1 μm (D). White arrowheads denote the juxtapositions between the GnRH-IR axon varicosities and the GnRH-IR perikarya. Five-pointed star marks the portal vessel. Abbreviations: AC, anterior commissure; Fx, fornix; MB, mammillary body; OCh, optic chiasm; OT, optic tract; PVN, paraventricular nucleus; SON, supraoptic nucleus. Scale bar, 20 μm. Reprinted with permission from Elsevier (Dudás & Merchenthaler, 2004).

Although numerous data suggest that galanin is one of the major modulators of reproductive functions in rat (Lopez et al., 1991; Sahu et al., 1994), little is known about the role galanin plays in the regulation of gonadal functions of humans. It has been suggested that galanin participates in the generation of the GnRH surge (Pau & Spies, 1997; Zdrojewicz & Sowinska, 2000). In contrast to known action in the hypothalamus (Zdrojewicz & Sowinska, 2000), galanin has not been shown to stimulate basal or GnRH-stimulated LH concentrations in the hypophysis of humans (Arvat et al., 1995; Giustina et al., 1994).

The galaninergic control of the hypothalamic GnRH secretion is supported by previous studies reporting galanin-immunoreactive (galanin-IR) fiber varicosities abutting GnRH-IR perikarya in the preoptic area of the rat (Merchenthaler et al., 1991) mouse (Rajendren & Li, 2001) and human (Dudás & Merchenthaler, 2004) brain, suggesting a direct synaptic control on hypothalamic GnRH secretion. In addition to the presence of these galaninergic-GnRH juxtapositions, galanin receptor subtype 1 (GAL-R1) is also expressed in a subpopulation of GnRH neurons in the female rat (Mitchell et al., 1999). Moreover, the expression of GAL-R1 within GnRH neurons is present only in proestrous rats or in ovariectomized rats treated with estrogen, and progesterone blocks GAL-R1 expression (Mitchell et al., 1999). Although not shown in humans, other types of galanin receptors are also present in the rodent preoptic area (Floren et al., 2000) and therefore, could be involved in galanin-regulated GnRH neuronal activity. Endogenous or intracerebroventricularly administered galanin probably stimulates GnRH-mediated release via these receptors. The receptor-mediated action of galanin is further supported by the findings that galantide, a specific partial antagonist of galanin receptors, blocks galanin-induced LH release (Sahu et al., 1994). These observations provide further support for galanin as a crucial factor in the initiation of the GnRH and subsequent LH surges prior to ovulation in the rat and possibly in humans. Moreover, these finding support the concept that the galaninergic fiber varicosities abutting on GnRH neurons may represent the morphological substrate of galaninergic control on GnRH secretion.

In the human hypothalamus, the vast majority of the galanin-IR perikarya are concentrated posteriorly to the lamina terminalis in four distinct subdivisions. (1) The infundibulum contains densely-packed galanin-IR cell bodies that are often associated with the portal vessels (Figure 4C). (2) Galanin-IR perikarya are detected in a narrow zone at the basal surface of the tuberal region extending from the infundibular nucleus to the optic tract. (3) Numerous perikarya are located periventricularly, in the preoptic and tuberal regions (Figure 4I-L) including the periventricular zone of the PVN. (4) Finally, in the posterior hypothalamus, the galanin-IR neurons are concentrated in the posterior subdivision of the periventricular area and in the tuberomammillary nucleus. In front of the lamina terminalis, scattered galanin-IR cell bodies can be observed along the diagonal band of Broca and few cells are found in the lamina terminalis itself. Galanin-IR fiber varicosities form a dense network in the infundibulum/median eminence (Figure 4B-J). Numerous axons can be detected periventricularly, in the preoptic and tuberal regions. Few galanin-IR fibers are observed along the diagonal band of Broca, around the anterior commissure and fornix, and in the lamina terminalis. In the posterior hypothalamus, fibers can be detected periventricularly and in the tuberomammillary nucleus.

The galaninergic and GnRH-IR neural elements overlap primarily in the infundibulum and the preoptic area. Indeed, the majority of juxtapositions between the galanin-IR axon varicosities and GnRH-IR perikarya can be observed in the infundibulum/median eminence of the human hypothalamus (Figure 4B-D). Here, the majority of the GnRH-IR neurons are densely surrounded by galanin fibers receiving more than 3 contacts (Dudás & Merchenthaler, 2004). Interestingly, numerous GnRH-IR cells receive both GnRH and galanin-IR axon varicosities in the medial basal hypothalamus (Figure 4H, J). Galanin-GnRH juxtapositions can also been found in the medial preoptic area (Figure 4A) and in the periventricular zone of the tuberal region, while few GnRH-IR perikarya are contacted by galanin-IR fibers in the posterior subdivision of the periventricular zone (Figure 4K), in the lamina terminalis and along the diagonal band of Broca. Close examination of semithin sections of these intimate associations reveale no gap between the juxtaposing GnRH-IR and galanin-IR neural elements (Figure 4D).

Interestingly, GnRH fibers also appear to form contacts with galaninergic perikarya suggesting a bi-directional communication between these two systems. Intimate associations between GnRH-IR nerve terminals and galanin-IR cell bodies can be observed mainly in the infundibulum/median eminence of the human hypothalamus. Here, numerous GnRH-IR perikarya in the infundibulum/median eminence appear to receive both GnRH-IR and galanin-IR axon varicosities. These multiple juxtapositions are not observed on the subpopulation of GnRH-IR neurons in the medial preoptic area and periventricular region, indicating that GnRH release in the infundibulum/median eminence may be uniquely modulated by multiple galanin/GnRH inputs.

Conclusion

Associations between the catecholaminergic system and the hypothalamic GnRH neurons may represent the morphological substrate of the catecholaminergic regulation of the gonadal functions. Additionally, catecholaminergic system may influence GnRH release via the hypothalamic NPY and galaninergic neurons. The density and morphology of these catecholaminergic-GnRH and catecholaminegic-NPY/galanin-GnRH associations indicate that these juxtapositions may be functional synapses and stress may regulate the gonadal functions via these hypothalamic neuronal networks.

References

Abe, J., Okamura, H., Ibata, Y., Motoyama, A., Wakabayashi, I., Ling, N. et al. (1990). Immunocytochemical demonstration of GAP-like immunoreactive neuronal elements in the human hypothalamus and pituitary. *Histochemistry, 94,* 127-133.

Adler, B. A., Johnson, M. D., Lynch, C. O., & Crowley, W. R. (1983). Evidence that norepinephrine and epinephrine systems mediate the stimulatory effects of ovarian hormones on luteinizing hormone and luteinizing hormone-releasing hormone. *Endocrinology, 113,* 1431-1438.

Arvat, E., Gianotti, L., Ramunni, J., Grottoli, S., Brossa, P. C., Bertagna, A. et al. (1995). Effect of galanin on basal and stimulated secretion of prolactin, gonadotropins, thyrotropin, adrenocorticotropin and cortisol in humans. *Eur.J Endocrinol, 133,* 300-304.

Barnes, R. B., Artal, R., & Lobo, R. A. (1987). Peripheral dopamine metabolism in polycystic ovary syndrome. *Obstet.Gynecol., 70,* 153-156.

Barraclough, C. A., Wise, P. M., & Selmanoff, M. K. (1984). A role for hypothalamic catecholamines in the regulation of gonadotropin secretion. *Recent Prog.Horm.Res., 40,* 487-529.

Barry, J. (1976). Characterization and topography of LH-RH neurons in the human brain. *Neurosci.Lett., 3,* 287-291.

Barry, J. (1977). Immunofluorescence study of LRF neurons in man. *Cell Tissue Res, 181,* 1-14.

Bennet, W. M., Hill, S. F., Ghatei, M. A., & Bloom, S. R. (1991). Galanin in the normal human pituitary and brain and in pituitary adenomas. *J Endocrinol, 130,* 463-467.

Bloch, B., Gaillard, R. C., Culler, M. D., & Negro-Vilar, A. (1992). Immunohistochemical detection of proluteinizing hormone-releasing hormone peptides in neurons in the human hypothalamus. *J.Clin.Endocrinol.Metab, 74,* 135-138.

Branchek, T. A., Smith, K. E., Gerald, C., & Walker, M. W. (2000). Galanin receptor subtypes. *Trends Pharmacol.Sci., 21,* 109-117.

Brann, D. W. & Mahesh, V. B. (1991). Detailed examination of the mechanism and site of action of progesterone and corticosteroids in the regulation of gonadotropin secretion: hypothalamic gonadotropin-releasing hormone and catecholamine involvement. *Biol.Reprod., 44,* 1005-1015.

Bukiia, N. G., Babichev, V. N., & Adamskaia, E. I. (1986). Participation of catecholamines in the regulation of an induced wave of gonadotropins in ovariectomized rats. *Probl.Endokrinol.(Mosk), 32,* 47-51.

Carey, D. G., Iismaa, T. P., Ho, K. Y., Rajkovic, I. A., Kelly, J., Kraegen, E. W. et al. (1993). Potent effects of human galanin in man: growth hormone secretion and vagal blockade. *J Clin Endocrinol.Metab, 77,* 90-93.

Chabot, J. G., Enjalbert, A., Pelletier, G., Dubois, P. M., & Morel, G. (1988). Evidence for a direct action of neuropeptide Y in the rat pituitary gland. *Neuroendocrinology, 47,* 511-517.

Coen, C. W. & Coombs, M. C. (1983). Effects of manipulating catecholamines on the incidence of the preovulatory surge of of luteinizing hormone and ovulation in the rat: evidence for a necessary involvement of hypothalamic adrenaline in the normal or 'midnight' surge. *Neuroscience, 10,* 187-206.

Collu, R., Gibb, W., & Ducharme, J. R. (1984). Effects of stress on the gonadal function. *J.Endocrinol.Invest, 7,* 529-537.

Collu, R., Tache, Y., & Ducharme, J. R. (1979). Hormonal modifications induced by chronic stress in rats. *J.Steroid Biochem., 11,* 989-1000.

Corder, R., Pralong, F. P., Muller, A. F., & Gaillard, R. C. (1990). Regional distribution of neuropeptide Y-like immunoreactivity in human hypothalamus measured by immunoradiometric assay: possible influence of chronic respiratory failure on tissue levels. *Neuroendocrinology, 51,* 23-30.

Crawley, J. N. (1995). Biological actions of galanin. *Regul.Pept., 59,* 1-16.

Crowley, W. R., Hassid, A., & Kalra, S. P. (1987). Neuropeptide Y enhances the release of luteinizing hormone (LH) induced by LH-releasing hormone. *Endocrinology, 120,* 941-945.

Crowley, W. R. & Kalra, S. P. (1987). Neuropeptide Y stimulates the release of luteinizing hormone-releasing hormone from medial basal hypothalamus in vitro: modulation by ovarian hormones. *Neuroendocrinology, 46,* 97-103.

Crowley, W. R. & Kalra, S. P. (1988). Regulation of luteinizing hormone secretion by neuropeptide Y in rats: hypothalamic and pituitary actions. *Synapse, 2,* 276-281.

Crowley, W. R., Shah, G. V., Carroll, B. L., Kennedy, D., Dockter, M. E., & Kalra, S. P. (1990). Neuropeptide-Y enhances luteinizing hormone (LH)-releasing hormone-induced LH release and elevations in cytosolic Ca2+ in rat anterior pituitary cells: evidence for involvement of extracellular Ca2+ influx through voltage-sensitive channels. *Endocrinology, 127,* 1487-1494.

Danger, J. M., Tonon, M. C., Jenks, B. G., Saint-Pierre, S., Martel, J. C., Fasolo, A. et al. (1990). Neuropeptide Y: localization in the central nervous system and neuroendocrine functions. *Fundam.Clin Pharmacol., 4,* 307-340.

Drouva, S. V. & Gallo, R. V. (1976). Catecholamine involvement in episodic luteinizing hormone release in adult ovariectomized rats. *Endocrinology, 99,* 651-658.

Dudás, B. & Merchenthaler, I. (2001). Catecholaminergic axons innervate LH-releasing hormone immunoreactive neurons of the human diencephalon. *J.Clin.Endocrinol.Metab, 86,* 5620-5626.

Dudás, B. & Merchenthaler, I. (2004). Bi-directional associations between galanin and luteinizing hormone-releasing hormone neuronal systems in the human diencephalon. *Neuroscience, 127,* 695-707.

Dudás, B. & Merchenthaler, I. (2006). Three-dimensional representation of the neurotransmitter systems of the human hypothalamus: inputs of the gonadotrophin hormone-releasing hormone neuronal system. *J.Neuroendocrinol., 18,* 79-95.

Dufourny, L., Schofield, N., & Skinner, D. C. (2003). Immunoreactive galanin expression in ovine gonadotropin-releasing hormone neurones: no effects of gender or reproductive status. *J Neuroendocrinol., 15,* 1062-1069.

Elsaesser, F. (2001). Stimulation of porcine pituitary luteinizing hormone release by galanin: putative auto/paracrine regulation. *Neuroendocrinology, 74,* 288-299.

Evans, J. J. (1999). Modulation of gonadotropin levels by peptides acting at the anterior pituitary gland. *Endocr.Rev., 20,* 46-67.

Finn, P. D., Pau, K. Y., Spies, H. G., Cunningham, M. J., Clifton, D. K., & Steiner, R. A. (2000). Galanin's functional significance in the regulation of the neuroendocrine reproductive axis of the monkey. *Neuroendocrinology, 71,* 16-26.

Floren, A., Land, T., & Langel, U. (2000). Galanin receptor subtypes and ligand binding. *Neuropeptides, 34,* 331-337.

Gai, W. P., Geffen, L. B., & Blessing, W. W. (1990). Galanin immunoreactive neurons in the human hypothalamus: colocalization with vasopressin-containing neurons. *J Comp Neurol., 298,* 265-280.

Gazal, O. S., Leshin, L. S., Stanko, R. L., Thomas, M. G., Keisler, D. H., Anderson, L. L. et al. (1998). Gonadotropin-releasing hormone secretion into third-ventricle cerebrospinal fluid of cattle: correspondence with the tonic and surge release of luteinizing hormone and its tonic inhibition by suckling and neuropeptide Y. *Biol.Reprod., 59,* 676-683.

Gitler, M. S. & Barraclough, C. A. (1987). Effects of drugs which modify catecholamine activity on amplification of LH release induced by locus coeruleus electrical stimulation. *Brain Res., 437,* 332-338.

Giustina, A., Licini, M., Schettino, M., Doga, M., Pizzocolo, G., & Negro-Vilar, A. (1994). Physiological role of galanin in the regulation of anterior pituitary function in humans. *Am.J Physiol, 266,* E57-E61.

Grottoli, S., Arvat, E., Gianotti, L., Ramunni, J., Di Vito, L., Maccagno, B. et al. (1996). Galanin positively modulates prolactin secretion in normal women. *J Endocrinol.Invest, 19,* 739-744.

Gundlah, C., Lu, N. Z., & Bethea, C. L. (2002). Ovarian steroid regulation of monoamine oxidase-A and -B mRNAs in the macaque dorsal raphe and hypothalamic nuclei. *Psychopharmacology (Berl), 160,* 271-282.

Hartman, R. D., Petersen, S., & Barraclough, C. A. (1989). Limited responsiveness of LHRH neurons to norepinephrine may account for failure of locus coeruleus or medullary A1 electrical stimulation to increase plasma LH in estrogen-treated ovariectomized rats. *Brain Res., 476,* 35-44.

Havern, R. L., Whisnant, C. S., & Goodman, R. L. (1991). Hypothalamic sites of catecholamine inhibition of luteinizing hormone in the anestrous ewe. *Biol.Reprod., 44,* 476-482.

Herbison, A. E. (1997). Noradrenergic regulation of cyclic GnRH secretion. *Rev.Reprod., 2,* 1-6.

Herbison, A. E. (1998). Multimodal influence of estrogen upon gonadotropin-releasing hormone neurons. *Endocr.Rev., 19,* 302-330.

Hoffman, G. E. (1985). Organization of LHRH cells: differential apposition of neurotensin, substance P and catecholamine axons. *Peptides, 6,* 439-461.

Hokfelt, T., Xu, Z. Q., Shi, T. J., Holmberg, K., & Zhang, X. (1998). Galanin in ascending systems. Focus on coexistence with 5-hydroxytryptamine and noradrenaline. *Ann.N.Y.Acad.Sci., 863,* 252-263.

Ibata, Y., Watanabe, K., Kinoshita, H., Kubo, S., Sano, Y., Sin, S. et al. (1979). Detection of catecholamine and luteinizing hormone-releasing hormone (LH-RH) containing nerve endings in the median eminence and the organon vasculosum laminae terminalis by fluorescence histochemistry and immunohistochemistry on the same microscopic sections. *Neurosci.Lett., 11,* 181-186.

Kalra, P. S., Dube, M. G., & Kalra, S. P. (2000). Effects of centrally administered antisense oligodeoxynucleotides on feeding behavior and hormone secretion. *Methods Enzymol., 314,* 184-200.

Kalra, S. P. (1993). Mandatory neuropeptide-steroid signaling for the preovulatory luteinizing hormone-releasing hormone discharge. *Endocr.Rev., 14,* 507-538.

Kalra, S. P. & Crowley, W. R. (1992). Neuropeptide Y: a novel neuroendocrine peptide in the control of pituitary hormone secretion, and its relation to luteinizing hormone. *Front Neuroendocrinol., 13,* 1-46.

Kalra, S. P. & Kalra, P. S. (1983). Neural regulation of luteinizing hormone secretion in the rat. *Endocr.Rev., 4,* 311-351.

Kalra, S. P. & McCann, S. M. (1974). Effects of drugs modifying catecholamine synthesis on plasma LH and ovulation in the rat. *Neuroendocrinology, 15,* 79-91.

Kaplan, L. M., Gabriel, S. M., Koenig, J. I., Sunday, M. E., Spindel, E. R., Martin, J. B. et al. (1988). Galanin is an estrogen-inducible, secretory product of the rat anterior pituitary. *Proc.Natl.Acad.Sci.U.S.A, 85,* 7408-7412.

Kasuya, E., Mizuno, M., Watanabe, G., & Terasawa, E. (1998). Effects of an antisense oligodeoxynucleotide for neuropeptide Y mRNA on in vivo luteinizing hormone-releasing hormone release in ovariectomized female rhesus monkeys. *Regul.Pept., 75-76,* 319-325.

Kaynard, A. H., Pau, K. Y., Hess, D. L., & Spies, H. G. (1990). Third-ventricular infusion of neuropeptide Y suppresses luteinizing hormone secretion in ovariectomized rhesus macaques. *Endocrinology, 127,* 2437-2444.

Kaynard, A. H. & Spies, H. G. (1991). Immunoneutralization of neuropeptide Y suppresses luteinizing hormone secretion in rabbits. *Endocrinology, 128,* 2769-2775.

Khorram, O., Pau, K. Y., & Spies, H. G. (1988). Release of hypothalamic neuropeptide Y and effects of exogenous NPY on the release of hypothalamic GnRH and pituitary gonadotropins in intact and ovariectomized does in vitro. *Peptides, 9,* 411-417.

Khorram, O., Roselli, C. E., Ellinwood, W. E., & Spies, H. G. (1987). The measurement of neuropeptide Y in discrete hypothalamic and limbic regions of male rhesus macaques with a human NPY-directed antiserum. *Peptides, 8,* 159-163.

King, J. C. & Anthony, E. L. (1984). LHRH neurons and their projections in humans and other mammals: species comparisons. *Peptides, 5 Suppl 1,* 195-207.

King, J. C., Anthony, E. L., Fitzgerald, D. M., & Stopa, E. G. (1985). Luteinizing hormone-releasing hormone neurons in human preoptic/hypothalamus: differential intraneuronal localization of immunoreactive forms. *J.Clin.Endocrinol.Metab, 60,* 88-97.

Koshiyama, H., Shimatsu, A., Kato, Y., Assadian, H., Hattori, N., Ishikawa, Y. et al. (1990). Galanin-induced prolactin release in rats: pharmacological evidence for the involvement of alpha-adrenergic and opioidergic mechanisms. *Brain Res., 507,* 321-324.

Krajewski, S. J., Abel, T. W., Voytko, M. L., & Rance, N. E. (2003). Ovarian steroids differentially modulate the gene expression of gonadotropin-releasing hormone neuronal subtypes in the ovariectomized cynomolgus monkey. *J.Clin.Endocrinol.Metab, 88,* 655-662.

Latimer, V. S., Rodrigues, S. M., Garyfallou, V. T., Kohama, S. G., White, R. B., Fernald, R. D. et al. (2000). Two molecular forms of gonadotropin-releasing hormone (GnRH-I and GnRH-II) are expressed by two separate populations of cells in the rhesus macaque hypothalamus. *Brain Res.Mol.Brain Res., 75,* 287-292.

Le, W. W., Berghorn, K. A., Smith, M. S., & Hoffman, G. E. (1997). Alpha1-adrenergic receptor blockade blocks LH secretion but not LHRH cFos activation. *Brain Res., 747,* 236-245.

Leranth, C., MacLusky, N. J., Shanabrough, M., & Naftolin, F. (1988). Catecholaminergic innervation of luteinizing hormone-releasing hormone and glutamic acid decarboxylase immunopositive neurons in the rat medial preoptic area. An electron-microscopic double immunostaining and degeneration study. *Neuroendocrinology, 48,* 591-602.

Leshin, L. S., Kraeling, R. R., Kineman, R. D., Barb, C. R., & Rampacek, G. B. (1996). Immunocytochemical distribution of catecholamine-synthesizing neurons in the hypothalamus and pituitary gland of pigs: tyrosine hydroxylase and dopamine-beta-hydroxylase. *J.Comp Neurol., 364,* 151-168.

Leupen, S. M., Besecke, L. M., & Levine, J. E. (1997). Neuropeptide Y Y1-receptor stimulation is required for physiological amplification of preovulatory luteinizing hormone surges. *Endocrinology, 138,* 2735-2739.

Leupen, S. M. & Levine, J. E. (1999). Role of protein kinase C in facilitation of luteinizing hormone (LH)-releasing hormone-induced LH surges by neuropeptide Y. *Endocrinology, 140,* 3682-3687.

Li, C., Chen, P., & Smith, M. S. (1999). Morphological evidence for direct interaction between arcuate nucleus neuropeptide Y (NPY) neurons and gonadotropin-releasing hormone neurons and the possible involvement of NPY Y1 receptors. *Endocrinology, 140,* 5382-5390.

Li, P. H. (1989). Catecholamine inhibition of luteinizing hormone secretion in isolated pig pituitary cells. *Biol.Reprod., 40,* 914-919.

Liu, H. X., Brumovsky, P., Schmidt, R., Brown, W., Payza, K., Hodzic, L. et al. (2001). Receptor subtype-specific pronociceptive and analgesic actions of galanin in the spinal cord: selective actions via GalR1 and GalR2 receptors. *Proc.Natl.Acad.Sci.U.S.A, 98,* 9960-9964.

Lopez, F. J., Merchenthaler, I., Ching, M., Wisniewski, M. G., & Negro-Vilar, A. (1991). Galanin: a hypothalamic-hypophysiotropic hormone modulating reproductive functions. *Proc.Natl.Acad.Sci.U.S.A, 88,* 4508-4512.

Martin, A. I., Fernandez-Ruiz, J., & Lopez-Calderon, A. (1995). Effects of catecholamine synthesis inhibitors and adrenergic receptor antagonists on restraint-induced LH release. *J.Endocrinol., 144,* 511-515.

McDonald, J. K., Koenig, J. I., Gibbs, D. M., Collins, P., & Noe, B. D. (1987). High concentrations of neuropeptide Y in pituitary portal blood of rats. *Neuroendocrinology, 46,* 538-541.

Meister, B., Ceccatelli, S., Hokfelt, T., Anden, N. E., Anden, M., & Theodorsson, E. (1989). Neurotransmitters, neuropeptides and binding sites in the rat mediobasal hypothalamus: effects of monosodium glutamate (MSG) lesions. *Exp.Brain Res, 76,* 343-368.

Melander, T., Hokfelt, T., Nilsson, S., & Brodin, E. (1986a). Visualization of galanin binding sites in the rat central nervous system. *Eur.J Pharmacol., 124,* 381-382.

Melander, T., Hokfelt, T., & Rokaeus, A. (1986b). Distribution of galaninlike immunoreactivity in the rat central nervous system. *J Comp Neurol., 248,* 475-517.

Merchenthaler, I. (1991a). Neurons with access to the general circulation in the central nervous system of the rat: a retrograde tracing study with fluoro-gold. *Neuroscience, 44,* 655-662.

Merchenthaler, I. (1991b). The hypophysiotropic galanin system of the rat brain. *Neuroscience, 44,* 643-654.

Merchenthaler, I., Lopez, F. J., Lennard, D. E., & Negro-Vilar, A. (1991). Sexual differences in the distribution of neurons coexpressing galanin and luteinizing hormone-releasing hormone in the rat brain. *Endocrinology, 129,* 1977-1986.

Merchenthaler, I., Lopez, F. J., & Negro-Vilar, A. (1990). Colocalization of galanin and luteinizing hormone-releasing hormone in a subset of preoptic hypothalamic neurons: anatomical and functional correlates. *Proc.Natl.Acad.Sci.U.S.A, 87,* 6326-6330.

Merchenthaler, I., Lopez, F. J., & Negro-Vilar, A. (1993). Anatomy and physiology of central galanin-containing pathways. *Prog.Neurobiol, 40,* 711-769.

Mitchell, V., Bouret, S., Prevot, V., Jennes, L., & Beauvillain, J. C. (1999). Evidence for expression of galanin receptor Gal-R1 mRNA in certain gonadotropin releasing hormone neurones of the rostral preoptic area. *J Neuroendocrinol., 11,* 805-812.

Moguilevsky, J. A., Arias, P., Szwarcfarb, B., Carbone, S., & Rondina, D. (1990). Sexual maturation modifies the catecholaminergic control of gonadotrophin secretion and the effect of ovarian hormones on hypothalamic neurotransmitters in female rats. *Neuroendocrinology, 52,* 393-398.

Murakami, Y., Ohshima, K., Mochizuki, T., & Yanaihara, N. (1993). Effect of human galanin on growth hormone prolactin, and antidiuretic hormone secretion in normal men. *J Clin Endocrinol.Metab, 77,* 1436-1438.

Nagatani, S., Tsukamura, H., Murahashi, K., Bucholtz, D. C., Foster, D. L., & Maeda, K. (1996). Paraventricular norepinephrine release mediates glucoprivic suppression of pulsatile luteinizing hormone secretion. *Endocrinology, 137,* 3183-3186.

Norgren, R. B., Jr. & Lehman, M. N. (1989). A double-label pre-embedding immunoperoxidase technique for electron microscopy using diaminobenzidine and tetramethylbenzidine as markers. *J Histochem.Cytochem., 37,* 1283-1289.

Paradisi, R., Grossi, G., Venturoli, S., Capelli, M., Porcu, E., Fabbri, R. et al. (1988). Evidence for a hypothalamic alteration of catecholamine metabolism in polycystic ovary syndrome. *Clin.Endocrinol.(Oxf), 29,* 317-326.

Pau, K. Y., Berria, M., Hess, D. L., & Spies, H. G. (1993). Preovulatory gonadotropin-releasing hormone surge in ovarian-intact rhesus macaques. *Endocrinology, 133,* 1650-1656.

Pau, K. Y., Berria, M., Hess, D. L., & Spies, H. G. (1995). Hypothalamic site-dependent effects of neuropeptide Y on gonadotropin-releasing hormone secretion in rhesus macaques. *J Neuroendocrinol., 7,* 63-67.

Pau, K. Y., Hess, D. L., Kaynard, A. H., Ji, W. Z., Gliessman, P. M., & Spies, H. G. (1989). Suppression of mediobasal hypothalamic gonadotropin-releasing hormone and plasma luteinizing hormone pulsatile patterns by phentolamine in ovariectomized rhesus macaques. *Endocrinology, 124,* 891-898.

Pau, K. Y., Kaynard, A. H., Hess, D. L., & Spies, H. G. (1991). Effects of neuropeptide Y on the in vitro release of gonadotropin-releasing hormone, luteinizing hormone, and beta-endorphin and pituitary responsiveness to gonadotropin-releasing hormone in female macaques. *Neuroendocrinology, 53,* 396-403.

Pau, K. Y., Ma, Y. J., Yu, J. H., Yang, S. P., Airhart, N., & Spies, H. G. (1997). Topographic comparison of the expression of norepinephrine transporter, tyrosine hydroxylase and neuropeptide Y mRNA in association with dopamine beta-hydroxylase neurons in the rabbit brainstem. *Brain Res.Mol.Brain Res., 48,* 367-381.

Pau, K. Y. & Spies, H. G. (1997). Neuroendocrine signals in the regulation of gonadotropin-releasing hormone secretion. *Chin J Physiol, 40,* 181-196.

Pelletier, G., Desy, L., Kerkerian, L., & Cote, J. (1984). Immunocytochemical localization of neuropeptide Y (NPY) in the human hypothalamus. *Cell Tissue Res, 238,* 203-205.

Peng, C., Chang, J. P., Yu, K. L., Wong, A. O., Van, G. F., Peter, R. E. et al. (1993). Neuropeptide-Y stimulates growth hormone and gonadotropin-II secretion in the goldfish pituitary: involvement of both presynaptic and pituitary cell actions. *Endocrinology, 132,* 1820-1829.

Rajendren, G. & Gibson, M. J. (1999). Expression of galanin immunoreactivity in gonadotropin-releasing hormone neurons in mice: a confocal microscopic study. *Brain Res, 821,* 270-276.

Rajendren, G. & Li, X. (2001). Galanin synaptic input to gonadotropin-releasing hormone perikarya in juvenile and adult female mice: implications for sexual maturity. *Brain Res Dev.Brain Res, 131,* 161-165.

Rance, N., Wise, P. M., Selmanoff, M. K., & Barraclough, C. A. (1981). Catecholamine turnover rates in discrete hypothalamic areas and associated changes in median eminence luteinizing hormone-releasing hormone and serum gonadotropins on proestrus and diestrous day 1. *Endocrinology, 108,* 1795-1802.

Rance, N. E. & Uswandi, S. V. (1996). Gonadotropin-releasing hormone gene expression is increased in the medial basal hypothalamus of postmenopausal women. *J Clin Endocrinol Metab, 81,* 3540-3546.

Rance, N. E., Young, W. S., III, & McMullen, N. T. (1994). Topography of neurons expressing luteinizing hormone-releasing hormone gene transcripts in the human hypothalamus and basal forebrain. *J.Comp Neurol., 339,* 573-586.

Raum, W. J. & Swerdloff, R. S. (1986). The effect of hypothalamic catecholamine synthesis inhibition by alpha-methyltyrosine on gonadotropin secretion during sexual maturation in the male Wistar rat. *Endocrinology, 119,* 168-175.

Reimann, W., Englberger, W., Friderichs, E., Selve, N., & Wilffert, B. (1994). Spinal antinociception by morphine in rats is antagonised by galanin receptor antagonists. *Naunyn Schmiedebergs Arch.Pharmacol., 350,* 380-386.

Ren, J., Koenig, J. I., & Hooi, S. C. (1999). Stimulation of anterior pituitary galanin and prolactin gene expression in suckling rats. *Endocrine., 11,* 251-256.

Rettori, V., Seilicovich, A., Goijman, S., & Debeljuk, L. (1981). Effect of inhibitors of catecholamine synthesis on the pituitary response to LH-RH. *Arch.Androl, 6,* 151-154.

Sahu, A. (1998). Absence of increased hypothalamic nitric oxide synthase gene expression during the preovulatory LH surge in middle-aged rats. *Neuroreport, 9,* 4019-4023.

Sahu, A., Crowley, W. R., & Kalra, S. P. (1995). Evidence that hypothalamic neuropeptide Y gene expression increases before the onset of the preovulatory LH surge. *J Neuroendocrinol., 7,* 291-296.

Sahu, A. & Kalra, S. P. (1998). Absence of increased neuropeptide Y neuronal activity before and during the luteinizing hormone (LH) surge may underlie the attenuated preovulatory LH surge in middle-aged rats. *Endocrinology, 139,* 696-702.

Sahu, A., Xu, B., & Kalra, S. P. (1994). Role of galanin in stimulation of pituitary luteinizing hormone secretion as revealed by a specific receptor antagonist, galantide. *Endocrinology, 134,* 529-536.

Sapolsky, R. M. & Krey, L. C. (1988). Stress-induced suppression of luteinizing hormone concentrations in wild baboons: role of opiates. *J.Clin.Endocrinol.Metab, 66,* 722-726.

Sawchenko, P. E., Swanson, L. W., Grzanna, R., Howe, P. R., Bloom, S. R., & Polak, J. M. (1985). Colocalization of neuropeptide Y immunoreactivity in brainstem catecholaminergic neurons that project to the paraventricular nucleus of the hypothalamus. *J Comp Neurol., 241,* 138-153.

Schussler, N., Bayet, M. C., Frain, O., Peillon, F., & Biguet, N. F. (1992). Evidence of tyrosine hydroxylase mRNA in the anterior and neurointermediate lobes of female rat pituitary. *Biochem.Biophys.Res.Commun., 189,* 1716-1724.

Schwartzberg, M., Unger, J., Weindl, A., & Lange, W. (1990). Distribution of neuropeptide Y in the prosencephalon of man and cotton-head tamarin (Saguinus oedipus): colocalization with somatostatin in neurons of striatum and amygdala. *Anat.Embryol.(Berl), 181,* 157-166.

Servin, A. L., Amiranoff, B., Rouyer-Fessard, C., Tatemoto, K., & Laburthe, M. (1987). Identification and molecular characterization of galanin receptor sites in rat brain. *Biochem.Biophys.Res Commun., 144,* 298-306.

Shoupe, D. & Lobo, R. A. (1984). Evidence for altered catecholamine metabolism in polycystic ovary syndrome. *Am.J.Obstet.Gynecol., 150,* 566-571.

Silverman, A. J., Antunes, J. L., Ferin, M., & Zimmerman, E. A. (1977). The distribution of luteinizing hormone-releasing hormone (LHRH) in the hypothalamus of the rhesus monkey. Light microscopic studies using immunoperoxidase technique. *Endocrinology, 101,* 134-142.

Silverman, A. J., Livne, I., & Witkin, J. W. (1994). The gonadohormone (GnRH), neuronal systems: immunocytochemistry and in situ hybridization. In E.Knobil & J. D. Neill (Eds.), *The physiology of reproduction* (pp. 1683-1709). New York: Raven Press.

Simonian, S. X., Spratt, D. P., & Herbison, A. E. (1999). Identification and characterization of estrogen receptor alpha-containing neurons projecting to the vicinity of the gonadotropin-releasing hormone perikarya in the rostral preoptic area of the rat. *J Comp Neurol., 411,* 346-358.

Skofitsch, G. & Jacobowitz, D. M. (1985). Immunohistochemical mapping of galanin-like neurons in the rat central nervous system. *Peptides, 6,* 509-546.

Steiner, R. A., Hohmann, J. G., Holmes, A., Wrenn, C. C., Cadd, G., Jureus, A. et al. (2001). Galanin transgenic mice display cognitive and neurochemical deficits characteristic of Alzheimer's disease. *Proc.Natl.Acad.Sci.U.S.A, 98,* 4184-4189.

Stopa, E. G., Koh, E. T., Svendsen, C. N., Rogers, W. T., Schwaber, J. S., & King, J. C. (1991). Computer-assisted mapping of immunoreactive mammalian gonadotropin-releasing hormone in adult human basal forebrain and amygdala. *Endocrinology, 128,* 3199-3207.

Tanoh, T., Shimatsu, A., Ishikawa, Y., Ihara, C., Yanaihara, N., & Imura, H. (1993). Galanin-induced growth hormone secretion in conscious rats: evidence for a possible involvement of somatostatin. *J Neuroendocrinol., 5,* 183-187.

Tatemoto, K., Rokaeus, A., Jornvall, H., McDonald, T. J., & Mutt, V. (1983). Galanin - a novel biologically active peptide from porcine intestine. *FEBS Lett., 164,* 124-128.

Tsuruo, Y., Kawano, H., Kagotani, Y., Hisano, S., Daikoku, S., Chihara, K. et al. (1990). Morphological evidence for neuronal regulation of luteinizing hormone-releasing hormone-containing neurons by neuropeptide Y in the rat septo-preoptic area. *Neurosci.Lett., 110,* 261-266.

Verney, C., el, A. A., & Zecevic, N. (1996). Comigration of tyrosine hydroxylase- and gonadotropin-releasing hormone-immunoreactive neurons in the nasal area of human embryos. *Brain Res.Dev.Brain Res., 97,* 251-259.

Walsh, K. M. & Kuenzel, W. J. (1997). Effect of sulfamethazine on sexual precocity and neuropeptide Y neurons within the tuberoinfundibular region of the chick brain. *Brain Res Bull., 44,* 707-713.

Walter, A., Mai, J. K., & Jimenez-Hartel, W. (1990). Mapping of neuropeptide Y-like immunoreactivity in the human forebrain. *Brain Res Bull., 24,* 297-311.

Watanobe, H., Nigawara, T., Anzai, J., Sakihara, S., Kageyama, K., Nasushita, R. et al. (1994). Neuropeptide Y potentiates the luteinizing hormone (LH) response to LH-releasing hormone in men. *Biochem.Biophys.Res Commun., 200,* 1111-1117.

Weiner, R. I., Findell, P. R., & Kordon, C. (1988). Role of classic and peptide neuromediators in the neuroendocrine regulation of LH and prolactin. In E.Knobil & J. Neill (Eds.), *The Physiology of Reproduction* (pp. 1235-1281). New York: Raven Press.

Williams, T. D., Lightman, S. L., Johnson, M. R., Carmichael, D. J., & Bannister, R. (1989). Selective defect in gonadotrophin secretion in patients with autonomic failure. *Clin.Endocrinol.(Oxf), 30,* 285-292.

Woller, M. J. & Terasawa, E. (1991). Infusion of neuropeptide Y into the stalk-median eminence stimulates in vivo release of luteinizing hormone-release hormone in gonadectomized rhesus monkeys. *Endocrinology, 128,* 1144-1150.

Wright, D. E. & Jennes, L. (1993). Origin of noradrenergic projections to GnRH perikarya-containing areas in the medial septum-diagonal band and preoptic area. *Brain Res., 621,* 272-278.

Wynick, D., Thompson, S. W., & McMahon, S. B. (2001). The role of galanin as a multi-functional neuropeptide in the nervous system. *Curr.Opin.Pharmacol., 1,* 73-77.

Xu, X. J., Hokfelt, T., Bartfai, T., & Wiesenfeld-Hallin, Z. (2000). Galanin and spinal nociceptive mechanisms: recent advances and therapeutic implications. *Neuropeptides, 34,* 137-147.

Yanagisawa, M., Yagi, N., Otsuka, M., Yanaihara, C., & Yanaihara, N. (1986). Inhibitory effects of galanin on the isolated spinal cord of the newborn rat. *Neurosci.Lett., 70,* 278-282.

Zdrojewicz, Z. & Sowinska, E. (2000). [The significance of galanin in physiologic and pathologic processes in humans]. *Postepy Hig.Med.Dosw., 54,* 819-833.

In: The Central Catecholaminergic System
Editor: Bertalan Dudás

ISBN: 978-1-63117-937-2

Chapter 5

Central Catecholaminergic Regulation of Growth

Bertalan Dudás and István Merchenthaler

Stress and Growth

The growth of the body is controlled by growth hormone (GH) released by the anterior lobe of the hypophysis. GH exerts its effects via somatomedins that regulate metabolism at the cellular level. The single major regulator of GH secretion is a 44 amino acid peptide, growth hormone-releasing hormone (GHRH) released by the hypothalamus. GHRH reaches the hypophysis via the hypothalamo-hypophyseal portal circulation. In addition to GHRH, hypothalamic neurons also release somatostatin, a 14-28 amino acid peptide, into the portal circulation. Somatostatin acts as an antagonist of GHRH inhibiting the release of GH at the hypophyseal level.

Numerous studies indicate that stress plays a crucial role in the regulation of growth. Prolonged activation of the hypothalamo-hypophyseal-adrenal (HPA) axis leads to suppression of GH release, possibly via modulating GHRH secretion (Dieguez et al., 1988; Stratakis et al., 1995). Psychological harassment often results in psychosocial dwarfism with delayed puberty, short stature and depression (Dieguez et al., 1988; Dorn & Chrousos, 1993; Frisch et al., 1979; Green et al., 1984; Money, 1977; Mouridsen & Nielsen, 1990; Powell et al., 1967; Reinhart & Drash, 1969; Saenger et al., 1977; Stanhope et al., 1988; Stanhope et al., 1994). This condition is independent of the food intake and characterized by decreased GH secretion that is reversible after the removal of the stressful environment (Albanese et al., 1994; Frisch et al., 1979; Mouridsen & Nielsen, 1990; Reinhart & Drash, 1969; Saenger et al., 1977; Stanhope et al., 1988). Immobilization stress suppresses GH secretion in rats (Armario et al., 1993) and the stimulatory effect of GHRH on GH secretion is reduced in patients with panic disorder (Uhde et al., 1992). Moreover, GH secretion decreases in critically ill patients in response to decreased hypothalamic activity (Van den, 2000; Van den, 2002; Van den & Shalet, 2002).

Although little is known about the exact mechanism of the stress-suppressed GH release, it has been previously suggested that the catecholaminergic regulation of the GHRH system plays a pivotal role in the impact of stress on growth, either directly, or via other neurotransmitter systems.

The Morphology of the Hypothalamic GHRH System

GHRH-immunoreactive (IR) perikarya form a well-circumscribed cell group in the basal hypothalamus, located almost exclusively in the basal part of the infundibular region (Figures 1,2). Here, perikarya form four well-defined subdivisions: (1) The majority of the GHRH-IR cell bodies is located in the infundibulum/median eminence (Figure 2A) and (2) in the basal part of the periventricular zone (Figure 2B). (3) A group of neurons can be observed in the dorsomedial subdivision of the ventromedial nucleus (Figure 2C) and (4) in the basal perifornical area of the tuberal region (Figure 2D).

The majority of GHRH neurons possess fusiform cell bodies with processes emanating from the opposite poles of the cells. Few GHRH-IR perikarya can be detected in the medial preoptic area and in the posterior hypothalamus and none in the lateral hypothalamus. In the basal part of the infundibulum, GHRH-IR axonal varicosities form a dense network; fibers can also be detected in the basal periventricular area, with their numbers decreasing dorsally. Numerous axons are located in the basal part of the medial hypothalamus, oriented parallel with the pial surface; fibers can also be found around the fornix in the preoptic and tuberal regions. Few labeled axon varicosities can be detected in the basal zone of the lateral hypothalamus, in the lamina terminalis, around the medial part of the mamillary body and in medial and lateral zones of the paraventricular nucleus. No GHRH-IR fibers can be observed in the supraoptic nucleus.

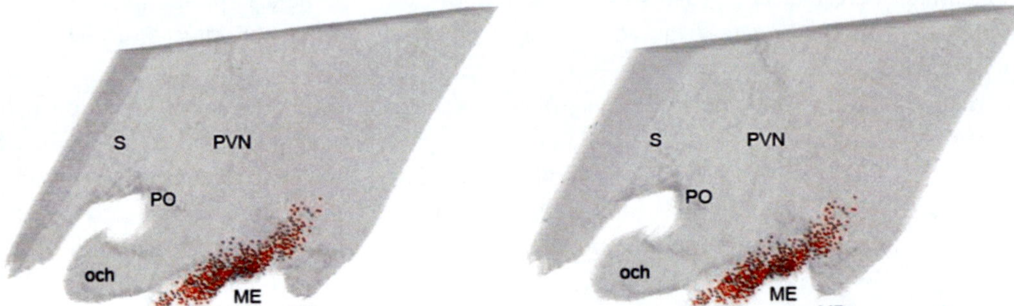

Figure 1. Stereoscopic images of the human hypothalamus illustrating the distribution of the GHRH perikarya denoted by red dots. Stereoscopic images can be observed using U or parallel vision. The eyes are relaxed to look into the distance until the pair of the images fuse, and then refocused by the brain. With this technique a 3D hypothalamus can be seen on the figure, floating in front of the paper, with the immunolabeled perikarya in it at different depth marked by the red dots. The optimal viewing distance is about 20 inches from the paper surface (average reading distance). Stereoscopic magnifier is suggested to readers unfamiliar with U or parallel vision. Abbreviations: Inf, infundibulum; ME, median eminence; MB, mamillary body; och, optic chiasm; PO, preoptic area; PVN, paraventricular nucleus; S, septum.

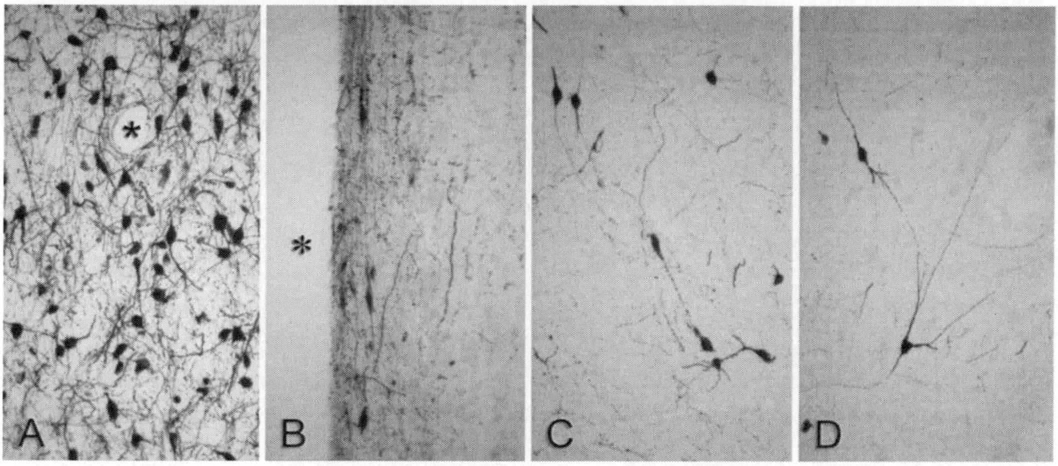

Figure 2. GHRH-IR neural elements in the human hypothalamus. GHRH-IR neurons are most abundant in the infundibulum/median eminence (A) and in the basal part of the periventricular area (B), where GHRH-IR perikarya are surrounded with dense GHRH-IR fiber network. The dorsomedial subdivision of the ventromedial nucleus (C) and the basal perifornical area (D) contain smaller number of GHRH-IR perikarya and axonal varicosities. Cross section of a portal vessel is denoted by a five-pointed star while a six-pointed star marks the 3rd ventricle. Magnification: 100x. Reprinted with permission from Elsevier (Anderson et al., 2010).

The Synchronized Activity of GHRH Neurons

The pulsatile release of GHRH is a well known phenomenon (Frohman et al., 1990; Mogi et al., 2004; Nakamura et al., 2003; Plotsky & Vale, 1985; Thomas et al., 2009) and it has been previously believed to be the single major factor driving the pulsatile secretion of GH that is released in 10-20 pulses in each 24-h cycle. However, the pulsatile pattern seems to be species-dependent. In cattle, the majority of the GH pulses are correlated to a preceding GHRH pulse indicating the crucial role of GHRH in the frequency control of the GH release (Thomas et al., 2009). Passive immunization with somatostatin antiserum does not alter pulsatile GH release, but immunization with antibodies raised against both somatostatin and GHRH abolishes GH bursts (Wehrenberg et al., 1983). In contrast to these findings, patients with an inactivating defect of the GHRH receptor gene maintain the regular frequency of the GH release with a diminished total 24-h GH production rate, suggesting that GH pulses are under the control of intermittent somatostatin withdrawal while the amplitude of GH pulses is driven by GHRH (Roelfsema et al., 2001). The fundamental role of somatostatin in the GH pulse generation has been supported by previous data describing that most of the descending phase of somatostatin pulses are associated with the initiation of GH pulses in goats (Mogi et al., 2004). Although the exact function of the pulsatile release of GHRH remains to be elusive, there is a general consensus that this phenomenon is based on the synchronized activity of the GHRH-IR neurons, suggesting communication between the GHRH-IR neural elements, either directly, via synaptic connections, or indirectly, via other neurotransmitter systems. Indeed, our previous studies revealed juxtapositions between the GHRH elements in the human hypothalamus (Anderson et al., 2010) (Figure 3). These juxtapositions may represent the morphological substrate of the synchronized activity of GHRH neurons that may result in the pulsatile GHRH and the consequent GH release.

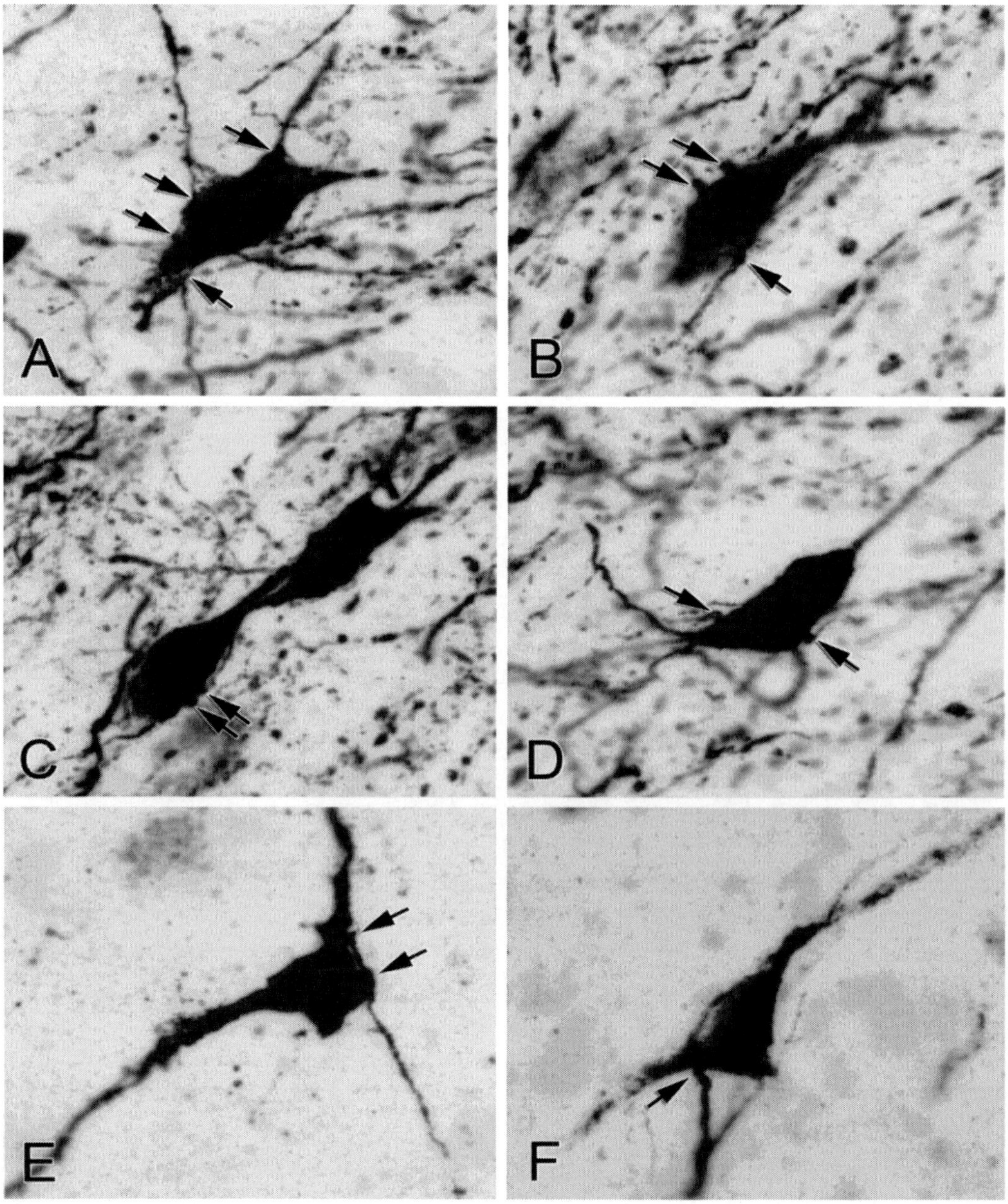

Figure 3. Juxtapositions between the GHRH-IR elements in the human hypothalamus. These GHRH-GHRH associations are characteristically *en passant* juxtapositions where GHRH-IR fibers abut GHRH-IR perikarya forming multiple contacts and typically exhibiting axonal swellings at the site of the contacts. The GHRH-GHRH juxtapositions are most dense in the infundibulum/median eminence (A,B) and in the basal part of the periventricular area (C,D), while juxtapositions are less numerous in the the dorsomedial subdivision of the ventromedial nucleus (E) and the basal perifornical area (F). Some of the juxtapositions are denoted by arrowheads. Magnification: 400x. Reprinted with permission from Elsevier (Anderson et al., 2010).

The Hypothalamic Somatostatinergic System

Somatostatin is a 14-28 amino acid peptide that is located in multiple sites of the human brain. The inhibitory effect of somatostatin on GH secretion of the hypophysis is a well known phenomenon. Somatostatin produced in the hypothalamus reaches the anterior hypophysis via the hypophyseal portal circulation. In the hypothalamus, the majority of the somatostatin-IR perikarya can be observed in the infundibulum/median eminence (arcuate nucleus) and in the periventricular area of the preoptic and infundibular regions (Figures 4,5). Somatostatin-IR neurons can also be found in the suprachiasmatic and ventromedial nuclei and in the the nucleus of the diagonal band of Broca. Scattered perikarya are also present around the mammillary nuclei and in the supramammillary nucleus, as well as in the tuberal region surrounding the fornix. The paraventricular nuclei also contain several perikarya, while only negligible amount of somatostatinergic axonal varicosities without apparent perikarya can be detected in the supraoptic nucleus. A number of cell bodies can be observed in the lateral hypothalamus, particularly at the infundibular and posterior hypothalamic regions. Few perikarya along with fiber varicosities are located in the lamina terminalis.

Somatostatin-IR axonal varicosities are abundant in the infundibulum and periventricular area of the preoptic and infundibular regions, while the medial hypothalamic regions contain only few somatostatin-IR fibers. Although the subdivisions of the hypothalamic somatostatinergic neurons that project to the portal vessels has not been identified yet in human, the abundance of the somatostatinergic elements in the human hypothalamus indicate that somatostatin, apart from its endocrine function to regulate GH secretion, may play a fundamental role in the regulation of other hypothalamic functions as well as a neurotransmitter/neuromodulator.

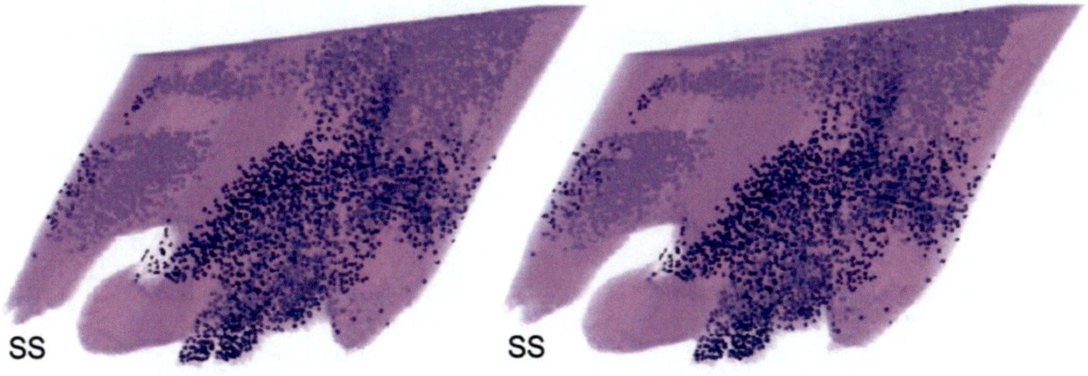

Figure 4. Stereoscopic images of the human hypothalamus illustrating the distribution of the somatostatinergic perikarya denoted by dots. Stereoscopic images can be seen using U or parallel vision. The eyes are relaxed to look into the distance until the pair of the images fuse, and then refocused by the brain. With this technique a 3D hypothalamus can be seen on the figure, floating in front of the paper, with the immunolabeled perikarya in it at different depth marked by the dots. The optimal viewing distance is about 20 inches from the paper surface (average reading distance). Stereoscopic magnifier is suggested to readers unfamiliar with U or parallel vision.

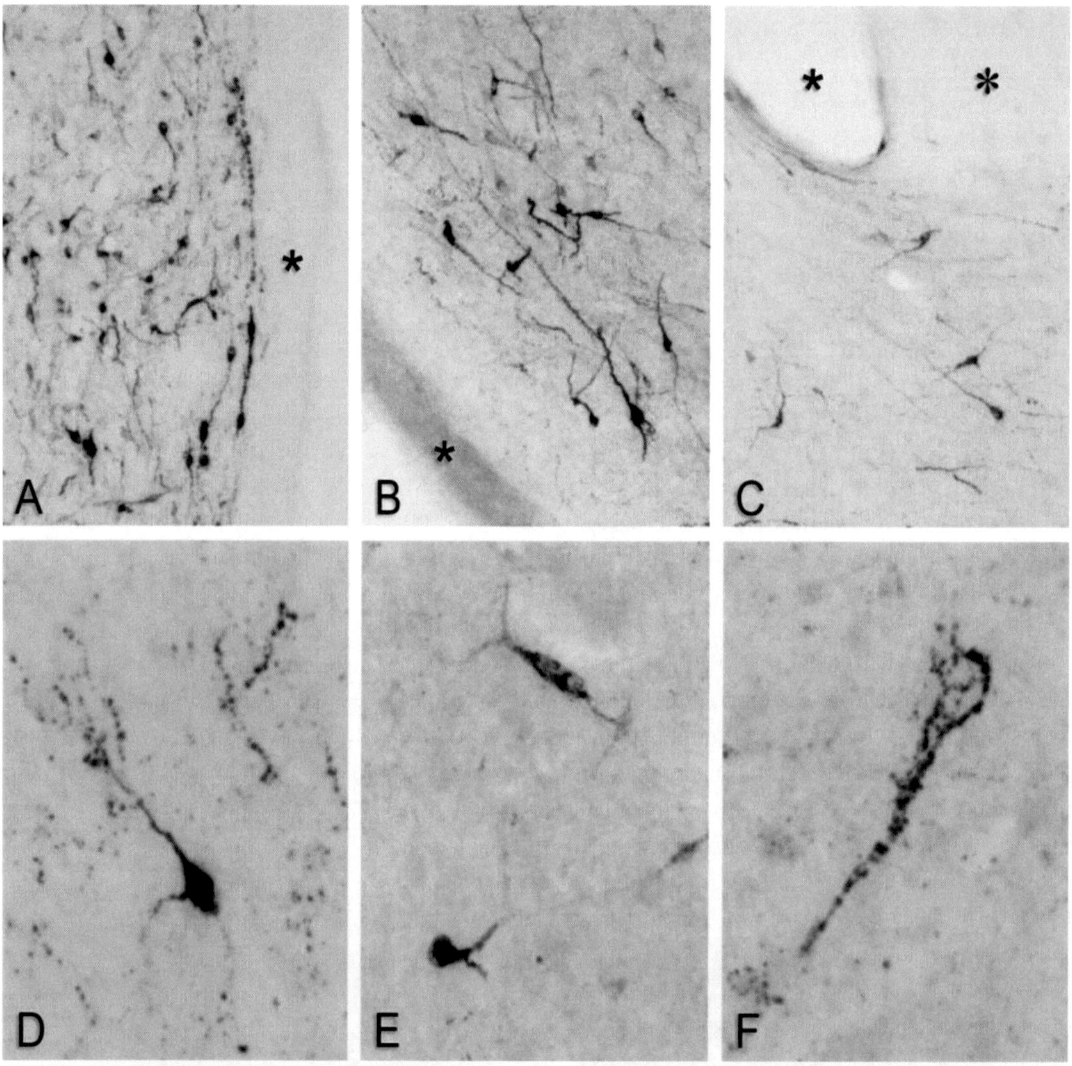

Figure 5. Somatostatinergic neural elements in the human hypothalamus. (A) PVN contains large number of somatostatin-IR perikarya. Asterisk denotes the 3rd ventricle. (B) Somatostatinergic perikarya are common in the infundibulum. The pial surface is marked by asterisk. (C) Fusiform somatostatin-IR neurons surround the fornix (six-pointed asterisk) and their processes are in close proximity of vessels (five-pointed asterisk). Somatostatin-IR cells are also located in the suprachiasmatic nucleus (D) and around the mammillary body (E). Somatostinergic fiber varicosities occasionally form well defined terminal fields around neurons that are not immunoreactive for somatostatin (F). Magnification: A-C: 200x; D-F: 400x.

Direct Catecholaminergic Control of GHRH Release

There is a common consensus that catecholaminergic neurons play a pivotal role in the stress-related physiological effects. We have previously reported that gonadotropin-releasing hormone (GnRH, also called luteinizing hormone-releasing hormone: LHRH) neurons appear to be innervated by catecholaminergic fiber varicosities in the human hypothalamus. These catecholaminergic-GnRH juxtapositions may be considered as the morphological substrate of the stress-suppressed gonadal functions. Similarly to these findings, catecholaminergic system may also participate, in addition to the NPY system, in the innervation of hypothalamic GHRH neurons and thus may represent one of the major factors of the stress-suppressed growth in human. Indeed, disruption of dopaminergic D_2 receptors impairs body growth in adult male mice by altering the GHRH-GH-IGF-I axis at the hypothalamic level (Garcia-Tornadu et al., 2006). Moreover, juxtapositions has been described previously between the noradrenergic and GHRH-IR neuronal elements in sheep (Iqbal et al., 2005b). Despite the previous animal data, the presence of the dopaminergic, adrenergic or noradrenergic input on the human GHRH neurons has only been recently confirmed in detail (Rotoli et al., 2011).

Tyrosine hydroxylase (TH), rate-limiting enzyme of the catecholaminergic synthesis represents each of the three catecholamines in all classes of catecholaminergic neurons. Dopamine, noradrenaline and adrenaline can be visualized by the presence of the key, rate-limiting enzymes of dopamine, noradrenaline and adrenaline synthesis, such as TH, dopamine-beta hydroxylase (DBH) and phenylethanolamine N-methyltransferase (PNMT), respectively. The majority of the GHRH neurons that appear to be heavily innervated by TH-IR elements are located in the basal periventricular area of the tuberal region (Figure 6A-D) and in the infundibular nucleus/median eminence (Figure 6F-G), while the lightly innervated GHRH cells or the perikarya without apparent TH-IR innervation are more characteristic to the dorsomedial subdivision of the ventromedial nucleus and to the perifornical area of the tuberal region. GHRH-IR neurons are typically surrounded by a dense TH-IR fiber network in the periventricular zone of the tuberal area (Figure 6A-D) where TH-IR fiber varicosities abut on virtually every GHRH cells forming multiple *en passant* type contacts with both the GHRH-IR perikarya and the GHRH-IR axons emanating from the cell bodies (Figure 6A-D). Catecholaminergic fibers frequently form well-defined fiber baskets around these GHRH neurons (Figure 6A-D) covering typically a significant surface area of the GHRH neurons. In the infundibular nucleus, mostly thin TH-IR axons form contacts with the densely packed GHRH-IR neurons (Figure 6F-G); here the number of contacting TH-IR elements per GHRH cells is less than that in the periventricular area. In addition to the periventricular zone and the infundibular nucleus, catecholaminergic-GHRH juxtapositions can also be observed in the dorsomedial subdivision of the ventromedial nucleus (Figure 6E,H) where relatively few GHRH neurons receive abutting TH-IR fibers, although occasionally GHRH neurons appear to be heavily innervated by the catecholaminergic fiber varicosities in this area receiving multiple, well-defined contacts on their surface (Figure 6E,H). In contrast, TH-GHRH juxtapositions are uncommon in the basal perifornical area, where TH-IR axons devoid the close vicinity of the GHRH neurons. Close examination of the hypothalamic TH-GHRH juxtapositions with high magnification utilizing oil immersion objectives typically does not reveal any gaps between the contacting elements. GHRH perikarya occasionally receive contacting DBH-IR fiber varicosities in *en passant* fashion, although these juxtapositions appear to be far less abundant than TH-GHRH associations. Sporadic DBH-GHRH contacts can be observed in the periventricular area of the tuberal region and in the infundibular nucleus (Figure 6J-K). PNMT-IR fiber varicosities can not be observed in the close vicinity of the GHRH perikarya.

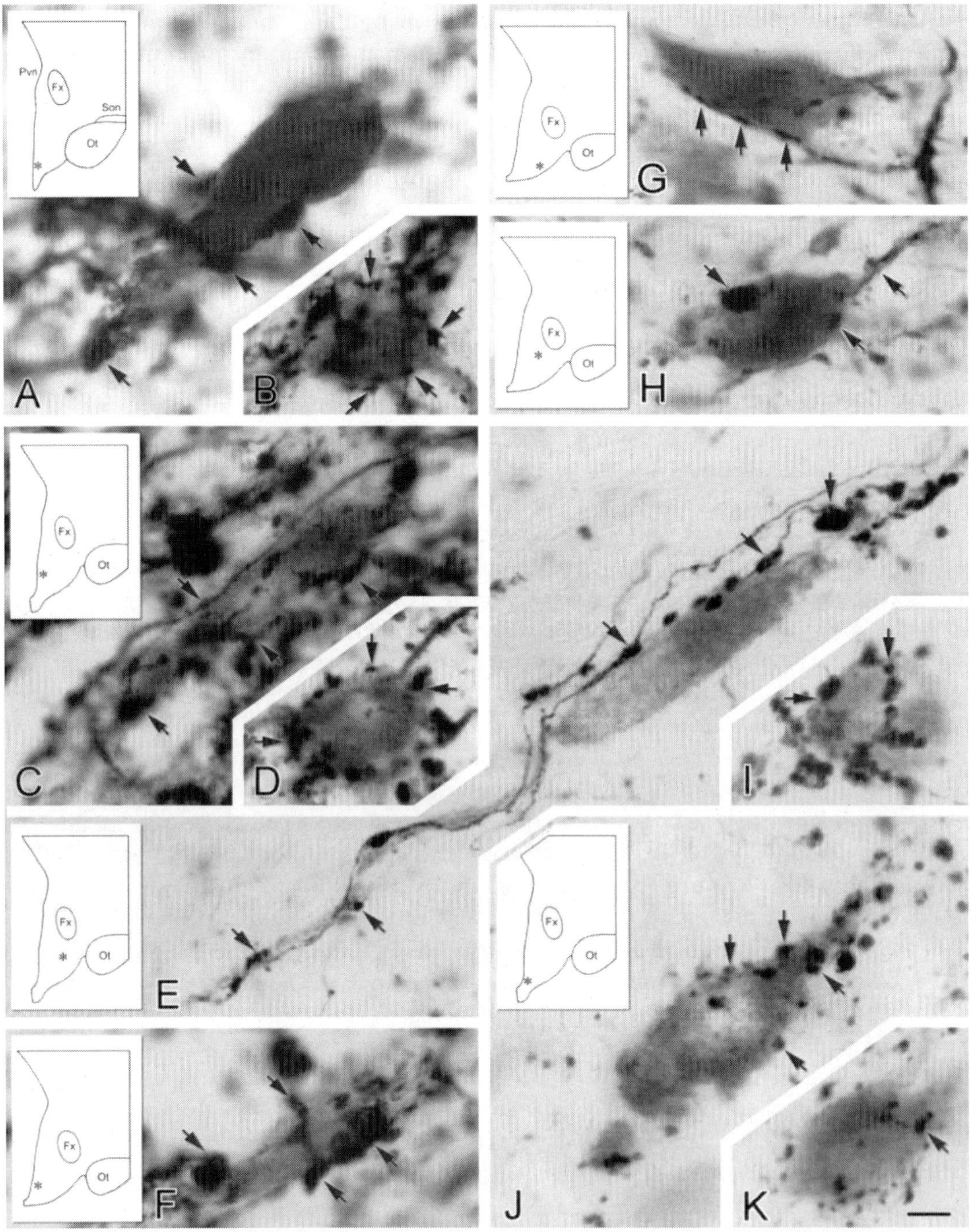

Figure 6. Double-label immunohistochemistry reveals juxtapositions (arrowheads) between the catecholaminergic (black) and GHRH-IR (brown) neural elements in the human diencephalon. Occasional juxtapositions between the DBH-IR and GHRH-IR neuronal elements were also observed primarily in the basal part of the infundibulum (J-K). The positions of the demonstrated GHRH-IR neurons are marked by asterisks on the coronal sections of the diencephalon in the corners of the micrographs. Scale bar: 10 μm. Abbreviations: fx, fornix; mb, mammillary body; pvn, paraventricular nucleus; ot, optic tract; son, supraoptic nucleus.

Catecholaminergic Regulation of GHRH via Neuropeptide Y (NPY)

Several studies indicate the catecholaminergic control of neuropeptide Y (NPY) and its central role in the stress response (for review see Chapter 2). Therefore, NPY should be considered a stress molecule (Carrasco & Van de Kar, 2003; Kakui & Kitamura, 2007; Zukowska-Grojec et al., 1988; Zukowska-Grojec & Vaz, 1988; Zukowska-Grojec et al., 1991; Zukowska-Grojec, 1995; Zukowska-Grojec et al., 1996). Indeed, plasma NPY levels rise significantly after exposure to numerous stressors (Castagne et al., 1987; Zukowska-Grojec et al., 1988; Zukowska-Grojec & Vaz, 1988). Plasma NPY levels are also raised by hemorrhagic stress (Morris et al., 1987; Morris et al., 1997; Rudehill et al., 1987), active orthostatism (Puybasset et al., 1993) and cold water exposure (Zukowska-Grojec & Vaz, 1988). This phenomenon can be blocked by NPY Y1 receptor antagonists that also attenuate stress-induced tachycardia (Zhang et al., 1997; Zukowska-Grojec et al., 1996). NPY levels are also increased in medical students under academic stress (Al-Ayadhi, 2005). Since increased NPY levels can be detected after handling control and adrenalectomized rats (Castagne et al., 1987), the stress-induced NPY secretion appears to be independent from the activation of the HPA axis. Restraint stress also increases NPY levels in the paraventricular nucleus in rats (Rybkin et al., 1997).

Since NPY is believed to play a key role in mediating the stress-related metabolic changes in human, the NPY system may be a crucial factor influencing GH secretion. Lesions in the periventricular preoptic area diminish GH release, indicating that in addition to GHRH, other neuropeptides may also be involved in the control of GH secretion (Critchlow et al., 1981; Rice et al., 1978). Although NPY can directly inhibit GH secretion in human hypophyseal cells (Adams et al., 1987; Barb & Barrett, 2005), there is a general consensus that NPY modulates GH release via the hypothalamic GHRH system (Bluet-Pajot et al., 1998). Indeed, previous studies indicate that stress suppresses GH and GHRH secretion, following an initial increase in NPY levels. Pulsatile GHRH secretion has shown to decrease in fasting diabetic male rats, while NPY levels were increased during fasting (Park et al., 2004). In fasting mice, GHRH secretion has been reported to decrease after a notable increase in NPY and corticotropin–releasing hormone (CRH) levels (Luque et al., 2007). After food withdrawal, hypothalamic GHRH mRNA levels were significantly elevated in mice with a preceding rise in NPY mRNA levels (Luque et al., 2007). Intracerebroventricular administration of NPY also causes bone loss possibly via the suppression of the hypothalamic GHRH and the subsequent GH release. Indeed, NPY Y2 receptor-deficient mice have an increased trabecular bone volume (Baldock et al., 2002). Moreover, preliminary results suggest that NPY neurons in the arcuate nucleus express GH receptor, suggesting that NPY also plays a physiological role in the feedback of regulation of GH secretion (Chan et al., 1996b; Chan et al., 1996a).

The morphology and distribution of NPY-IR neuronal elements in the human hypothalamus have already been described (Dudás et al., 2000; Dudás & Merchenthaler, 2006). Numerous papers reported on the pattern of GHRH-IR neurons in the brain of several species, including human (Bloch et al., 1983a; Bloch et al., 1983b; Bloch et al., 1984; Ciofi et al., 1988; Goldstone et al., 2003; Jacobowitz et al., 1983; Merchenthaler et al., 1984b; Merchenthaler et al., 1984a; Miki et al., 1994; Rao et al., 1996; Sawchenko et al., 1985; Smith et al., 1984), and recently a high-resolution 3D map of the GHRH-IR neuronal elements in the human brain has been published (Deltondo et al., 2008).

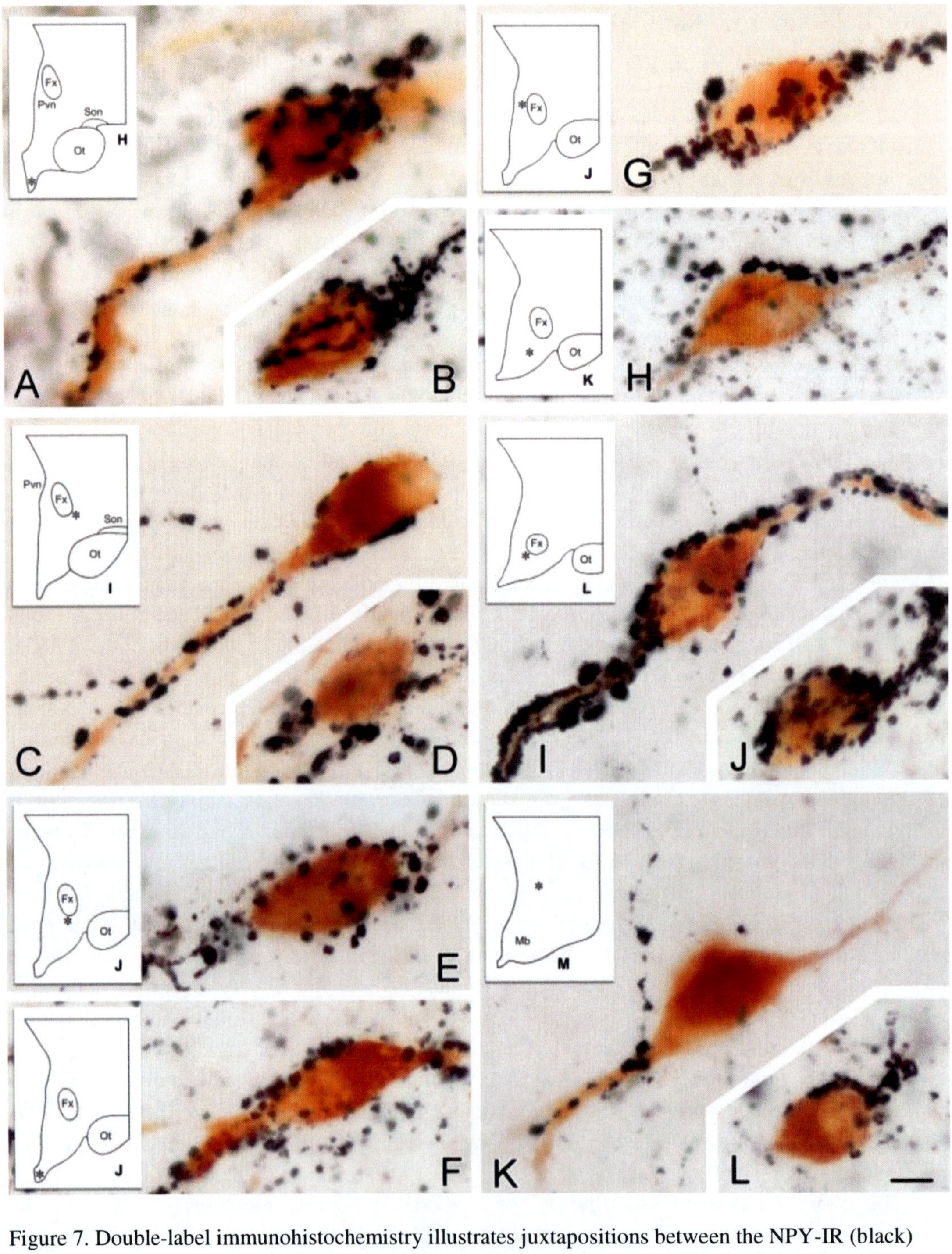

Figure 7. Double-label immunohistochemistry illustrates juxtapositions between the NPY-IR (black) and GHRH-IR (brown) neural elements in the human diencephalon. The NPY-IR fiber varicosities often covered a significant surface area of the GHRH neurons forming numerous *en passant* type contacts. The positions of the demonstrated GHRH-IR neurons are marked by asterisks on the coronal sections of the diencephalon in the corners of the micrographs. The thickness of the sections is 30 µm. Scale bar: 20 µm. Abbreviations: Fx, fornix; Mb, mammillary body; Pvn, paraventricular nucleus; Ot, optic tract; Son, supraoptic nucleus. Reprinted with permission from Elsevier (delTondo et al., 2010).

Juxtapositions between the NPY-IR fiber varicosities and GHRH-IR perikarya can be observed mainly in the infundibular nucleus (Figure 7A,B,F), where GHRH-IR neurons are densely packed. Numerous NPY-GHRH juxtapositions can be seen in the basal perifornical area of the tuberal region (Figure 7C,D,E), in the periventricular zone of the tuberal area (Figure 7G), and in the ventromedial nucleus (Figure 7H). Few juxtapositions can be found at the rostral part of the posterior hypothalamus (Figure 7K,L). In these areas, NPY-IR fiber varicosities surround GHRH-IR neurons, typically forming numerous *en passant* type contacts with both of the GHRH-IR cell bodies and the GHRH-IR axons emanating from the perikarya. Close examination of these juxtapositions with high magnification utilizing oil immersion objectives does not reveal any gaps between the contacting elements. The majority of the observed GHRH-IR perikarya (52%) appear to be heavily innervated by NPY-IR fiber varicosities that often form well-defined fiber baskets around the GHRH neurons with more than six contacts/cell and cover a significant surface area of the GHRH neuron (Figure 7A,B,G,I,J). The rest of the GHRH neurons are lightly innervated (41% of the counted neurons), receiving 1-6 contacting NPY-IR axon varicosities, or does not appear to have any contacts with NPY fibers (7% of the counted neurons). The majority of the heavily innervated GHRH cells are located in the infundibular nucleus/median eminence, while the lightly innervated cells or the cells without apparent innervation are more characteristic to the periventricular zone, perifornical area of the tuberal region, ventromedial nucleus and the posterior hypothalamus.

Other Neurotransmitter/Hormonal Systems Influencing Growth

Previous studies revealed that additional neurotransmitters/neuromodulators including endogenous opiates, tachykinin, substance P (SP), bombesin, orexin and ghrelin, calcitonin gene-related peptide (CGRP), histamine, and hormones including calcitonin appear to participate in the regulation of GHRH secretion and the consequent GH release (Estienne & Barb, 2005; Pugliese et al., 1992; Villa et al., 1997; Iqbal et al., 2005a; Estienne & Barb, 2005; Muccioli et al., 1998; Netti et al., 1989; Grilli et al., 1996; Ceda et al., 1989). Indeed, our recent studies revealed that SP-IR and endogenous opiate-containing axonal varicosities abut on the surface of GHRH perikarya in humans forming multiple contacts that appear to be synapses, while passing by. These morphological findings have been supported by physiologic data suggesting the control of these neurotransmitter sytem in the GHRH secretion. Similar to NPY, these systems may be regulated by catecholamines, therefore, in addition to the direct catecholaminergic-GHRH and the indirect catecholaminergic-NPY-GHRH interactions, catecholamines may control of GHRH secretion via these neurotransmitter systems.

References

Adams, E. F., Venetikou, M. S., Woods, C. A., Lacoumenta, S., & Burrin, J. M. (1987). Neuropeptide Y directly inhibits growth hormone secretion by human pituitary somatotropic tumours. *Acta Endocrinol.(Copenh), 115,* 149-154.

Al-Ayadhi, L. Y. (2005). Neurohormonal changes in medical students during academic stress. *Ann.Saudi.Med., 25,* 36-40.

Albanese, A., Hamill, G., Jones, J., Skuse, D., Matthews, D. R., & Stanhope, R. (1994). Reversibility of physiological growth hormone secretion in children with psychosocial dwarfism. *Clin.Endocrinol.(Oxf), 40,* 687-692.

Anderson, D., Baker, M., Grignol, G., Hu, W., Merchenthaler, I., & Dudás, B. (2010). Distribution and morphology of the juxtapositions between growth hormone-releasing hormone-(ghrh)-immunoreactive neuronal elements. *Growth Horm.IGF.Res., 20,* 356-359.

Armario, A., Marti, O., Gavalda, A., Giralt, M., & Jolin, T. (1993). Effects of chronic immobilization stress on GH and TSH secretion in the rat: response to hypothalamic regulatory factors. *Psychoneuroendocrinology, 18,* 405-413.

Baldock, P. A., Sainsbury, A., Couzens, M., Enriquez, R. F., Thomas, G. P., Gardiner, E. M. et al. (2002). Hypothalamic Y2 receptors regulate bone formation. *J.Clin.Invest, 109,* 915-921.

Barb, C. R. & Barrett, J. B. (2005). Neuropeptide Y modulates growth hormone but not luteinizing hormone secretion from prepuberal gilt anterior pituitary cells in culture. *Domest.Anim Endocrinol., 29,* 548-555.

Bloch, B., Brazeau, P., Bloom, F., & Ling, N. (1983a). Topographical study of the neurons containing hpGRF immunoreactivity in monkey hypothalamus. *Neurosci.Lett., 37,* 23-28.

Bloch, B., Brazeau, P., Ling, N., Bohlen, P., Esch, F., Wehrenberg, W. B. et al. (1983b). Immunohistochemical detection of growth hormone-releasing factor in brain. *Nature, 301,* 607-608.

Bloch, B., Gaillard, R. C., Brazeau, P., Lin, H. D., & Ling, N. (1984). Topographical and ontogenetic study of the neurons producing growth hormone-releasing factor in human hypothalamus. *Regul.Pept., 8,* 21-31.

Bluet-Pajot, M. T., Epelbaum, J., Gourdji, D., Hammond, C., & Kordon, C. (1998). Hypothalamic and hypophyseal regulation of growth hormone secretion. *Cell Mol.Neurobiol., 18,* 101-123.

Carrasco, G. A. & Van de Kar, L. D. (2003). Neuroendocrine pharmacology of stress. *Eur.J.Pharmacol., 463,* 235-272.

Castagne, V., Corder, R., Gaillard, R., & Mormede, P. (1987). Stress-induced changes of circulating neuropeptide Y in the rat: comparison with catecholamines. *Regul.Pept., 19,* 55-63.

Ceda, G. P., Denti, L., Ceresini, G., Rastelli, G., Dotti, C., Cavalieri, S. et al. (1989). Calcitonin inhibition of growth hormone-releasing hormone-induced GH secretion in normal men. *Acta Endocrinol.(Copenh), 120,* 416-422.

Chan, Y. Y., Clifton, D. K., & Steiner, R. A. (1996a). Role of NPY neurones in GH-dependent feedback signalling to the brain. *Horm.Res., 45 Suppl 1,* 12-14.

Chan, Y. Y., Steiner, R. A., & Clifton, D. K. (1996b). Regulation of hypothalamic neuropeptide-Y neurons by growth hormone in the rat. *Endocrinology, 137,* 1319-1325.

Ciofi, P., Croix, D., & Tramu, G. (1988). Colocalization of GHRF and NPY immunoreactivities in neurons of the infundibular area of the human brain. *Neuroendocrinology, 47,* 469-472.

Critchlow, V., Abe, K., Urman, S., & Vale, W. (1981). Effect of lesions in the periventricular nucleus of the preoptic-anterior hypothalamus on growth hormone and thyrotropin secretion and brain somatostatin. *Brain Res., 222,* 267-276.

Deltondo, J., Por, I., Hu, W., Merchenthaler, I., Semeniken, K., Jojart, J. et al. (2008). Associations between the human growth hormone-releasing hormone- and neuropeptide-Y-immunoreactive systems in the human diencephalon: a possible morphological substrate of the impact of stress on growth. *Neuroscience, 153,* 1146-1152.

Dieguez, C., Page, M. D., & Scanlon, M. F. (1988). Growth hormone neuroregulation and its alterations in disease states. *Clin.Endocrinol.(Oxf), 28,* 109-143.

Dorn, L. D. & Chrousos, G. P. (1993). The endocrinology of stress and stress system disorders in adolescence. *Endocrinol.Metab Clin.North Am., 22,* 685-700.

Dudás, B. & Merchenthaler, I. (2006). Three-dimensional representation of the neurotransmitter systems of the human hypothalamus: inputs of the gonadotrophin hormone-releasing hormone neuronal system. *J.Neuroendocrinol., 18,* 79-95.

Dudás, B., Mihaly, A., & Merchenthaler, I. (2000). Topography and associations of luteinizing hormone-releasing hormone and neuropeptide Y-immunoreactive neuronal systems in the human diencephalon. *J.Comp Neurol., 427,* 593-603.

Estienne, M. J. & Barb, C. R. (2005). The control of adenohypophysial hormone secretion by amino acids and peptides in swine. *Domest.Anim Endocrinol., 29,* 34-42.

Frisch, H., Granditsch, G., & Wurst, E. (1979). [Psychosomal dwarfism with reversible growth hormone deficiency (author's transl)]. *Wien.Klin.Wochenschr., 91,* 726-731.

Frohman, L. A., Downs, T. R., Clarke, I. J., & Thomas, G. B. (1990). Measurement of growth hormone-releasing hormone and somatostatin in hypothalamic-portal plasma of unanesthetized sheep. Spontaneous secretion and response to insulin-induced hypoglycemia. *J.Clin.Invest, 86,* 17-24.

Garcia-Tornadu, I., Rubinstein, M., Gaylinn, B. D., Hill, D., Arany, E., Low, M. J. et al. (2006). GH in the dwarf dopaminergic D2 receptor knockout mouse: somatotrope population, GH release, and responsiveness to GH-releasing factors and somatostatin. *J.Endocrinol., 190,* 611-619.

Goldstone, A. P., Unmehopa, U. A., & Swaab, D. F. (2003). Hypothalamic growth hormone-releasing hormone (GHRH) cell number is increased in human illness, but is not reduced in Prader-Willi syndrome or obesity. *Clin.Endocrinol.(Oxf), 58,* 743-755.

Green, W. H., Campbell, M., & David, R. (1984). Psychosocial dwarfism: a critical review of the evidence. *J.Am.Acad.Child Psychiatry, 23,* 39-48.

Grilli, R., Sibilia, V., Torsello, A., Pagani, F., Guidi, M., Luoni, M. et al. (1996). Role of the neuronal histaminergic system in the regulation of somatotropic function: comparison between the neonatal and the adult rat. *J.Endocrinol., 151,* 195-201.

Iqbal, J., Manley, T. R., Ciofi, P., & Clarke, I. J. (2005a). Reduction in adiposity affects the extent of afferent projections to growth hormone-releasing hormone and somatostatin neurons and the degree of colocalization of neuropeptides in growth hormone-releasing hormone and somatostatin cells of the ovine hypothalamus. *Endocrinology, 146,* 4776-4785.

Iqbal, J., Manley, T. R., Yue, Q., Namavar, M. R., & Clarke, I. J. (2005b). Noradrenergic regulation of hypothalamic cells that produce growth hormone-releasing hormone and somatostatin and the effect of altered adiposity in sheep. *J.Neuroendocrinol., 17,* 341-352.

Jacobowitz, D. M., Schulte, H., Chrousos, G. P., & Loriaux, D. L. (1983). Localization of GRF-like immunoreactive neurons in the rat brain. *Peptides, 4,* 521-524.

Kakui, N. & Kitamura, K. (2007). Direct evidence that stimulation of neuropeptide Y Y5 receptor activates hypothalamo-pituitary-adrenal axis in conscious rats via both corticotropin-releasing factor- and arginine vasopressin-dependent pathway. *Endocrinology, 148,* 2854-2862.

Luque, R. M., Park, S., & Kineman, R. D. (2007). Severity of the catabolic condition differentially modulates hypothalamic expression of growth hormone-releasing hormone in the fasted mouse: potential role of neuropeptide Y and corticotropin-releasing hormone. *Endocrinology, 148,* 300-309.

Merchenthaler, I., Thomas, C. R., & Arimura, A. (1984a). Immunocytochemical localization of growth hormone releasing factor (GHRF)-containing structures in the rat brain using anti-rat GHRF serum. *Peptides, 5,* 1071-1075.

Merchenthaler, I., Vigh, S., Schally, A. V., & Petrusz, P. (1984b). Immunocytochemical localization of growth hormone-releasing factor in the rat hypothalamus. *Endocrinology, 114,* 1082-1085.

Miki, N., Ono, M., sakawa-Yasumoto, K., Aoki, T., Murata, Y., Ishituka, Y. et al. (1994). Characterization and localization of mouse hypothalamic growth hormone-releasing factor and effect of gold thioglucose-induced hypothalamic lesions. *J.Neuroendocrinol., 6,* 71-78.

Mogi, K., Yonezawa, T., Chen, D. S., Li, J. Y., Suzuki, M., Yamanouchi, K. et al. (2004). Relationship between growth hormone (GH) pulses in the peripheral circulation and GH-releasing hormone and somatostatin profiles in the cerebrospinal fluid of goats. *J Vet.Med Sci., 66,* 1071-1078.

Money, J. (1977). The syndrome of abuse dwarfism (psychosocial dwarfism or reversible hyposomatotropism). *Am.J.Dis.Child, 131,* 508-513.

Morris, M., Kapoor, V., & Chalmers, J. (1987). Plasma neuropeptide Y concentration is increased after hemorrhage in conscious rats: relative contributions of sympathetic nerves and the adrenal medulla. *J.Cardiovasc.Pharmacol., 9,* 541-545.

Morris, M. J., Cox, H. S., Lambert, G. W., Kaye, D. M., Jennings, G. L., Meredith, I. T. et al. (1997). Region-specific neuropeptide Y overflows at rest and during sympathetic activation in humans. *Hypertension, 29,* 137-143.

Mouridsen, S. E. & Nielsen, S. (1990). Reversible somatotropin deficiency (psychosocial dwarfism) presenting as conduct disorder and growth hormone deficiency. *Dev.Med.Child Neurol., 32,* 1093-1098.

Muccioli, G., Ghe, C., Ghigo, M. C., Papotti, M., Arvat, E., Boghen, M. F. et al. (1998). Specific receptors for synthetic GH secretagogues in the human brain and pituitary gland. *J.Endocrinol., 157,* 99-106.

Nakamura, S., Mizuno, M., Katakami, H., Gore, A. C., & Terasawa, E. (2003). Aging-related changes in in vivo release of growth hormone-releasing hormone and somatostatin from the stalk-median eminence in female rhesus monkeys (Macaca mulatta). *J Clin.Endocrinol.Metab, 88,* 827-833.

Netti, C., Guidobono, F., Sibilia, V., Pagani, F., Braga, P. C., & Pecile, A. (1989). Evidence of a central inhibition of growth hormone secretion by calcitonin gene-related peptide. *Neuroendocrinology, 49,* 242-247.

Park, S., Sohn, S., & Kineman, R. D. (2004). Fasting-induced changes in the hypothalamic-pituitary-GH axis in the absence of GH expression: lessons from the spontaneous dwarf rat. *J.Endocrinol., 180,* 369-378.

Plotsky, P. M. & Vale, W. (1985). Patterns of growth hormone-releasing factor and somatostatin secretion into the hypophysial-portal circulation of the rat. *Science, 230,* 461-463.

Powell, G. F., Brasel, J. A., Raiti, S., & Blizzard, R. M. (1967). Emotional deprivation and growth retardation simulating idiopathic hypopituitarism. II. Endocrinologic evaluation of the syndrome. *N.Engl.J.Med., 276,* 1279-1283.

Pugliese, M. T., Abdenur, J., Fort, P., & Lifshitz, F. (1992). The relationship between beta-endorphin and the growth hormone (GH) response to GH releasing hormone in prepubertal children. *Endocr.Res., 18,* 41-50.

Puybasset, L., Lacolley, P., Laurent, S., Mignon, F., Billaud, E., Cuche, J. L. et al. (1993). Effects of clonidine on plasma catecholamines and neuropeptide Y in hypertensive patients at rest and during stress. *J.Cardiovasc.Pharmacol., 21,* 912-919.

Rao, S. D., Rao, P. D., & Peter, R. E. (1996). Growth hormone-releasing hormone immunoreactivity in the brain, pituitary, and pineal of the goldfish, Carassius auratus. *Gen.Comp Endocrinol., 102,* 210-220.

Reinhart, J. B. & Drash, A. L. (1969). Psychosocial dwarfism: environmentally induced recovery. *Psychosom.Med., 31,* 165-172.

Rice, R. W., Abe, K., & Critchlow, V. (1978). Abolition of plasma growth hormone response to stress and of the circadian rhythm in pituitary-adrenal function in female rats with preoptic-anterior hypothalamic lesions. *Brain Res., 148,* 129-141.

Roelfsema, F., Biermasz, N. R., Veldman, R. G., Veldhuis, J. D., Frolich, M., Stokvis-Brantsma, W. H. et al. (2001). Growth hormone (GH) secretion in patients with an inactivating defect of the GH-releasing hormone (GHRH) receptor is pulsatile: evidence for a role for non-GHRH inputs into the generation of GH pulses. *J Clin.Endocrinol.Metab, 86,* 2459-2464.

Rotoli, G., Grignol, G., Hu, W., Merchenthaler, I., & Dudás, B. (2011). Catecholaminergic axonal varicosities appear to innervate growth hormone-releasing hormone-immunoreactive neurons in the human hypothalamus: the possible morphological substrate of the stress-suppressed growth. *J Clin.Endocrinol.Metab, 96,* E1606-E1611.

Rudehill, A., Olcen, M., Sollevi, A., Hamberger, B., & Lundberg, J. M. (1987). Release of neuropeptide Y upon haemorrhagic hypovolaemia in relation to vasoconstrictor effects in the pig. *Acta Physiol Scand., 131,* 517-523.

Rybkin, I. I., Zhou, Y., Volaufova, J., Smagin, G. N., Ryan, D. H., & Harris, R. B. (1997). Effect of restraint stress on food intake and body weight is determined by time of day. *Am.J.Physiol, 273,* R1612-R1622.

Saenger, P., Levine, L. S., Wiedemann, E., Schwartz, E., Korth-Schutz, S., Pareira, J. et al. (1977). Somatomedin and growth hormone in psychosocial dwarfism. *Padiatr.Padol.Suppl,* 1-12.

Sawchenko, P. E., Swanson, L. W., Rivier, J., & Vale, W. W. (1985). The distribution of growth-hormone-releasing factor (GRF) immunoreactivity in the central nervous system of the rat: an immunohistochemical study using antisera directed against rat hypothalamic GRF. *J.Comp Neurol., 237,* 100-115.

Smith, R. M., Howe, P. R., Oliver, J. R., & Willoughby, J. O. (1984). Growth hormone releasing factor immunoreactivity in rat hypothalamus. *Neuropeptides, 4,* 109-115.

Stanhope, R., Adlard, P., Hamill, G., Jones, J., Skuse, D., & Preece, M. A. (1988). Physiological growth hormone (GH) secretion during the recovery from psychosocial dwarfism: a case report. *Clin.Endocrinol.(Oxf), 28,* 335-339.

Stanhope, R., Wilks, Z., & Hamill, G. (1994). Failure to grow: lack of food or lack of love? *Prof.Care Mother.Child, 4,* 234-237.

Stratakis, C. A., Gold, P. W., & Chrousos, G. P. (1995). Neuroendocrinology of stress: implications for growth and development. *Horm.Res., 43,* 162-167.

Thomas, M. G., Amstalden, M., Hallford, D. M., Silver, G. A., Garcia, M. D., Keisler, D. H. et al. (2009). Dynamics of GHRH in third-ventricle cerebrospinal fluid of cattle: relationship with serum concentrations of GH and responses to appetite-regulating peptides. *Domest.Anim Endocrinol., 37,* 196-205.

Uhde, T. W., Tancer, M. E., Rubinow, D. R., Roscow, D. B., Boulenger, J. P., Vittone, B. et al. (1992). Evidence for hypothalamo-growth hormone dysfunction in panic disorder: profile of growth hormone (GH) responses to clonidine, yohimbine, caffeine, glucose, GRF and TRH in panic disorder patients versus healthy volunteers. *Neuropsychopharmacology, 6,* 101-118.

Van den, B. G. (2000). Novel insights into the neuroendocrinology of critical illness. *Eur.J.Endocrinol., 143,* 1-13.

Van den, B. G. (2002). Dynamic neuroendocrine responses to critical illness. *Front Neuroendocrinol., 23,* 370-391.

Van den, B. G. & Shalet, S. M. (2002). Critical illness as a model of hypothalamic ageing. *Novartis.Found.Symp., 242,* 205-215.

Villa, P., Fulghesu, A. M., De, M. L., Valle, D., Mancini, A., Pavone, V. et al. (1997). Impact of long-term naltrexone treatment on growth hormone and insulin secretion in hyperandrogenic and normal obese patients. *Metabolism, 46,* 538-543.

Wehrenberg, W. B., Brazeau, P., Luben, R., Ling, N., & Guillemin, R. (1983). A noninvasive functional lesion of the hypothalamo-pituitary axis for the study of growth hormone-releasing factor. *Neuroendocrinology, 36,* 489-491.

Zhang, W., Lundberg, J. M., & Thoren, P. (1997). Neuropeptide Y Y1 receptor antagonist (BIBP 3226) attenuates stress evoked tachycardia in conscious spontaneously hypertensive rats. *Cardiovasc.Drugs Ther., 11,* 801-806.

Zukowska-Grojec, Z. (1995). Neuropeptide Y. A novel sympathetic stress hormone and more. *Ann.N.Y.Acad.Sci., 771,* 219-233.

Zukowska-Grojec, Z., Dayao, E. K., Karwatowska-Prokopczuk, E., Hauser, G. J., & Doods, H. N. (1996). Stress-induced mesenteric vasoconstriction in rats is mediated by neuropeptide Y Y1 receptors. *Am.J.Physiol, 270,* H796-H800.

Zukowska-Grojec, Z., Konarska, M., & McCarty, R. (1988). Differential plasma catecholamine and neuropeptide Y responses to acute stress in rats. *Life Sci., 42,* 1615-1624.

Zukowska-Grojec, Z., Shen, G. H., Capraro, P. A., & Vaz, C. A. (1991). Cardiovascular, neuropeptide Y, and adrenergic responses in stress are sexually differentiated. *Physiol Behav., 49,* 771-777.

Zukowska-Grojec, Z. & Vaz, A. C. (1988). Role of neuropeptide Y (NPY) in cardiovascular responses to stress. *Synapse, 2,* 293-298.

In: The Central Catecholaminergic System
Editor: Bertalan Dudás

ISBN: 978-1-63117-937-2

Chapter 6

Catecholaminergic Regulation of the Magnocellular Neurosecretory System

Bertalan Dudás and István Merchenthaler

The Magnocellular System

The magnocellular system is composed of neurons with relatively large perikarya occupying the paraventricular (PVN) and supraoptic nuclei (SON). These neurons are responsible for the formation of neurohormones oxytocin and vasopressin, which are structurally related to each other; in non- mammalian vertebrates the hormone vasotocin exhibits both oxytocin- and vasopressin-like functions. Oxytocinergic and vasopressinergic neurons project into the neurohypophysis through the hypophyseal stalk as the hypothalamo-hypophyseal tract. The PVN consists of magno- and parvocellular compartments. In humans, the magnocellular part of the PVN is located mostly in the medial hypothalamus, while the periventricular part is filled mostly with smaller, more lightly stained neurons (parvocellular part). In the magnocellular part, there is also some distinction between the localization of the oxytocin and vasopressin producing neurons; vasopressin-positive perikarya tend to congregate in the ventrolateral zone of the paraventricular nucleus, forming a dense cluster of cells, while oxytocin-immunoreactive cells generally avoid this zone and form a loose network in the nucleus (Saper, 2004).

Similar to the PVN, the SON is composed of mostly large, intensely-stained neurons occupying the area in the lateral hypothalamus adjacent to the optic tract (Figure 1). Additional cell clusters of magnocellular neurons are also detectable along the medial border of the optic tract, and in the preoptic area scattered between the paraventricular and supraoptic nuclei (Figure 2B); these cells are also oxytocin- or vasopressin-positive and project to the neurohypophysis. Since both the PVN and SON are highly vascularized, neurons of the magnocellular system tend to be associated with blood vessels.

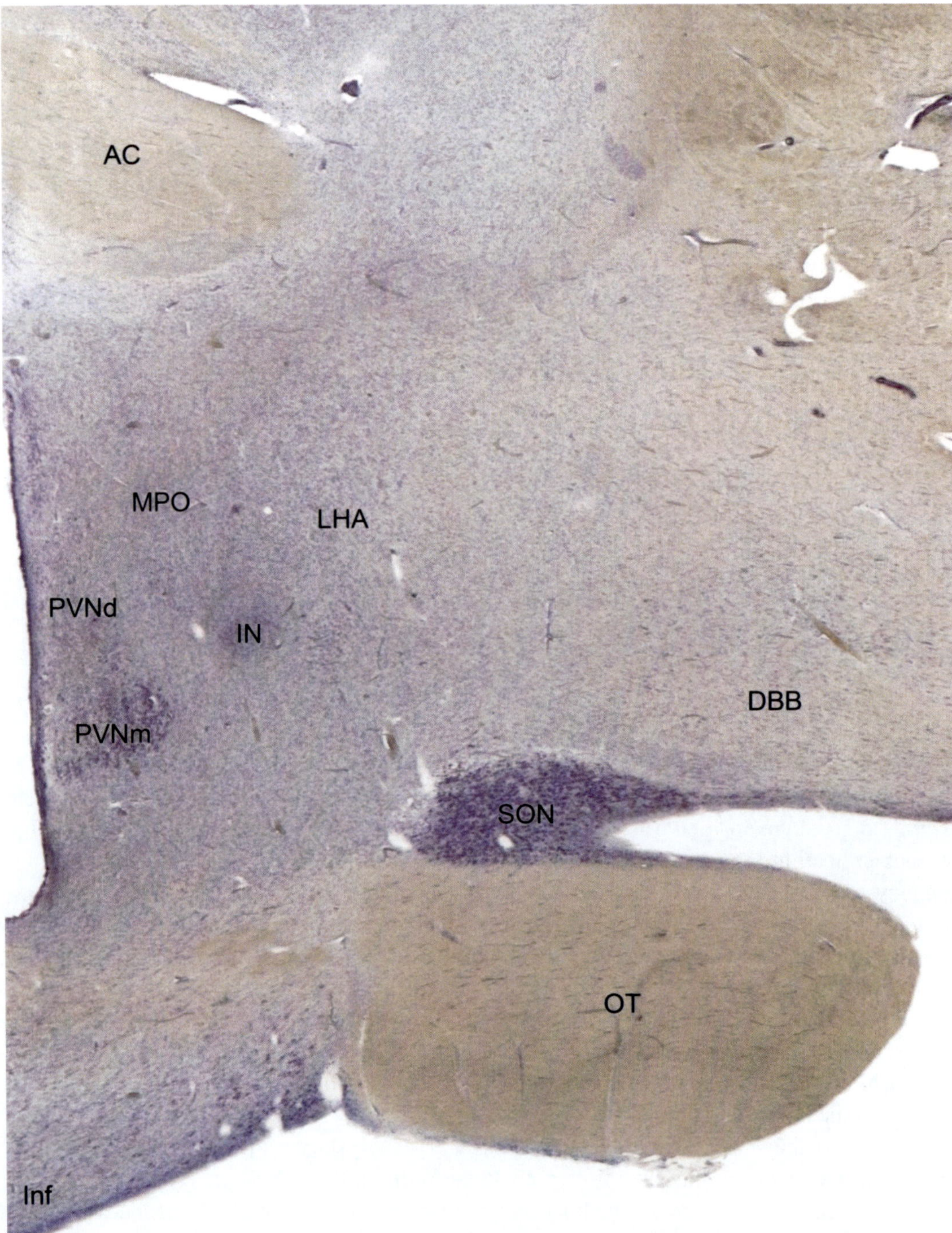

Figure 1. Frontal section of the infundibular region of the hypothalamus illustrating the most discernible structures with Nissl staining. Abbreviations: AC, anterior commissure; DBB, diagonal band of Broca; IN, intermediate nucleus; Inf, infundibulum; LHA, lateral hypothalamic area; MPO, medial preoptic area; OT, optic tract; PVNd, paraventricular nucleus, dorsal part; PVNm, paraventricular nucleus, magnocellular part; SON, supraoptic nucleus.

Magnocellular Neurotransmitters: Oxytocin and Vasopressin

Oxytocin is a nonapeptide with both hormone and neurotransmitter/neuromodulator attributes. Oxytocin plays a key role in parturition and lactation in both humans and animals (Amico et al., 2004; Blanks & Thornton, 2003; Carrasco & Van de Kar, 2003; Carter & Lightman, 1987b; Chatterton, Jr. et al., 2000; Douglas et al., 2000; Douglas et al., 2002; Kasting, 1988; Kendrick et al., 1991; Neumann et al., 1995). Although the physiologic effects of oxytocin in smooth muscle contraction are well established (Duridanova et al., 1997; Maigaard et al., 1986; Mironneau, 1976; Oishi et al., 1991; Sakai et al., 1981), several studies reported that oxytocin plays a major regulatory role in complex neural functions including memory and behavior (Argiolas & Melis, 2004; de Oliveira et al., 2007; Engelmann et al., 2000; Frasch et al., 1995; Herbert, 1994; Hughes et al., 1987; Insel et al., 1997; Van Wimersma Greidanus et al., 1986).

The vast majority of the oxytocin-immunoreactive (IR) perikarya are located in the PVN and SON and accessory nuclei scattered between. In these nuclei perikarya are densely packed (Figures 1,2A); a small number of oxytocinergic cell bodies are found in the basal part of the periventricular zone of the tuberal part of hypothalamus and in the infundibular region. Oxytocinergic neurons are either fusiform in shape with two processes emanating from the opposite poles of the cells or multipolar cells with large, round-shaped perikarya (Figure 4). Oxytocin–IR fibers are located mainly in the PVN, SON, and in the periventricular zone and infundibular region. These fibers are frequently oriented parallel to the ventricular and basal surface of the hypothalamus, typically running towards the hypophyseal stalk. No oxytocinergic perikarya can be observed in front of the lamina terminalis, in the lateral hypothalamic zone and in the posterior hypothalamus.

Vasopressin is a nonapeptide structurally similar to oxytocin. Vasopressin is secreted mainly by the magnocellular system of hypothalamo-hypophyseal axis. In addition to the water retentive effect, vasopressin also mediates peripheral vasoconstriction resulting in increased blood pressure and it is also considered as a neurotransmitter/neuromodulator. Similar to the oxytocinergic system, vasopressin-IR perikarya are densely packed in the PVN and SON (Figure 3), while few perikarya can detected in the infundibular region (Figure 3) and the periventricular zone of preoptic and tuberal part of hypothalamus. Although the detected vasopressin-IR neurons are typically large, multipolar cells with rounded cell bodies and centrally positioned nuclei (Figure 6D-F), numerous fusiform cells can also be detected with processes emanating from the opposite poles of the perikarya (Figure 6A-C). In addition to the magnocellular system in the PVN and SON, vasopressin is also synthesized by small neurons in the suprachiasmatic muclei. The majority of the vasopressin–IR fibers can be found in the infundibular region apparently projecting towards the hypophyseal stalk (hypothalamo-hypophyseal tract). Vasopressin-IR axonal varicosities can also be observed in the periventricular zone of the preoptic and tuberal regions, and in the PVN and SON. Although few periventricularly-arranged immunoreactive fibers can also be seen in the mamillary region, no vasopressin-IR perikarya can be detected in the posterior hypothalamus.

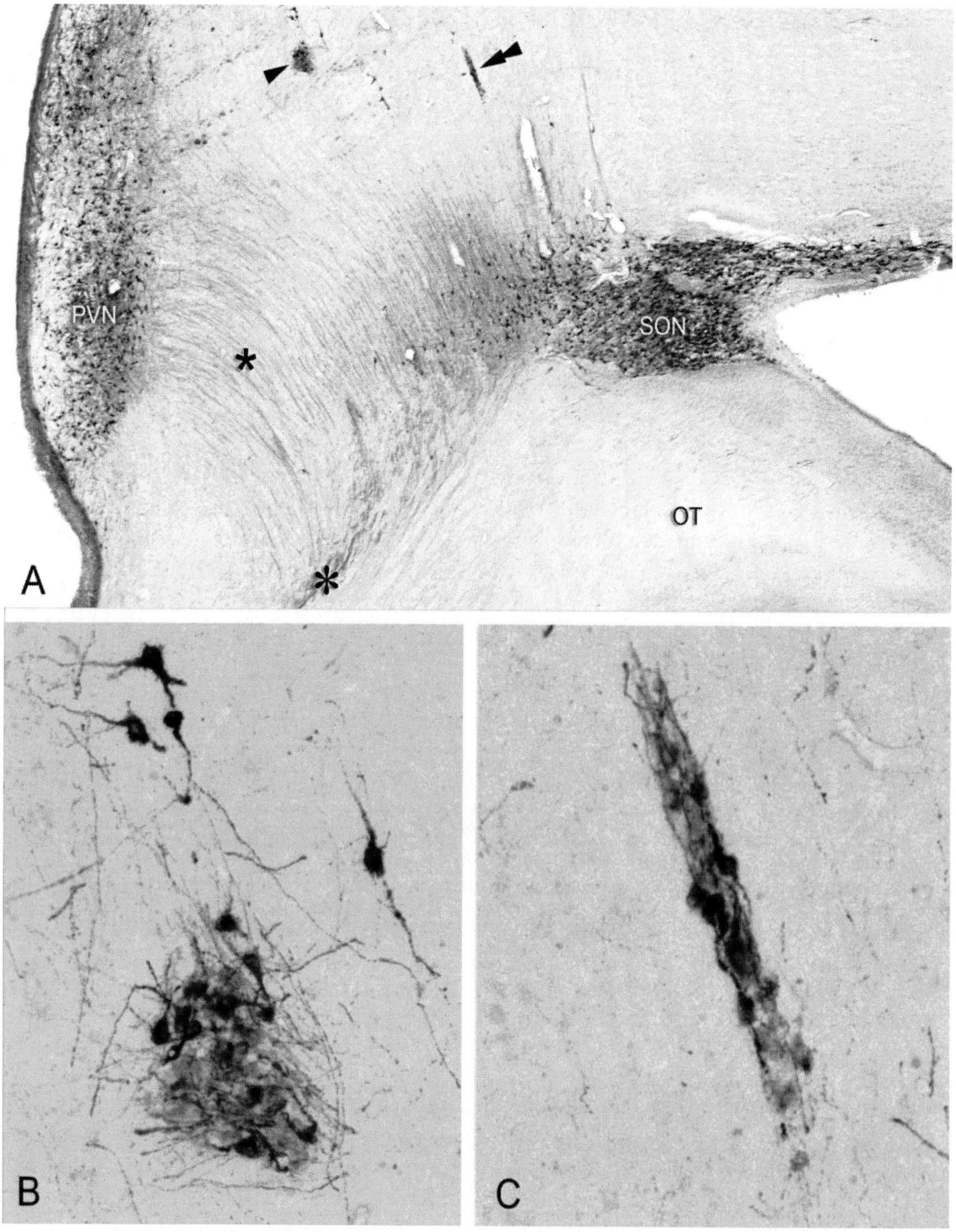

Figure 2. Oxytocinergic elements in the human hypothalamus. (A) OT immunostaining delineates the paraventricular (PVN) and supraoptic nuclei (SON) and the fiber connections between them (five-pointed asterisk). Six-pointed asterisk marks the hypothalamo-hypophyseal tract. OT: optic tract. Additional clusters of OT-immunoreactive neurons are detectable in the preoptic area scattered between the PVN and SON (arrowhead, also illustrated on insert B). Oxytocinergic neurons tend to be associated with blood vessels (double arrowhead, also illustrated on insert C).

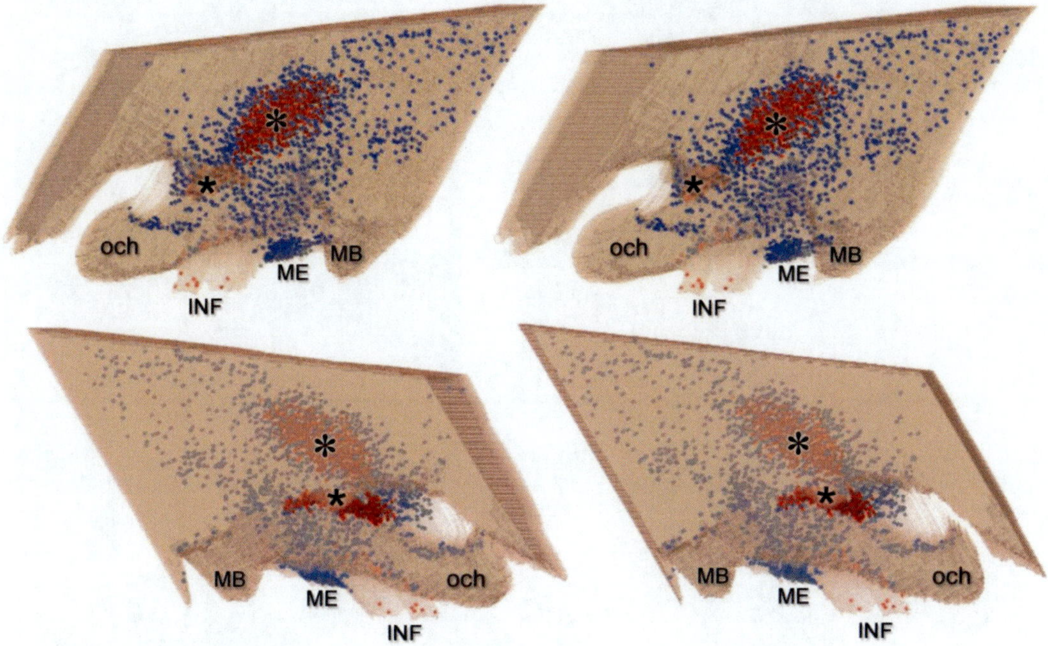

Figure 3. Stereoscopic images of the human hypothalamus illustrating catecholaminergic (blue dots) and vasopressin-IR perikarya (red dots). The overlapping sites between these systems are primarily located in the paraventricular and supraoptic nuclei. Stereoscopic images can be seen using U or parallel vision. The eyes are relaxed to look into the distance until the pair of the images fuse, and then refocused by the brain. With this technique a 3D hypothalamus can be seen on the figure, floating in front of the paper, with the immunolabeled perikarya in it at different depth marked by blue and red dots. The optimal viewing distance is about 20 inches from the paper surface (average reading distance). If the separation is too great for the eyes (double vision), move further away from the picture and the required angle will decrease. Abbreviations: INF, infundibulum; MB, mamillary body; ME, median eminence; och, optic chiasm; five-pointed star, supraoptic nucleus; six-pointed star, paraventricular nucleus. Reprinted with permission from Wiley (Dudás et al., 2006).

Stress and Oxytocin

A number of studies suggest that oxytocin is involved in the regulation of the stress response. Immobilization stress increases plasma oxytocin levels in rats (Carter & Lightman, 1987b). Psychological stress, such as exposure to uncontrollable noise results in significant increases in plasma oxytocin levels in humans (Sanders et al., 1990). In contrast, acute physical and mental stress can impair the milk ejection reflex by reducing the release of oxytocin in brestfeeding women (Dewey, 2001). Interestingly, emotional stress does not affect plasma oxytocin levels while it increases hypothalamic oxytocin release in rats (Engelmann et al., 1999). Similar to emotional stress, application of shaker stress (Nishioka et al., 1998) also increases the release of oxytocin in the hypothalamus. These findings suggest that hypothalamic oxytocinergic neurons play a crucial role in the stress-induced oxytocin release.

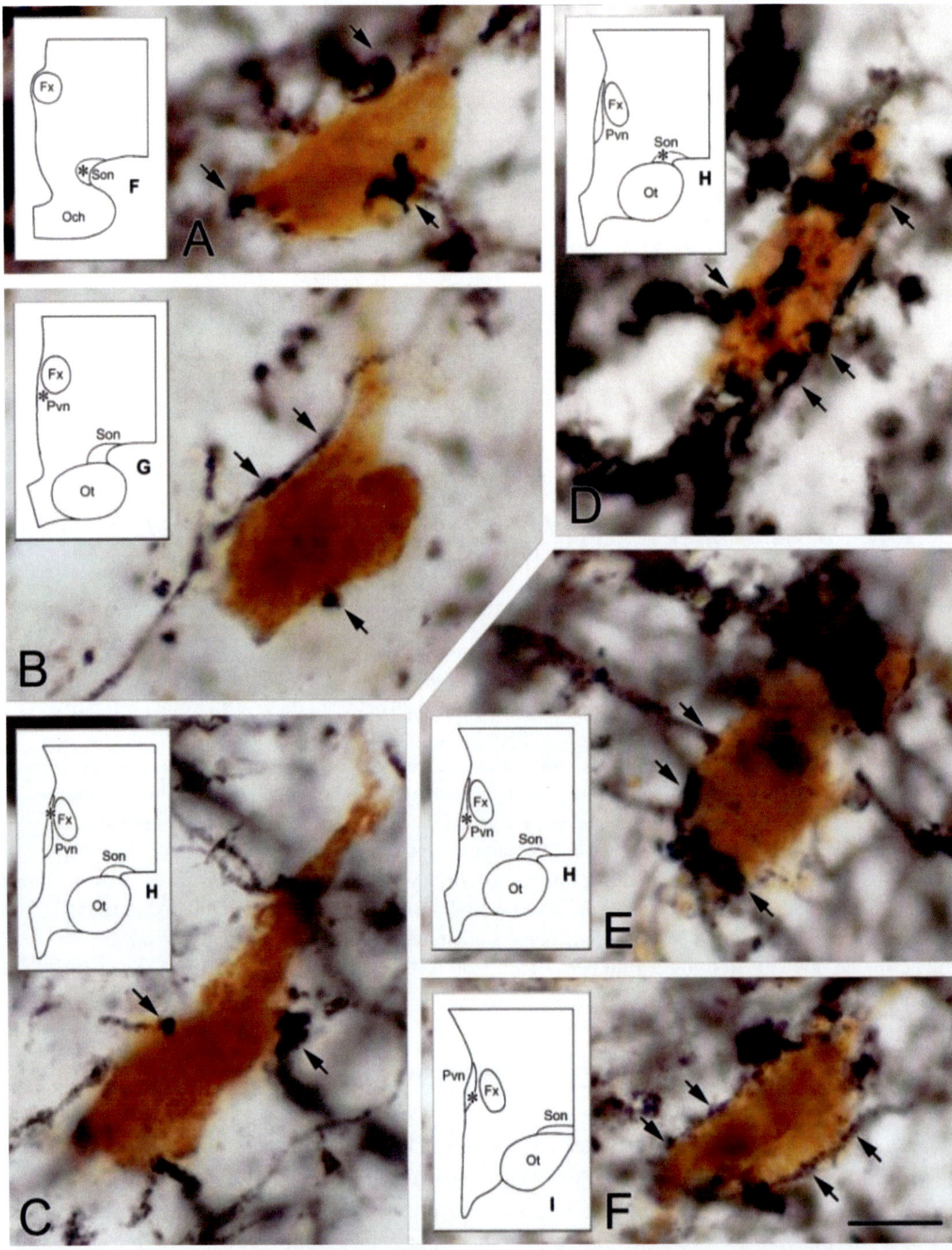

Figure 4. Juxtapositions between catecholaminergic, TH-IR fiber varicosities (black) and oxytocin-IR perikarya (brown) in the human supraoptic (A,D) and paraventricular nuclei (B,C,E,F). The schematic drawings at the upper corner of the micrographs represent the frontal hypothalamic sections with the positions of the demonstrated oxytocin-IR neurons denoted by asterisks. Arrowheads point to the juxtapositions between the catecholaminergic and oxytocin-IR elements. Scale bar, 20 μm. Abbreviations: Fx, fornix; Pvn, paraventricular nucleus; Och, optic chiasm; Ot, optic tract; Son, supraoptic nucleus. Reprinted with permission from Elsevier (Semeniken et al., 2009).

Although it has been established that oxytocin plays a major role in the mediation of the stress response in numerous species including humans (Callahan et al., 1989; Callahan et al., 1992; Carter & Lightman, 1987b; Chatterton, Jr. et al., 2000; Douglas et al., 2000; Engelmann et al., 1999; Jezova et al., 1995; Sanders et al., 1990; Windle et al., 1997; Windle et al., 2004), the exact mechanism of this modulation has not been elucidated yet. The central oxytocinergic system appears to mediate the cardiovascular response to acute stress in rats (Callahan et al., 1989; Callahan et al., 1992). Since lesioning the PVN attenuates stress-induced tachycardia in rats (Callahan et al., 1992), the integrity of oxytocinergic neurons in the PVN appears to be crucial in the response to stress. In contrast to these findings, a number of animal studies indicate that oxytocin plays a major role in the attenuation of the stress response (Cook, 1997; Legros, 2002; Uvnas-Moberg, 1997; Windle et al., 1997; Windle et al., 2004). Administration of oxytocin to rats subjected to noise significantly reduces the stress response, suggesting an endogenous anxiolytic-like function of oxytocin (Windle et al., 1997).

Previous studies indicate that the effect of oxytocin on stress responses may be species-dependent. Jezova et al. (1995) observed that oxytocin has a stimulatory effect on ACTH release in rats, while inhibiting ACTH release in humans. The discrepancy between the effects of oxytocin in rats versus humans suggests significant species differences in the mechanisms that play role in the oxytocin release. Such divergence therefore, may prevent the extrapolation of research data revealed in rat brains to humans and make human neuroendocrine studies absolute crucial.

Catecholamines and Oxytocin

Although several neurotransmitter systems appear to regulate hypothalamic oxytocin secretion, it is a general consensus that catecholaminergic system plays a pivotal role in the stress-mediated oxytocin secretion. Central administration of noradrenaline stimulates oxytocin release (Onaka, 2004) and selective lesion of the hypothalamic noradrenergic system decreases the stress-induced oxytocin secretion in male rats (Carter & Lightman, 1987a). Indeed, the key enzyme of the catecholamine synthesis, tyrosine hydroxylase (TH) had been found to co-localize with oxytocin in the PVN and SON in humans (Panayotacopoulou et al., 1994). Moreover, both PVN and SON receive a dense catecholaminergic fiber network (Figures 4, 5AB), often forming well-defined, catecholaminergic, basket-like terminal fields (Dudás & Merchenthaler, 2001; Dudás et al., 2006). These axon terminals indicate that catecholamines may influence neurotransmitter systems located in the PVN and SON by direct synaptic contact (Dudás & Merchenthaler, 2001). Indeed, catecholaminergic-oxytocinergic juxtapositions have been previously described in rats (Michaloudi et al., 1997). These associations have also been confirmed in human (Semeniken et al., 2009) and they are believed to represent functional synapses, which in turn, may represent the morphological substrate of stress-regulated oxytocin release via the catecholaminergic system. As expected, the majority of the associations detected between the oxytocinergic perikarya and catecholaminergic, TH-IR fiber varicosities are located in the SON (Figure 4A,D) and PVN (Figure 4B,C,E,F). Few intimate catecholaminergic-oxytocinergic juxtapositions can be observed in the infundibulum. The majority of the detected oxytocinergic neurons are densely associated (more than 3 contacts) with catecholaminergic fibers in the PVN (91%) and SON (86%). The rest of the oxytocinergic neurons in this region receive a lighter density of abutting catecholaminergic fibers (1-3 contacts) or no apparent associations at all. The basal part of the periventricular zone at the infundibulum contains few oxytocinergic cell bodies with either dense or light catecholaminergic associations. The majority of the detected juxtapositions are *en passant* type contacts, i.e., catecolaminergic axons contacts oxytocinergic perikarya at multiple sites while passing by forming axon varicosities at the contacts. Close examination of these catecholaminergic-oxytocinergic juxtapositions using oil immersion objective generally reveals no gaps between the contacting elements.

In addition to the catecholamine-oxytocinergic associations, the vast majority of the TH-IR perikarya appear to receive multiple abutting TH-IR fiber varicosities in the PVN (Figure 5C) and SON (Figure 5D). Most of these associations are *en passant type* contacts (Fig. 1C,D). Numerous contacts can be observed between catecholaminergic axons as well. The TH-IR perikarya receiving abutting fiber varicosities appear to be equally distributed in the PVN and SON. Catecholamines are known to co-localize with oxytocin in the PVN/SON in the human hypothalamus (Panayotacopoulou et al., 1994). Indeed, after using double-label immunohistochemistry for TH and oxytocin, the number of oxytocinergic perikarya in the PVN and SON appears to be significantly reduced when compared to data of single label immunohistochemistry against oxytocin. Since the chromogen labeling the TH-IR structures covers not only the recognition sites of the TH antibodies but also the antigenic site of oxytocin within the same neuron, the primary antibodies of the second label cannot find their target. This phenomenon indicates that some of the TH-IR neural elements may also be oxytocinergic. Thus, the TH-TH associations described in the human PVN (Figure 5C) and SON (Figure 5D) may actually represent additional catecholaminergic-oxytocinergic interactions.

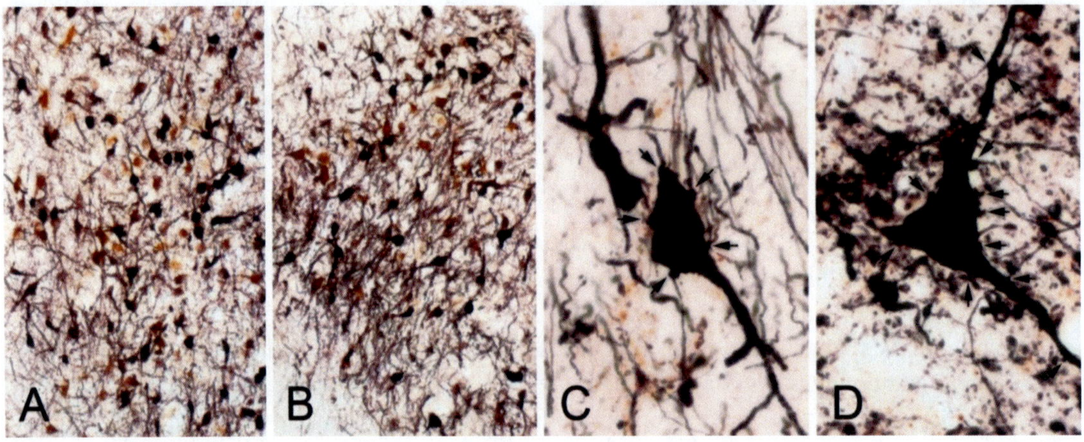

Figure 5. The distribution of the catecholaminergic TH-IR (black) and oxytocinergic (brown) neuronal elements in the paraventricular (A) and supraoptic nuclei (B). Numerous TH-IR neurons receive abutting TH-IR fiber varicosities (arrowheads) in the paraventricular (C) and supraoptic nuclei (D). Since TH has been reported to co-localize with oxytocin in human, these associations (C,D) may represent catecholaminergic-oxytocinergic juxtapositions. Scale bar, 100 μm (A,B) and 20 μm (C,D). Reprinted with permission from Elsevier (Semeniken et al., 2009).

Since TH is the key, rate-limiting enzyme of the catecholamine synthesis, TH immunoreactivity can indicate the presence of dopamine, noradrenaline or adrenaline. In human, PNMT-IR axons are extremely rare suggesting that most of the fiber varicosities that may innervate the oxytocinergic neurons are either dopaminergic or noradrenergic. Previous studies revealed that the vast majority of the TH-IR structures represent dopaminergic elements due to the relative scarcity of the DBH-immunoreactivity in the human hypothalamus; therefore, most of the described catecholoaminergic-oxytocinergic juxtapositions are considered to represent dopaminergic associations.

Stress and Vasopressin

Physical and emotional stress has a substantial impact on water and electrolyte balance. Although the mechanism of this phenomenon is not entirely understood, there is a general agreement that vasopressin plays a pivotal role in the stress–induced hemodynamic and osmotic changes (Aguilera et al., 1993; Aguilera & Rabadan-Diehl, 2000; Baylis, 1989; Carrasco & Van de Kar, 2003; Gauquelin-Koch et al., 1996; Glasgow et al., 2000; Husain et al., 1979; Jezova et al., 1995; Morgan et al., 1980; Robertson, 1976; von Bormann et al., 1985; Weidler et al., 1981; Weidler et al., 1982).

The primary stimuli of vasopressin release are stressors that trigger changes in plasma osmolality and volume (Aguilera et al., 1993; Morgan et al., 1980; Robertson, 1976). Additionally, these stimuli are reported to increase vasopressin gene expression in the rat SON (Glasgow et al., 2000; Zemo & McCabe, 2002). Hypertonic saline injection, representing a complex stress stimulus with osmotic and physical-psychological components, induces vasopressin secretion in rats (Jezova et al., 1995). Moreover, hemorrhage and water deprivation also increase vasopressin release (Aguilera et al., 1993; Kelly et al., 1983; Kiss et al., 1994). It is generally believed that in addition to direct regulation of the vasopressin release by osmotic changes of the blood, these phenomena also involve catecholaminergic influence on the vasopressin system (Jezova et al., 1995; Kanda et al., 1993; Kiss et al., 1994; Meyerhoff et al., 1990).

Several studies have reported the modulation of vasopressin release by nonosmotic stressors. Exercise and insulin-induced hypoglycaemia induces vasopressin release (Whitnall, 1989; Wittert et al., 1992). Surgical stress and nausea are known to increase vasopressin secretion in human (Amano et al., 1993; de Lange et al., 1982; Furuya et al., 1993; Koch, 1999). Moreover, vasopressin secretion is induced by emotional stress. These data suggest that catecholamines may also play a fundamental role in the modulation of water and electrolyte balance via vasopressin release (Hydbring-Sandberg et al., 2004; Wotjak et al., 1996). Indeed, catecholamine-induced vasopressin increase has been suggested as a critical factor of the pathogenesis of hypertension in stress (Zimmerman & Frohlich, 1990). In contrast to these findings, a number of studies found decrease of vasopressin levels in the plasma following various stressors. Low temperature combined with fluid and food deprivation reduces vasopressin release in human (Wittert et al., 1992). Acute emotional stress decreases plasma vasopressin levels of dehydrated rats (Keil & Severs, 1977; Onaka & Yagi, 1993). To complicate the question even more, prolonged immobilization was found to decrease vasopressin secretion in rats after an initial increase (Michajlovskij et al., 1988).

In addition to the peripheral water retentive effect, vasopressin is also considered as a neurotransmitter/neuromodulator. This hypothesis is supported by previous studies demonstrating that vasopressin appears to be involved in numerous psychiatric conditions involving stress (Scantamburlo et al., 2001), while stress also increases vasopressin levels in the blood by releasing vasopressin from the posterior lobe of the hypophysis (Aguilera et al., 1993; Morgan et al., 1980; Robertson, 1976). However, the exact role that the centrally released vasopressin plays in the stress response remains to be reconciled.

Catecholaminergic Control of Vasopressin Release

The notion of direct connection between stress stimuli and the vasopressin-modulated water and electrolyte balance is generally accepted. Since one of the central coordinators of the stress response is the catecholaminergic system, it is a general consensus that catecholaminergic axons may influence vasopressin release by directly innervating vasopressinergic neurons in the hypothalamus (McNeill & Sladek, Jr., 1980; Nakada & Nakai, 1985; Silverman et al., 1983; Sladek, Jr. & McNeill, 1980). Indeed, increased TH immunoreactivity was reported in the PVN and SON in illnesses associated with prolonged osmotic and nonosmotic stimulation of the vasopressin release (Panayotacopoulou et al., 2002) indicating that stress-induced catecholamine release may directly participate in the regulation of hypothalamic vasopressin secretion. Similarly to the catecholamine control of the oxytocin release, this modulation may occur via direct catecholaminergic-vasopressinergic associations, which may represent human synapses and may be the morphological substrate of catecholaminergic-modulated vasopressin release. Indeed, previous studies revealed that catecholaminergic fibers form well-defined terminal fields in the PVN and SON (Dudás & Merchenthaler, 2001; Dudás et al., 2006), and TH has been reported to co-localize with both vasopressin and oxytocin in these nuclei (Panayotacopoulou et al., 1994). Indeed, simultaneous presence of TH immunoreactivity and vasopressin mRNA was described in neurons of the human PVN and SON (Panayotacopoulou et al., 2000). Since previous studies reported that vasopressin-TH colocalization is not significant in adult human brain (Panayotacopoulou et al., 1994), vasopressin release may be primarily influenced by the catecholaminergic system via direct synaptic mechanisms. Indeed, the vast majority of the vasopressin-IR perikarya in the human hypothalamus appear to receive catecholaminergic abutting fiber varicosities with synapse-like contacts. These juxtapositions between the vasopressin-IR perikarya and catecholaminergic elements can be observed mainly in the PVN and SON, where black, silver impregnated, Ni-DAB-stained TH-IR axonal varicosities abut on vasopressin-IR perikarya visualized with brown DAB chromogen (Figure 6). These juxtapositions are usually *en passant* type contacts with TH-IR fibers innervating apparently more than one vasopressin-IR neurons while passing by, but numerous terminal type contacts can also be detected. Close examination of these juxtapositions with oil immersion reveals no gap between the contacting elements. Few juxtapositions can also be observed in the infundibulum (Figure 6F). In the PVN, the vast majority (98%) of the detected vasopressin-IR neurons appear to be heavily innervated (more than 3 contacts) by catecholaminergic fibers (Figure 6A-B).

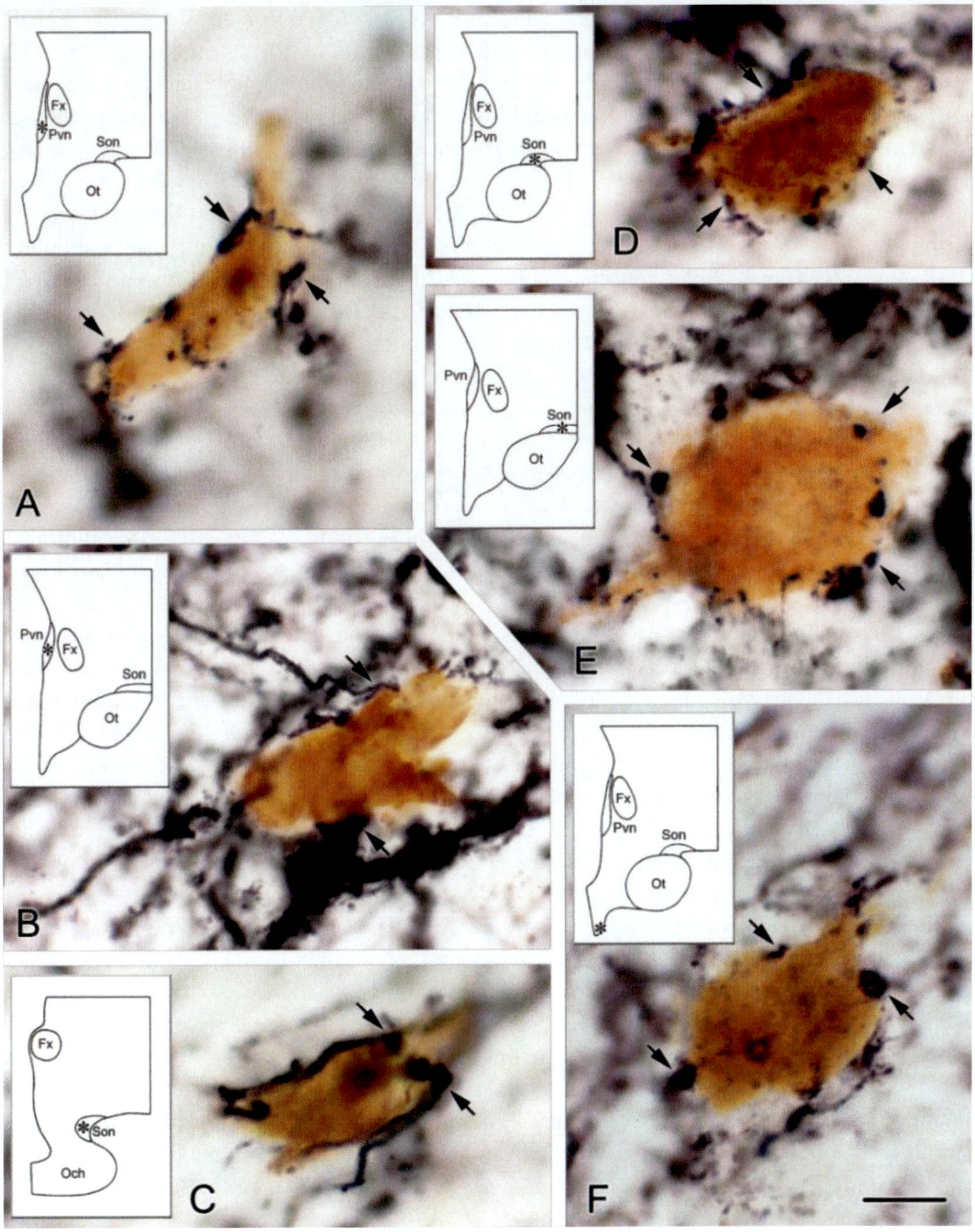

Figure 6. Double-label immunohistochemistry illustrates juxtapositions between the catecholaminergic, TH-IR (black), and vasopressin-IR (brown) neural elements in the human hypothalamus. The position of the demonstrated vasopressin-IR neurons is shown by asterisks on the coronal sections of the diencephalon in the corners of the micrographs. The thickness of the sections is 30 μm, the pictures were taken with oil immersion with an objective of 100 X. Arrowheads point to juxtapositions between the catecholaminergic and vasopressinergic elements. Scale bar: 20 μm. Abbreviations: ac, anterior commissure; fx, fornix; pvn, paraventricular nucleus; och, optic chiasm; ot, optic tract; son, supraoptic nucleus. Reprinted with permission from Wiley (Dudás et al., 2006).

The remaining perikarya are lightly innervated (1-3 contacts) or do not receive TH-IR fiber varicosities. The amount of vasopressin-IR perikarya in the PVN without apparent TH-IR juxtapositions is insignificant. The size of the vast majority of the heavily innervated vasopressin-IR perikarya in the PVN appears to be similar to the volume of the magnocellular vasopressin-IR neurons in the SON. In the SON, catecholaminergic fiber varicosities heavily innervate (more than 3 contacts) 82% of the detected vasopressin-IR perikarya (Figure 6C-E). The rest of the vasopressin-IR neurons are lightly (1-3 contact) or not innervated. Few vasopressin-IR neurons can be detected in the periventricular zone and in the infundibulum with light or heavy catecholaminergic innervation (Fig.6F). No juxtapositions can be found between vasopressin-IR and TH-IR axonal varicosities, except the proximal part of the vasopressinergic fibers in the close vicinity of the cell body.

Magnocellular neurons in the PVN appear to respond to stress differently than those in SON. Cold exposure and isolation stress increases vasopressin mRNA levels in magnocellular neurons of the PVN but not in the SON (Angulo et al., 1991). On the other hand, the vast majority of the vasopressin-IR perikarya in the SON appear to be heavily innervated by abutting TH-IR axonal varicosities, and these juxtapositions are morphologically similar to those in the PVN. These findings suggest that additional neurotransmitter systems may participate in the modulation of the vasopressin release in the PVN and SON.

Previous data suggest that catecholamine-induced vasopressin release may play a crucial role in the mechanism of depression. Plasma levels of vasopressin and oxytocin appear to be increased in patients with major depression, indicating that vasopressin and/or vasopressin-mediated functions influence the activity of the hypothalamic-hypophyseal-adrenal (HPA) axis (van Londen et al., 1997). Indeed, increased levels of vasopressin was found in depressed individuals along with significant disregulation of the HPA axis (Scott & Dinan, 1998) and significant increase in vasopressin mRNA in the PNV was reported in the rat model of depression, as compared to controls (Nakase et al., 1998). Moreover, vasopressin levels are decreased in patients after receiving antidepressant treatment (Scott & Dinan, 1998). These data indicate that magnocellular vasopressin release plays a pivotal role in the regulation of the HPA axis in numerous species, including human. The principal symptoms in melancholic depression include tachycardia and hypertension indicating that vasopressin release in depression may be induced by the increased catecholaminergic release. Since the vasopressinergic system is suggested to be one of the main future targets of antidepressant drug development (Scott & Dinan, 2002), modulation of catecholamine-induced vasopressin secretion may open an entirely new avenue in the treatment of depression. Consequently, the catecholaminergic-vasopressinergic juxtapositions described above may be functional synapses and may represent the morphological substrate of the catecholamine-regulated vasopressin release in human.

Conclusion

Catecholaminergic fibers terminating on the surface of the oxytocin- and vasopressin-IR neurons may represent functional synapses and may form the morphological substrate of an interaction between these systems. According to these findings, these juxtapositions may represent the sites of the stress-induced oxytocin and vasopressin release in humans. Consequently, the central catecholaminergic system may regulate water balance and blood pressure as well as smooth muscle contraction and complex behavioral effects centrally via modulating vasopressin and oxytocin release from the human diencephalon. The negligible amount of adrenergic elements in the human hypothalamus and the relative scarcity of the noradrenergic elements compared to the dopaminergic structures suggest that these juxtapositions are dopaminergic. The large number of the catecholaminergic-oxytocin and catecholaminergic-vasopressin juxtapositions in the PVN/SON suggests that these regions may play a pivotal role in mediating stress response by releasing oxytocin and vasopressin in humans.

References

Aguilera, G., Lightman, S. L., & Kiss, A. (1993). Regulation of the hypothalamic-pituitary-adrenal axis during water deprivation. *Endocrinology, 132,* 241-248.

Aguilera, G. & Rabadan-Diehl, C. (2000). Vasopressinergic regulation of the hypothalamic-pituitary-adrenal axis: implications for stress adaptation. *Regul.Pept., 96,* 23-29.

Amano, J., Suzuki, A., & Sunamori, M. (1993). Antidiuretic hormone and cardiovascular responses during and after coronary artery bypass surgery. *Thorac.Cardiovasc.Surg., 41,* 297-300.

Amico, J. A., Mantella, R. C., Vollmer, R. R., & Li, X. (2004). Anxiety and stress responses in female oxytocin deficient mice. *J.Neuroendocrinol., 16,* 319-324.

Angulo, J. A., Ledoux, M., & McEwen, B. S. (1991). Genomic effects of cold and isolation stress on magnocellular vasopressin mRNA-containing cells in the hypothalamus of the rat. *J.Neurochem., 56,* 2033-2038.

Argiolas, A. & Melis, M. R. (2004). The role of oxytocin and the paraventricular nucleus in the sexual behaviour of male mammals. *Physiol Behav., 83,* 309-317.

Baylis, P. H. (1989). Regulation of vasopressin secretion. *Baillieres Clin.Endocrinol.Metab, 3,* 313-330.

Blanks, A. M. & Thornton, S. (2003). The role of oxytocin in parturition. *BJOG., 110 Suppl 20,* 46-51.

Callahan, M. F., Kirby, R. F., Cunningham, J. T., Eskridge-Sloop, S. L., Johnson, A. K., McCarty, R. et al. (1989). Central oxytocin systems may mediate a cardiovascular response to acute stress in rats. *Am.J.Physiol, 256,* H1369-H1377.

Callahan, M. F., Thore, C. R., Sundberg, D. K., Gruber, K. A., O'Steen, K., & Morris, M. (1992). Excitotoxin paraventricular nucleus lesions: stress and endocrine reactivity and oxytocin mRNA levels. *Brain Res., 597,* 8-15.

Carrasco, G. A. & Van de Kar, L. D. (2003). Neuroendocrine pharmacology of stress. *Eur.J.Pharmacol., 463,* 235-272.

Carter, D. A. & Lightman, S. L. (1987a). Modulation of oxytocin secretion by ascending noradrenergic pathways: sexual dimorphism in rats. *Brain Res., 406,* 313-316.

Carter, D. A. & Lightman, S. L. (1987b). Oxytocin responses to stress in lactating and hyperprolactinaemic rats. *Neuroendocrinology, 46,* 532-537.

Chatterton, R. T., Jr., Hill, P. D., Aldag, J. C., Hodges, K. R., Belknap, S. M., & Zinaman, M. J. (2000). Relation of plasma oxytocin and prolactin concentrations to milk production in mothers of preterm infants: influence of stress. *J.Clin.Endocrinol.Metab, 85,* 3661-3668.

Cook, C. J. (1997). Oxytocin and prolactin suppress cortisol responses to acute stress in both lactating and non-lactating sheep. *J.Dairy Res., 64,* 327-339.

de Lange, S., Boscoe, M. J., Stanley, T. H., de Bruijin, N., Philbin, D. M., & Coggins, C. H. (1982). Antidiuretic and growth hormone responses during coronary artery surgery with sufentanil-oxygen and alfentanil-oxygen anesthesia in man. *Anesth.Analg., 61,* 434-438.

de Oliveira, L. F., Camboim, C., Diehl, F., Consiglio, A. R., & Quillfeldt, J. A. (2007). Glucocorticoid-mediated effects of systemic oxytocin upon memory retrieval. *Neurobiol.Learn.Mem., 87,* 67-71.

Dewey, K. G. (2001). Maternal and fetal stress are associated with impaired lactogenesis in humans. *J.Nutr., 131,* 3012S-3015S.

Douglas, A. J., Johnstone, H., Brunton, P., & Russell, J. A. (2000). Sex-steroid induction of endogenous opioid inhibition on oxytocin secretory responses to stress. *J.Neuroendocrinol., 12,* 343-350.

Douglas, A. J., Leng, G., & Russell, J. A. (2002). The importance of oxytocin mechanisms in the control of mouse parturition. *Reproduction., 123,* 543-552.

Dudás, B. & Merchenthaler, I. (2001). Catecholaminergic axons innervate LH-releasing hormone immunoreactive neurons of the human diencephalon. *J.Clin.Endocrinol.Metab, 86,* 5620-5626.

Dudás, B., Semeniken, K. R., & Merchenthaler, I. (2006). Morphological substrate of the catecholaminergic input of the vasopressin neuronal system in humans. *J.Neuroendocrinol., 18,* 895-901.

Duridanova, D. B., Nedelcheva, M. D., & Gagov, H. S. (1997). Oxytocin-induced changes in single cell K+ currents and smooth muscle contraction of guinea-pig gastric antrum. *Eur.J.Endocrinol., 136,* 531-538.

Engelmann, M., Ebner, K., Landgraf, R., Holsboer, F., & Wotjak1 CT (1999). Emotional stress triggers intrahypothalamic but not peripheral release of oxytocin in male rats. *J.Neuroendocrinol., 11,* 867-872.

Engelmann, M., Wotjak, C. T., Ebner, K., & Landgraf, R. (2000). Behavioural impact of intraseptally released vasopressin and oxytocin in rats. *Exp.Physiol, 85 Spec No,* 125S-130S.

Frasch, A., Zetzsche, T., Steiger, A., & Jirikowski, G. F. (1995). Reduction of plasma oxytocin levels in patients suffering from major depression. *Adv.Exp.Med.Biol., 395,* 257-258.

Furuya, K., Shimizu, R., Hirabayashi, Y., Ishii, R., & Fukuda, H. (1993). Stress hormone responses to major intra-abdominal surgery during and immediately after sevoflurane-nitrous oxide anaesthesia in elderly patients. *Can.J.Anaesth., 40,* 435-439.

Gauquelin-Koch, G., Blanquie, J. P., Viso, M., Florence, G., Milhaud, C., & Gharib, C. (1996). Hormonal response to restraint in rhesus monkeys. *J.Med.Primatol., 25,* 387-396.

Glasgow, E., Murase, T., Zhang, B., Verbalis, J. G., & Gainer, H. (2000). Gene expression in the rat supraoptic nucleus induced by chronic hyperosmolality versus hyposmolality. *Am.J.Physiol Regul.Integr.Comp Physiol, 279,* R1239-R1250.

Herbert, J. (1994). Oxytocin and sexual behaviour. *BMJ, 309,* 891-892.

Hughes, A. M., Everitt, B. J., Lightman, S. L., & Todd, K. (1987). Oxytocin in the central nervous system and sexual behaviour in male rats. *Brain Res., 414,* 133-137.

Husain, M. K., Manger, W. M., Rock, T. W., Weiss, R. J., & Frantz, A. G. (1979). Vasopressin release due to manual restraint in the rat: role of body compression and comparison with other stressful stimuli. *Endocrinology, 104,* 641-644.

Hydbring-Sandberg, E., von Walter, L. W., Hoglund, K., Svartberg, K., Swenson, L., & Forkman, B. (2004). Physiological reactions to fear provocation in dogs. *J.Endocrinol., 180,* 439-448.

Insel, T. R., Young, L., & Wang, Z. (1997). Central oxytocin and reproductive behaviours. *Rev.Reprod., 2,* 28-37.

Jezova, D., Skultetyova, I., Tokarev, D. I., Bakos, P., & Vigas, M. (1995). Vasopressin and oxytocin in stress. *Ann N Y Acad Sci, 771,* 192-203.

Kanda, K., Omori, S., Yamamoto, C., Miyamoto, N., Kawano, S., Murata, Y. et al. (1993). Urinary excretion of stress hormones of rats in tail-suspension. *Environ.Med., 37,* 39-41.

Kasting, N. W. (1988). Simultaneous and independent release of vasopressin and oxytocin in the rat. *Can.J.Physiol Pharmacol., 66,* 22-26.

Keil, L. C. & Severs, W. B. (1977). Reduction in plasma vasopressin levels of dehydrated rats following acute stress. *Endocrinology, 100,* 30-38.

Kelly, R. T., Rose, J. C., Meis, P. J., Hargrave, B. Y., & Morris, M. (1983). Vasopressin is important for restoring cardiovascular homeostasis in fetal lambs subjected to hemorrhage. *Am.J.Obstet.Gynecol., 146,* 807-812.

Kendrick, K. M., Keverne, E. B., Hinton, M. R., & Goode, J. A. (1991). Cerebrospinal fluid and plasma concentrations of oxytocin and vasopressin during parturition and vaginocervical stimulation in the sheep. *Brain Res.Bull., 26,* 803-807.

Kiss, A., Jezova, D., & Aguilera, G. (1994). Activity of the hypothalamic pituitary adrenal axis and sympathoadrenal system during food and water deprivation in the rat. *Brain Res., 663,* 84-92.

Koch, K. L. (1999). Illusory self-motion and motion sickness: a model for brain-gut interactions and nausea. *Dig.Dis.Sci., 44,* 53S-57S.

Legros, J. J. (2002). [Oxytocin: a natural means of treating psychological stress]. *Bull.Mem.Acad.R.Med.Belg., 157,* 383-389.

Maigaard, S., Forman, A., & Andersson, K. E. (1986). Differential effects of angiotensin, vasopressin and oxytocin on various smooth muscle tissues within the human uteroplacental unit. *Acta Physiol Scand., 128,* 23-31.

McNeill, T. H. & Sladek, J. R., Jr. (1980). Simultaneous monoamine histofluorescence and neuropeptide immunocytochemistry: II. Correlative distribution of catecholamine varicosities and magnocellular neurosecretory neurons in the rat supraoptic and paraventricular nuclei. *J.Comp Neurol., 193,* 1023-1033.

Meyerhoff, J. L., Oleshansky, M. A., Kalogeras, K. T., Mougey, E. H., Chrousos, G. P., & Granger, L. G. (1990). Neuroendocrine responses to emotional stress: possible interactions between circulating factors and anterior pituitary hormone release. *Adv.Exp.Med.Biol., 274:91-111.,* 91-111.

Michajlovskij, N., Lichardus, B., Kvetnansky, R., & Ponec, J. (1988). Effect of acute and repeated immobilization stress on food and water intake, urine output and vasopressin changes in rats. *Endocrinol.Exp., 22,* 143-157.

Michaloudi, H. C., el, M. M., Poulain, D. A., Papadopoulos, G. C., & Theodosis, D. T. (1997). The noradrenergic innervation of identified hypothalamic magnocellular somata and its contribution to lactation-induced synaptic plasticity. *J.Neuroendocrinol., 9,* 17-23.

Mironneau, J. (1976). Effects of oxytocin on ionic currents underlying rhythmic activity and contraction in uterine smooth muscle. *Pflugers Arch., 363,* 113-118.

Morgan, R. J., Martyn, J. A., Philbin, D. M., Coggins, C. H., & Burke, J. F. (1980). Water metabolism and antidiuretic hormone (ADH) response following thermal injury. *J.Trauma, 20,* 468-472.

Nakada, H. & Nakai, Y. (1985). Electron microscopic examination of the catecholaminergic innervation of neurophysin- or vasopressin-containing neurons in the rat hypothalamus. *Brain Res., 361,* 247-257.

Nakase, S., Kitayama, I., Soya, H., Hamanaka, K., & Nomura, J. (1998). Increased expression of magnocellular arginine vasopressin mRNA in paraventricular nucleus of stress-induced depression-model rats. *Life Sci., 63,* 23-31.

Neumann, I., Pittman, Q. J., & Landgraf, R. (1995). Release of oxytocin within the supraoptic nucleus. Mechanisms, physiological significance and antisense targeting. *Adv.Exp.Med.Biol., 395:173-83.,* 173-183.

Nishioka, T., Anselmo-Franci, J. A., Li, P., Callahan, M. F., & Morris, M. (1998). Stress increases oxytocin release within the hypothalamic paraventricular nucleus. *Brain Res., %19;781,* 56-60.

Oishi, K., Takano-Ohmuro, H., Minakawa-Matsuo, N., Suga, O., Karibe, H., Kohama, K. et al. (1991). Oxytocin contracts rat uterine smooth muscle in Ca2(+)-free medium without any phosphorylation of myosin light chain. *Biochem.Biophys.Res.Commun., 176,* 122-128.

Onaka, T. (2004). Neural pathways controlling central and peripheral oxytocin release during stress. *J.Neuroendocrinol., 16,* 308-312.

Onaka, T. & Yagi, K. (1993). Effects of novelty stress on vasopressin and oxytocin secretion by the pituitary in the rat. *J.Neuroendocrinol., 5,* 365-369.

Panayotacopoulou, M. T., Goudsmit, E., Van, H., & Swaab, D. F. (2000). Simultaneous detection of tyrosine hydroxylase-immunoreactivity and vasopressin mRNA in neurons of the human paraventricular and supraoptic nucleus. *Brain Res, 855,* 181-185.

Panayotacopoulou, M. T., Malidelis, Y. I., Fliers, E., Bouras, C., Ravid, R., & Swaab, D. F. (2002). Increased expression of tyrosine hydroxylase immunoreactivity in paraventricular and supraoptic neurons in illnesses with prolonged osmotic or nonosmotic stimulation of vasopressin release. *Neuroendocrinology, 76,* 254-266.

Panayotacopoulou, M. T., Raadsheer, F. C., & Swaab, D. F. (1994). Colocalization of tyrosine hydroxylase with oxytocin or vasopressin in neurons of the human paraventricular and supraoptic nucleus. *Brain Res Dev Brain Res, 83,* 59-66.

Robertson, G. L. (1976). The regulation of vasopressin function in health and disease. *Recent Prog.Horm.Res., 33:333-85.,* 333-385.

Sakai, K., Yamaguchi, T., & Uchida, M. (1981). Oxytocin-induced Ca-free contraction of rat uterine smooth muscle: effects of divalent cations and drugs. *Arch.Int.Pharmacodyn.Ther., 250,* 40-54.

Sanders, G., Freilicher, J., & Lightman, S. L. (1990). Psychological stress of exposure to uncontrollable noise increases plasma oxytocin in high emotionality women. *Psychoneuroendocrinology, 15,* 47-58.

Saper, C. B. (2004). Hypothalamus. In G.Paxinos & J. K. Mai (Eds.), *The human nervous system* (2 ed., pp. 513-550). Elsevier.

Scantamburlo, G., Ansseau, M., & Legros, J. J. (2001). [Role of the neurohypophysis in psychological stress]. *Encephale, 27,* 245-259.

Scott, L. V. & Dinan, T. G. (1998). Vasopressin and the regulation of hypothalamic-pituitary-adrenal axis function: implications for the pathophysiology of depression. *Life Sci., 62,* 1985-1998.

Scott, L. V. & Dinan, T. G. (2002). Vasopressin as a target for antidepressant development: an assessment of the available evidence. *J.Affect.Disord., 72,* 113-124.

Semeniken, K., Merchenthaler, I., Hu, W., & Dudás, B. (2009). Catecholaminergic input to the oxytocin neurosecretory system in the human hypothalamus. *J.Chem.Neuroanat., 37,* 229-233.

Silverman, A. J., Hou-Yu, A., & Oldfield, B. J. (1983). Ultrastructural identification of noradrenergic nerve terminals and vasopressin-containing neurons of the paraventricular nucleus in the same thin section. *J.Histochem.Cytochem., 31,* 1151-1156.

Sladek, J. R., Jr. & McNeill, T. H. (1980). Simultaneous monoamine histofluorescence and neuropeptide immunocytochemistry. IV. Verification of catecholamine-neurophysin interactions through single-section analysis. *Cell Tissue Res., 210,* 181-189.

Uvnas-Moberg, K. (1997). Oxytocin linked antistress effects--the relaxation and growth response. *Acta Physiol Scand.Suppl, 640:38-42.,* 38-42.

van Londen, L., Goekoop, J. G., van Kempen, G. M., Frankhuijzen-Sierevogel, A. C., Wiegant, V. M., van der Velde, E. A. et al. (1997). Plasma levels of arginine vasopressin elevated in patients with major depression. *Neuropsychopharmacology, 17,* 284-292.

Van Wimersma Greidanus, T. B., Burbach, J. P., & Veldhuis, H. D. (1986). Vasopressin and oxytocin. Their presence in the central nervous system and their functional significance in brain processes related to behaviour and memory. *Acta Endocrinol.Suppl (Copenh), 276,* 85-94.

von Bormann, B., Sturm, G., Kling, D., Scheld, H. H., Boldt, J., & Hempelmann, G. (1985). [Significance of endocrine parameters of stress]. *Anaesthesist, 34,* 280-286.

Weidler, B., von Bormann, B., Scheld, H., & Hempelmann, G. (1982). Plasma-ADH-levels--a reliable stress parameter? *Rinsho Kyobu Geka, 2,* 919-924.

Weidler, B., von, B. B., Lennartz, H., Dennhardt, R., & Hempelmann, G. (1981). [Plasma antidiuretic hormone level as an indicator of perioperative stress (Part I) (author's transl)]. *Anasth.Intensivther.Notfallmed., 16,* 315-318.

Whitnall, M. H. (1989). Stress selectively activates the vasopressin-containing subset of corticotropin-releasing hormone neurons. *Neuroendocrinology, 50,* 702-707.

Windle, R. J., Kershaw, Y. M., Shanks, N., Wood, S. A., Lightman, S. L., & Ingram, C. D. (2004). Oxytocin attenuates stress-induced c-fos mRNA expression in specific forebrain regions associated with modulation of hypothalamo-pituitary-adrenal activity. *J.Neurosci., 24,* 2974-2982.

Windle, R. J., Shanks, N., Lightman, S. L., & Ingram, C. D. (1997). Central oxytocin administration reduces stress-induced corticosterone release and anxiety behavior in rats. *Endocrinology, 138,* 2829-2834.

Wittert, G. A., Or, H. K., Livesey, J. H., Richards, A. M., Donald, R. A., & Espiner, E. A. (1992). Vasopressin, corticotrophin-releasing factor, and pituitary adrenal responses to acute cold stress in normal humans. *J.Clin.Endocrinol.Metab, 75,* 750-755.

Wotjak, C. T., Kubota, M., Liebsch, G., Montkowski, A., Holsboer, F., Neumann, I. et al. (1996). Release of vasopressin within the rat paraventricular nucleus in response to emotional stress: a novel mechanism of regulating adrenocorticotropic hormone secretion? *J.Neurosci., 16,* 7725-7732.

Zemo, D. A. & McCabe, J. T. (2002). Transcriptional responses of the rat vasopressin gene to acute and repeated acute osmotic stress. *Neurosci.Res., 44,* 45-50.

Zimmerman, R. S. & Frohlich, E. D. (1990). Stress and hypertension. *J.Hypertens.Suppl, 8,* S103-S107.

In: The Central Catecholaminergic System
Editor: Bertalan Dudás

ISBN: 978-1-63117-937-2

Chapter 7

Toxic Metabolites of Catecholamines in Parkinson's Disease

Thomas D. Corso and George Grignol

Introduction

Although tragic for the patients suffering from Parkinson's disease, progress in our understanding of this disorder starting with MPTP (1-methyl-4-phenyl-1,2,3,6-tetrahydropyridine) is a fascinating story. The emphasis of this chapter will be on toxins including MPTP and 6-hydroxydopamine (6-OH-DA) and the role of endogenous toxins either derived from the catecholamines or affecting catecholamine metabolism (Figure 1).

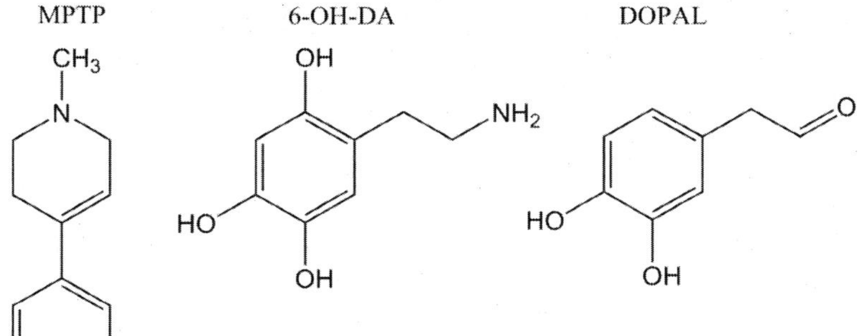

Figure 1. Three toxins known to selectively kill dopamine cells.

The dopamine metabolite DOPAL (3,4-dihydroxyphenylacetaldehyde) has been shown to be toxic to dopaminergic cells (Mattammal et al., 1993), and evidence has shown that DOPAL concentrations increase with impairment of mitochondrial function (Lamensdorf et al., 2000a; Lamensdorf et al., 2000b) or from oxidative stress (Florang et al., 2007; Rees et al., 2007). DOPAL has also been shown to cross-link the protein alpha-synuclein inducing aggregation of this protein (Burke et al., 2008). This is significant since alpha-synuclein aggregates are the primary component of Lewy bodies which are a histological hallmark of Parkinson's disease (Engelender, 2008).

Lewy Bodies, α-Synuclein and Parkin

The neurodegenerative movement disorder known as Parkinson's disease results from the death of dopamine cells in the region of the midbrain called the substantia nigra (Rubin & Strayer, 2012). The normally functioning dopamine cells in this area of the brain are visible to the eye because they are pigmented (Chapter 2, Figure 4). In Parkinson's disease these cells are largely absent. Another feature of the Parkinson's disease brain on autopsy is the presence of cellular inclusions called Lewy bodies (Rubin & Strayer, 2012). The primary components of Lewy bodies are aggregated proteins with the primary protein being aggregated alpha-synuclein (Engelender, 2008; Yasuda & Mochizuki, 2010). It is becoming common for authors to now refer to Parkinson's disease as one of the synucleinopathy disorders. There is mounting evidence that that aggregated alpha-synuclein induces apoptosis (Buttner et al., 2013). There is also indication that this aggregate resists degradation via the ubiquitin proteolytic pathway (Tanik et al., 2013), which would explain its occurrence as an inclusion material in the Lewy bodies. Progression of this cell death in Parkinson's disease may be due to the release of this aggregated alpha-synuclein to the extracellular space by both cell death and by other mechanisms, which then leads to toxicity of adjacent neurons and astrocytes via membrane receptor activation, calcium influx and nitric oxide-induced apoptosis (Kazmierczak et al., 2013). Alpha-synuclein has also been shown to bind to the protein Parkin, which is part of an ubiquitin-proteasome system involved in this targeting of proteins for degradation (Choi et al., 2001; Kawahara et al., 2008). Ubiquitin is an essential protein that is needed for the disposal of proteins (Nelson & Cox, 2000) and ubiquitin has been shown to be bound to alpha-synuclein aggregates in the Lewy bodies. Alpha-synuclein has a chaperon function and Parkin appears to be part of the protein turnover pathway with proper function of both being essential to cell survival since genetic defects of Parkin cause a form of early-onset Parkinsonism (Choi et al., 2001; Kawahara et al., 2008). Genetic defects of alpha-synuclein also cause Parkinsonism (Singleton et al., 2003). Since most cases of Parkinson's disease are not genetic, environmental causes are of primary concern. Since it has been demonstrated that DOPAL cross-links alpha-synuclein, inducing aggregation of this protein (Burke et al., 2008), a review of the factors that elevate DOPAL concentrations are of interest. Since there is evidence showing that DOPAL concentrations increase with either impairment of mitochondrial function (Lamensdorf et al., 2000a; Lamensdorf et al., 2000b) or from oxidative stress (Florang et al., 2007; Rees et al., 2007), a review of environmental agents that bring this about would support this evolving pathway.

Inhibition of the Electron Transport Chain (ETC) and Products of Oxidative Stress Elevate DOPAL Concentrations

Figure 2 shows the synthesis and oxidation of DOPAL. The pathway begins with the amino acid tyrosine being hydroxylated in a tetrahydrobiopterin (THB) requiring step to L-DOPA (levo-dihydroxy phenylalanine). L-DOPA is then decarboxylated to dopamine.

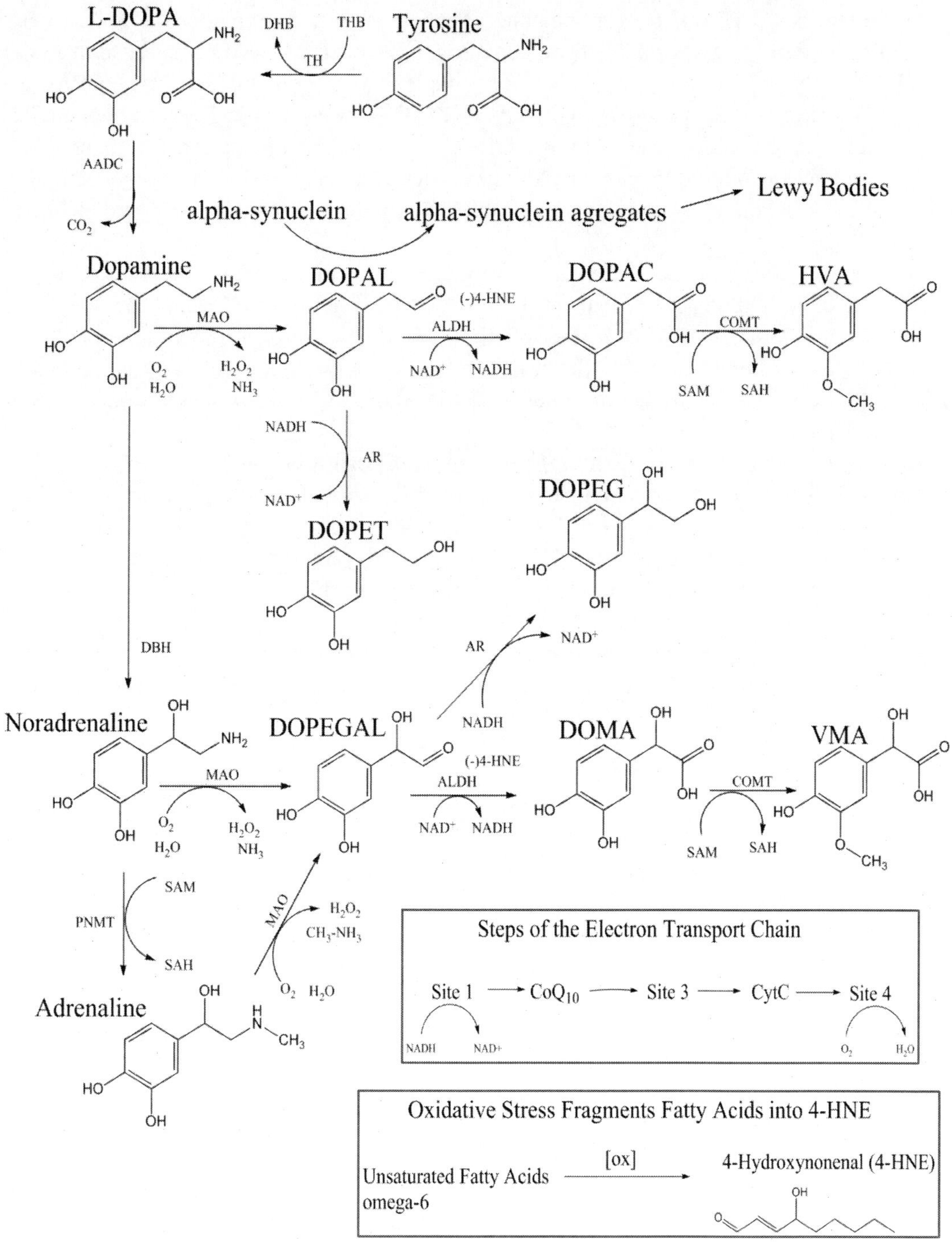

Figure 2. Oxidative stress on unsaturated fatty acids increases 4-HNE concentrations which inhibit ALDH. Inhibition of Site I of the electron transport chain increases the NADH:NAD$^+$ ratio, which will inhibit ALDH. DOPAL causes alpha synuclein to aggregate and create Lewy Bodies which are thought to be toxic to cells. It is presumed that DOPEGAL would do the same.

Dopamine is then oxidized via substrate channeling by a combination of 2 enzymes: monoamine oxidase (MAO) and aldehyde dehydrogenase (ALDH). MAO converts dopamine to DOPAL and then before DOPAL leaves the complex, ALDH quickly oxidizes DOPAL to DOPAC (dihydroxy phenylacetic acid). Lastly, DOPAC is methylated to HVA (homovanillic acid), which is excreted from the body. If DOPAL leaves the complex, there is evidence that DOPAL, and not the other dopamine metabolites, selectively reacts with alpha-synuclein and induces the formation of the toxic alpha-synuclein oligomers, both in vivo and in vitro (Galvin, 2006).

As a consequence of oxidative stress, products of membrane lipid oxidation, which include 4-HNE (4-hydroxy-2-nonenal) have been shown to inhibit ALDH and thus increase DOPAL levels (Florang et al., 2007; Rees et al., 2007). It has also been shown that inhibitors of the ETC also increase DOPAL (Lamensdorf et al., 2000a; Lamensdorf et al., 2000b), presumably due to ETC inhibitors increasing the NADH:NAD$^+$ ratio which would inhibit ALDH (see figure 2).

DOPAL has a parallel equivalent in the noradrenaline pathway which is DOPEGAL (3,4-dihydroxylphenylethyleneglycolaldehyde). Both of these short lived transient intermediates have been shown to be toxic to dopaminergic and noradrenergic cells respectively (Mattammal et al., 1993; Burke et al., 1996). This is relevant since Lewy bodies are also found in the noradrenaline cells of the locus ceruleus (Kim, 2013).

Recently, a study assessed the lifetime use of pesticides and herbicides of farm workers and found a correlation between the occurrence of Parkinson's disease and the exposure to those agents that inhibit site I of the mitochondrial electron transport chain and also for those that increase oxidative stress (Tanner et al., 2011).

Parkinson's Disease and the MPTP Story

In 1986, PBS aired a NOVA production called "The Case of the Frozen Addict", which presented very disturbing events relating to the topic of "designer drugs". At that time, the controlled substance laws in the United States listed only specific drug molecules but didn't regulate pharmacologically similar molecules that differed by only a minor functional group such as a methyl verse an ethyl. This story presented the tragic occurrences of young people with symptoms that looked like Parkinson's disease but at ages as young at 18. It was soon learned that all these young people had one thing in common; they were all IV drug users. These patients developed a Parkinsonism that was so advanced that they could not move and were thus called the "Frozen Addicts".

The first known case was identified in the late 1970's, when a 23-year-old man in Maryland showed debilitating signs of Parkinson's disease (Davis et al., 1979). This young man later died of an overdose and an autopsy revealed an almost complete loss of the pigmentation in the substantia nigra region of his brain, almost identical to idiopathic PD. An investigation showed that this student had a history of drug abuse and that he particularly liked the opioid drug meperidine (Demerol). His educational background included knowledge of synthetic organic chemistry and he engaged in the effort to synthesize a "designer drug" called 1-methyl-4-phenyl-4-propionoxypiperidine (MPPP). MPPP has similar pharmacological properties to meperidine, but the ester group is flipped, and at that time would thus not have been a controlled substance, thus exploiting a loophole in the drug laws that would permit getting high without breaking the law. Unfortunately, the placement of the ester group (see Figure 3) in this molecule was susceptible to an organic chemical reaction called an elimination reaction that under conditions of either too much acid or too much heat yielded a side product called MPTP (Davis et al., 1979). Tragically, a version of this story was repeated a few years later in California when several young people used what they thought was heroin or a heroin-like drug and they developed what looked like PD within a few days of injecting this drug (Langston et al., 1983). The same as the young man in Maryland, the California patients had taken MPPP that was contaminated with MPTP.

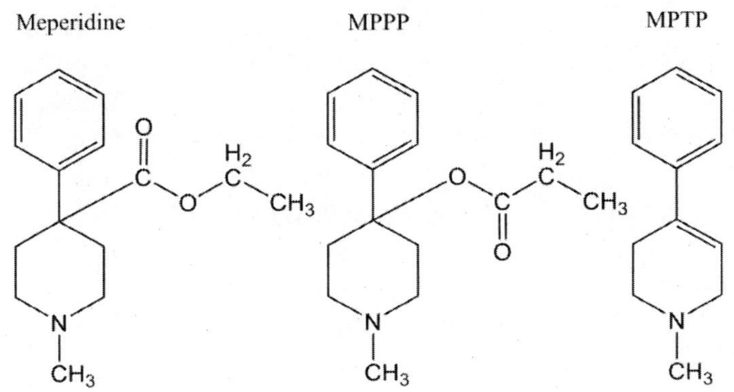

Figure 3. Comparison of the chemical structures Meperidine (Demerol), MPPP and the elimination product MPTP.

It was now clear that patients with MPTP-induced Parkinsonism were similar to patients with idiopathic Parkinson's disease (Langston & Ballard, 1984). MPTP is selectively toxic because it is able to cross the blood brain barrier and is then transformed into MPP^+ (Figure 4) mostly in glial cells by the enzyme MAO. MPP^+ is selectively taken up into dopaminergic cells via the dopamine transporter (DAT) and has been shown to be a site 1 inhibitor of the electron transport chain (Langston et al., 1984a; Langston & Ballard, 1984; Langston et al., 1984b; Ransom et al., 1987).

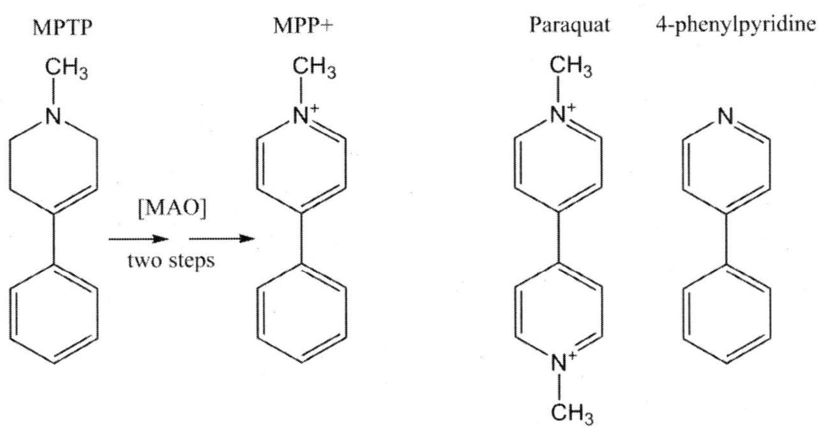

Figure 4. Conversion of MPTP to MPP^+ by MAO and the comparison of the structure of MPP^+ to that of paraquat and 4-phenyl pyridine.

More disturbing was a report of a research chemist who developed Parkinson's disease following bench work with MPTP (Langston & Ballard, Jr., 1983). This contributed to the growing belief that PD may be caused by toxins in the work place or environment (Calne & Langston, 1983). Although it's clear that MPTP causes a PD-like syndrome in the MPTP exposed patients, there is little evidence that this molecule is responsible for idiopathic PD. However, could similar molecules in the environment be responsible?

From early on, the herbicide paraquat (Figure 4) was suspected due to its similar structure to MPP^+. However, animal studies didn't result in much evidence for paraquat as a specific dopaminergic neurotoxin like MPTP except evidence did emerge that a synergistic mixture with the Manganese based insecticide called maneb (manganese ethylenebisdithiocarbamate), caused significant reductions of substantia nigra cells in mice (McCormack et al., 2002; Thiruchelvam et al., 2000a; Thiruchelvam et al., 2000b; Thiruchelvam et al., 2002). This correlates with evidence that Mn miners have a high rate of developing a Parkinsonian syndrome very similar to Parkinson's disease (Olanow, 2004). The one common feature of both Mn and MPP^+ is that they are both known to impair mitochondrial function. The study that assessed the lifetime use of pesticides and herbicides of farm workers and found a correlation between those agents that inhibit site I of the mitochondrial electron transport chain, also found a correlation for those that increase oxidative stress, including Paraquat (Tanner et al., 2011).

L-DOPA as a Treatment and a Toxin

L-DOPA is the most common treatment for PD, but there is debate regarding the possibility that it accelerates the progression of the disorder (Olney et al., 1990; Mytilineou et al. 1993; Lipski et al., 2011). Although there is debate regarding the direct toxicity of L-DOPA, there is growing evidence of its metabolites having toxic properties. The primary metabolite of L-DOPA is dopamine (Figure 2) and there is some evidence that excess dopamine has some degree of toxicity. It has been reported that methamphetamine, a drug that induces dopamine release, can cause the loss of dopaminergic fibers and cell bodies, and may actually predispose users to Parkinson's disease (Ares-Santos et al., 2013). These authors suggest the involvement of overstimulation at dopamine receptors. This would imply that an overdose or over use of L-DOPA, which is rapidly converted to dopamine could have toxic implications. However, increased dopamine concentrations would also lead to increased DOPAL concentrations.

Products of the MAO Enzymes May be Toxic

There are two major isozymes of monoamine oxidase (MAO), MAO-A and MAO-B. Dopamine is oxidized to DOPAL primarily by MAO-A in the astrocytes and MAO-B in dopaminergic neurons (Figure 2). DOPAL has been shown to be toxic in cell models and was found elevated in postmortem human Parkinson brain (Mattammal et al., 1995; Siegle et al., 1999; Burke et al., 2004). It's significant to note that the same enzyme that creates DOPAL (Figure 2) is also the same enzyme that converts MPTP to MPP^+ (Figure 4). In addition, MAO inhibitors (MAO-I's) were shown to be protective in monkeys against MPTP

(Langston et al., 1984b), and in human trials MAO-I's slowed down the progression of Parkinson's disease (Tetrud & Langston, 1987; Tetrud & Langston, 1989; Shoulson et al., 2002; Pardo et al., 1993). This would be consistent with the lowering of DOPAL levels.

As an additional interesting note, there is a negative correlation between Parkinson's disease patients and smoking (Tanner et al., 2002), possibly due to the fact that a component of cigarette smoke, 4-Phenylpyridine (Figure 4), is an MAO inhibitor (Irwin et al., 1987) which would decrease both the rate of MPTP conversion to MPP^+ as well as the conversion of Dopamine to DOPAL.

DOPAL and DOPEGAL are classified as catechol aldehydes. Catechols have a benzene ring with an ortho pair of phenolic hydroxyl (–OH) groups as depicted in Figure 5. Doorn and co-workers recently demonstrated that the molecules that contain both an aldehyde and a catechol are significantly more toxic than catechols or aldehydes alone (Rees et al., 2009). The normal concentrations of these catechol aldehydes are very low compared to the other intermediates due to the rapid oxidation by aldehyde dehydrogenase (Figure 2). However, this review will list the evidence showing that abnormal or prolonged elevation or both of these catechol aldehydes play at least some role in the degenerative process of dopaminergic and noradrenergic cells.

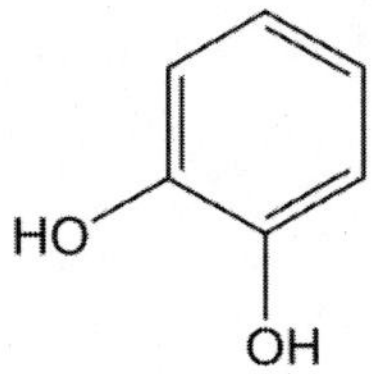

Figure 5. Structure of catechol

Concerns over the Activity of Aldehyde Dehydrogenase

One of the mechanism by which DOPAL can be toxic would certainly be associated with the fact that it's an aldehyde. It is well established that aldehydes are reactive with amines and can form condensation products. If the reactive aldehyde intermediates are a significant factor in Parkinson's disease, the next logical question would be why would they accumulate? One logical answer would be due to a decrease in their rate of elimination by the enzyme aldehyde dehydrogenase (Figure 2) to the product DOPAC. There was early evidence to suggest that disulfiram (an aldehyde dehydrogenase inhibitor) is toxic to cells (McCaffery & Drager, 1994) and more recently, disulfiram given along with L-DOPA, has been shown to increase DOPAL levels both *in vitro* and *in vivo* (Legros et al., 2004). This elevation did cause decreased cell survival *in vitro*, however they were unable to show any decrease in dopamine terminals in the striatum or a reduction in DA concentration in rats. To support this, there is evidence that substantia nigra cells actively expressing aldehyde dehydrogenase have a higher survival rate when transplanted (Haque et al., 1997). There is at least a partial correlation between genetic variation of aldehyde dehydrogenase genes and Parkinson's disease (Buervenich et al., 2000).

A study of SHSY5Y cells treated with 100 nM dopamine, 1 nM disulfiram (aldehyde dehydrogenase inhibitor) or both shows that 24 hour treatment followed by 24 hour of fresh media shows about 25% decreased cell viability using the MTT assay and over 50% decreased values when both DA and disulfiram were used synergistically (Bonnet et al., 2004). Treatment of male Sprague-Dawley rats with L-DOPA-benserizide (benserizide prevents the conversion of L-DOPA to dopamine outside the blood brain barrier) elevates dopamine and DOPAC levels but not DOPAL, but L-DOPA-benserizide plus disulfiram does significantly elevate DOPAL as well as DOPET (Bonnet et al., 2004; Legros et al., 2004; Legros et al., 2004).

Mice that are deficient in both ALDH1 and ALDH2 show age dependent decreases in motor function, which can be alleviated with L-DOPA/benserizide, but similar to Parkinson's disease, no significant effect on cognitive tests. These mice also showed decreases in tyrosine hydroxylase-immunopositive cells in the substantia nigra, reduced dopamine and dopamine metabolites, and elevated DOPAL and 4-HNE (Wey et al., 2012).

Mitochondrial Toxins May Increase Concentrations of DOPAL

Inhibition of site 1 of the electron transport chain (ETC) would result in a drop of the ATP:ADP ratio and an increase of the NADH:NAD^+ ratio. This increase in the NADH:NAD^+ ratio would affect the catabolism of DA metabolites and lead to an increase in the dopamine metabolite dihydroxy phenyl acetaldehyde (DOPAL) and an increase in the metabolite dihydroxy phenyl ethanol (DOPET). Figure 2 shows that DA is metabolized by MAO to DOPAL and that DOPAL is oxidized by aldehyde dehydrogenase (ALDH) to DOPAC. The reaction from DOPAL to DOPAC requires NAD^+ and produces NADH. If the ETC is inhibited, the increase of the NADH:NAD^+ ratio would slow down ALDH and cause a decrease in the conversion of DOPAL to DOPAC. This would then increase production of DOPET by a minor pathway.

In theory, the electron transport chain site I inhibitors (MPP^+ and rotenone) all should cause an increase in DOPAL levels as well as increased levels of alpha-synuclein aggregation. Rotenone was shown to increase DOPAL and DOPET levels in differentiated PC12 cells (Lamensdorf et al., 2000a; Lamensdorf et al., 2000b). This elevation of DOPAL was further increased by co-treatment with ALDH inhibitors and with aldehyde reductase (AR) inhibitors. MAO co-treatment decreased DOPAL levels. However this same group reported that MPP^+ reduced DOPAL levels. This counter-intuitive finding merits further study. However, since MPP^+ is a product of MAO from MPTP, it would be plausible for MPP^+ to exert feedback inhibition on MAO, decreasing the conversion of dopamine to DOPAL, while at the same time also inhibiting site I of the ETC.

Inhibition of any site in the ETC would also block site I. Blockade of Site IV would prevent the transfer of electrons from cytochrome C, and then working backwards would not be able to take electrons from site III, which would not take them from CoQ and thus could not take them form Site I (Figure 2). Cyanide is a site IV inhibitor and sublethal exposure is associated with a Parkinson-like syndrome (Zhang et al., 2009). Cyanide is not selective enough of a toxin to specifically call it a Parkisonian toxin like MPTP, but certainly inhibition at any site of the ETC should cause an increase of DOPAL.

CoQ and Parkinson's Disease

Site I of the ETC passes its electrons to CoQ_{10} (Figure 2), also known as CoQ and ubiquinone. Inhibition or deficiencies of CoQ_{10} would prevent site I from accepting electrons, so this should also increase DOPAL levels and increase alpha-synuclein aggregation. CoQ_{10} is a lipid soluble molecule with a hydrocarbon tail composed of 10 isoprenoids (Figure 6).

An isoprene is a 5 carbon molecule and is commonly polymerized in biological molecules including CoQ_{10}, Vitamin A, Vitamin E and Vitamin K (Nelson & Cox, 2000). So the tail on CoQ_{10} would have 50 carbons. The quinone portion of the molecule, which consists of the two carbonyl groups para to each other, can accept electrons one at a time to become the semiquinone (not shown) and then the quinol (shown in Figure 6). The quinol would then revert back to the quinone as it passes the electrons one at a time to site III of the ETC (Nelson & Cox, 2000).

An epidemiological study of Parkinson's patients showed that they had significantly greater odds of having a CoQ_{10} deficiency than age matched control subjects (Mischley et al., 2012). Complementing this is another recent study showing that antioxidants such as CoQ_{10} and aspirin are neuroprotective in Parkinson's disease, as are MAO-B inhibitors (Seidl & Potashkin, 2011). Statin drugs used to lower cholesterol are HMG-CoA reductase inhibitors. HMG-CoA reductase is the rate limiting step in the synthesis of the 5 carbon isoprenoid intermediates, which are then condensed into cholesterol (Nelson & Cox, 2000). The concern is that isoprenoids are also the precursors of CoQ_{10}, and patients taking statin drugs could be at higher risk of both CoQ_{10} deficiency and Parkinson's disease. However, a study in Parkinson's patients who are also taking statins did not show a worsening in the symptoms of PD (Lieberman et al., 2005), so this role of CoQ_{10} is still hypothetical. Because CoQ_{10} is an electron acceptor, it also functions as an antioxidant. In this capacity, it has been shown to attenuate iron-induced deleterious changes with pretreatment of CoQ_{10} (Kooncumchoo et al., 2006). The role of CoQ_{10} is still a subject of debate and more research is needed before its role in Parkinson's disease is commonly accepted.

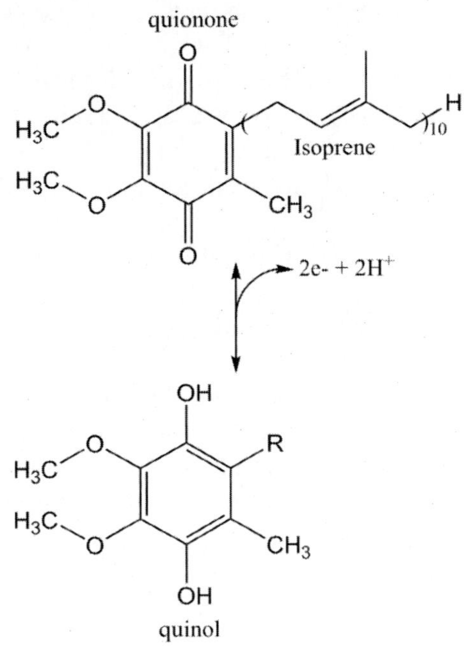

Figure 6. Structure of CoQ_{10}.

Toxicity of DOPAL

The suspicious link between DOPAL and PD was established when it was identified and shown to be elevated in post mortem substantia nigra of Parkinson's patients (Mattammal et al., 1993). Mattammal et al. demonstrated that 6.5μM DOPAL in cell culture was toxic to PC-12 cells, selectively toxic to dopamine cells in mesencephalic fetal rat cells cultures, and is taken up by the dopamine uptake system in synaptosomes (Mattammal et al., 1995). DOPAL is produced primarily by MAO in the astrocytes MAO-A and by neuronal MAO-B in the striatum, (as determined using microdialysis) (Fornai et al., 2000).

A study in PC12 cells showed that DOPAL is significantly more toxic than dopamine, L-DOPA, DOPAC or HVA (Kristal et al., 2001). This same paper also shows that DOPAL is 1000 time more toxic than dopamine to isolated energetically compromised mitochondria (Kristal et al., 2001). Inhibition of complex I or III increases levels of DOPAL and DOPET (Lamensdorf et al., 2000a; Lamensdorf et al., 2000b). Unilateral injections of DOPAL into the substantia nigra pars compacta of rats shows a decrease in tyrosine-hydroxylase immunopositive cells near the injection site and the appearance of argyrophilic cells, indicating cell death (Corso, 1998; Corso & Keller, 2000). These findings have been independently complemented and confirmed in work showing that unilateral injections of DOPAL increased rotational turning in the direction of the injection side similar to 6-hydroxydopamine or MPP^+ (Panneton et al., 2010). They also report a significant decrease in the number of cells in the substantia nigra, pars compacta region (mostly dopaminergic), and a decrease of tyrosine hydroxylase-positive cells in this same area when counted using stereological techniques.

In PC12 cells, DOPAL levels can be elevated by a combined inhibition of aldehyde dehydrogenase (ALDH) and aldehyde reductase (AR) (Figure 2), and this can potentiate rotenone-induced toxicity (Lamensdorf et al., 2000a; Lamensdorf et al., 2000b). It has also been shown in PC12 cells, that reserpine (which blocks the vesicular uptake of dopamine from the cytoplasm into the vesicle) resulted in an elevation of DOPAL along with eventual decrease in dopamine (Goldstein et al., 2012). This effect is enhanced with aldehyde dehydrogenase inhibitors and aldehyde reductase inhibitors (combination of both gave highest elevation) and the DOPAL was correlated with increased apoptosis and alpha-synuclein diamerization (Goldstein et al., 2012). Further fitting with the evolving model is a report that this toxicity can be reduced by either an antioxidant, like ascorbic acid, or by using the MAO inhibitor deprenyl (Pardo et al., 1993). Since rotenone is an inhibitor of the mitochondrial electron transport chain at site I (the same as MPP^+) and this leads to both a decrease of available NAD^+ (due to the buildup of NADH not being oxidized at site 1) and a subsequent decrease in ATP production. Recall that aldehyde dehydrogenase uses NAD^+ as its oxidizing agent and thus DOPAL concentrations would rise. Another toxin, 3-morpholinosydnoniminie, an agent that induces apoptosis, induces an increased rate of oxidation of dopamine to DOPAL, and this is attenuated in metallothionein-transgenic fetal stem cells (Sharma & Ebadi, 2003).

The toxicity of DOPAL is most certainly due to its higher chemical reactivity compared to the other dopamine metabolites. This is also why DOPAL cannot be purchased commercially since it is chemically unstable and must be synthesized by the researcher just prior to study. What makes DOPAL more reactive than the other dopamine metabolites is the aldehyde group (Figure 7). Standard organic chemistry textbooks describe aldehydes as being reactive with amines and DOPAL, as an aldehyde, primary reacts with amines (Rees et al., 2009).

However the reactivity of the aldehyde group in DOPAL towards amines is more reactive than other aldehydes and this appears to be due to the adjacent catechol on DOPAL. A comparison of the chemical reactivity of DOPAL to other groups (Figure 8) that don't have the intact catechol, such as phenyl acetaldehyde (PAL), or either of the 3-methoxy-4-hydroxy-phenylacetaldehyded (MOPAL) or dimethoxy phenylacetaldehyded (DMPAL), implying that DOPAL has the most reactive aldehyde (Rees et al., 2009).

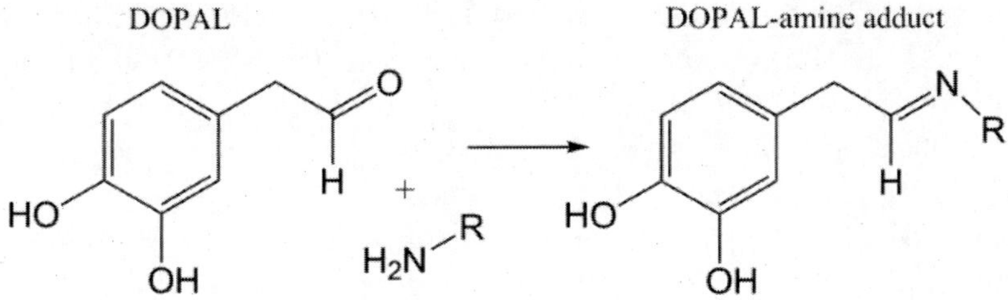

Figure 7. Reaction of the aldehyde with an amine.

DOPAL forms covalent adduct products with proteins, which was confirmed by MALDI-TOF mass spectroscopy by an increase in the molecular weight of a peptide by the same amount as the molecular weight of DOPAL or MOPAL, respectively. There is also indication that DOPAL cross-links proteins implying that the catechol is also reactive with proteins. This is blocked by reducing agents that keep the catechol in the reduced state (Rees et al., 2009).

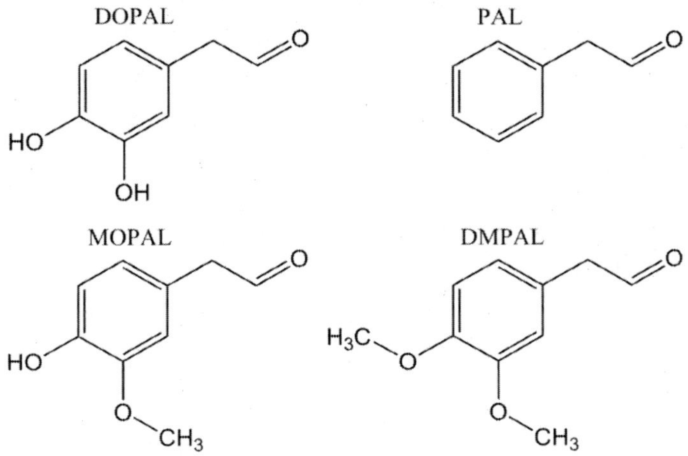

Figure 8. Comparison of structures between DOPAL and its analogous structures differing by either absence of catechol hydroxyl groups or containing methylated hydroxyl groups.

A measure of mitochondrial function using the MTT assay on PC6-3 cells shows that analogs of DOPAL that don't have the catechol (PAL), or the catechol is methylated (MOPAL and DMPAL), or the aldehyde is nitrated, show significantly less toxicity than DOPAL, meaning both the aldehyde and the catechol groups are required for toxicity (Vermeer et al., 2012). DOPAL also inhibits tyrosine hydroxylase activity, but the other analogs of DOPAL again do not show this same effect. DOPAL also induces an increase in the concentration of superoxide anion.

The drug L-threo-3,4-dihydroxyophenylserine (Figure 9), which is noradrenaline prodrug (Droxydopa) used to treat orthostatic hypotension has been shown to non-enzymatically decompose into DOPAL (Holmes et al., 2010). A clinical study of this drug, given orally to both healthy volunteers and to patients with Parkinson's disease with orthostatic hypotension, showed a low level of DOPAL in their blood of healthy patients 6 hours after the dose, but the Parkinson's patients showed very low, but detectable levels of DOPAL in the blood before taking the drug and then a significant elevation of DOPAL, 2 to 6 hours after taking the drug. The implication of this is that L-threo-3,4-dihydroxyophenylserine elevates DOPAL levels which are quickly degraded in healthy patients but this is not the case in Parkinson's patients. This implies impaired aldehyde dehydrogenase activity in these patients.

L-DOPS

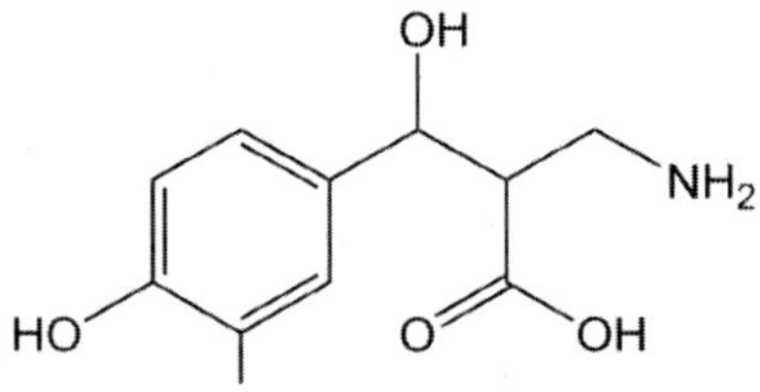

Figure 9. Structure of L-threo-3,4- dihydroxyophenylserine (L-DOPS)

Another study has shown that in postmortem Parkinson patients, the putamen had a significantly lower concentration of dopamine and all the dopamine metabolites compared to control but a significantly higher ratio of DOPAL:DA and DOPAL:DOPAC. The same trend was noticed in caudate, but the variance in the date resulted in a difference that did not achieve statistical significance (Goldstein et al., 2011).

Oxidative Stress

Oxidative stress can cause the formation of fatty acid decomposition products such as 4-hydroxy-2-nonenal (4HNE) and malondialdehyde (MDA). Both of these molecules have been shown to inhibit aldehyde dehydrogenase (Florang et al., 2007; Rees et al., 2007). Studies on isolated human recombinant aldehyde dehydrogenase 2 (hALDH2) show that DOPAL oxidation is slowed down in a dose dependent manner by 4HNE (Florang et al., 2007). Parallel studies on mitochondrial lysate and also on intact mitochondria demonstrate a decrease in DOPAC formation from dopamine when inhibited by 4HNE and more importantly the production of DOPAL increased in these same studies (Florang et al., 2007). Additional studies using synaptosomes demonstrated the same findings when inhibited with either 4HNE or MDA (Rees et al., 2007). More intriguing was their findings that using MALDI mass spectroscopy on peptides incubated with dopamine or DOPAL showed what appears to be amide adduct products of DOPAL but not dopamine (Rees et al., 2007). Incubation of synaptosomes with dopamine showed the formation of catechol adducts when co-incubated with the ALDH inhibitor 4HNE, and this was blocked by the MAO-I, pargyline (Rees et al., 2007). This implies that DOPAL modifies proteins when elevated by ALDH inhibitors. The cell viability of PC6-3 cells is significantly decreased when treated with 100μM 4-HNE via the MTT assay (Jinsmaa et al., 2009). However in the presence of 100μM DA, it only takes 10μM of 4-HNE, to cause a significant increase in DOPAL and DOPET, and a decrease in DOPAC formation (Jinsmaa et al., 2009). An amount of 10μM MDA causes a decrease in DOPAC, but it takes 50μM MDA to increase DOPAL. There is no increase in DOPET, implying that MDA also inhibits aldehyde reductase.

This all indicates that toxicity observed in cells following exposure to know inducers of oxidative stress may bring about some of their toxicity through DOPAL. Certainly additional studies confirming this link are merited.

Quinone Formation

When MAO converts dopamine to DOPAL, hydrogen peroxide is also produced (Figure 10). Catechols can be oxidized to quinones and hydrogen peroxide is one of the agents that induce this reaction (Li et al., 2001). Depicted in the central column of Figure 11 is the pathway for the L-DOPA to dopamine to DOPAL to DOPAC. DOPAL can also be reduced to DOPET (bottom center). All five of these intermediates can be oxidized to quinones (right column). All of these can also have their catechols stabilized via methylation (left column). All of the quinone products may also be toxic (Asanuma et al., 2003), however the combination of the aldehyde and quinone on the same molecule makes DOPAL-quinone the most toxic molecule on this table. Dopaquinone has been shown to be mutagenic by reacting with DNA via a 1,4-Michael addition to form predominantly depurinating adducts at the N-7 of guanine and the N-3 of adenine (Cavalieri et al., 2002). Dopaquinone also reacts with cysteine, forming 5-S-CyS-DA, and 5-S-CyS-DA which is further oxidized to 7-(2-aminoethyl)-3,4-dihydro-5-hydroxy-2H-1,4-benzothiazine-3-carboxylic acid which is rapidly accumulated by isolated intact rat brain mitochondria and selectively inhibits complex I respiration and the alpha-ketoglutarate dehydrogenase (alpha-KGDH) complex (Li & Dryhurst, 2001).

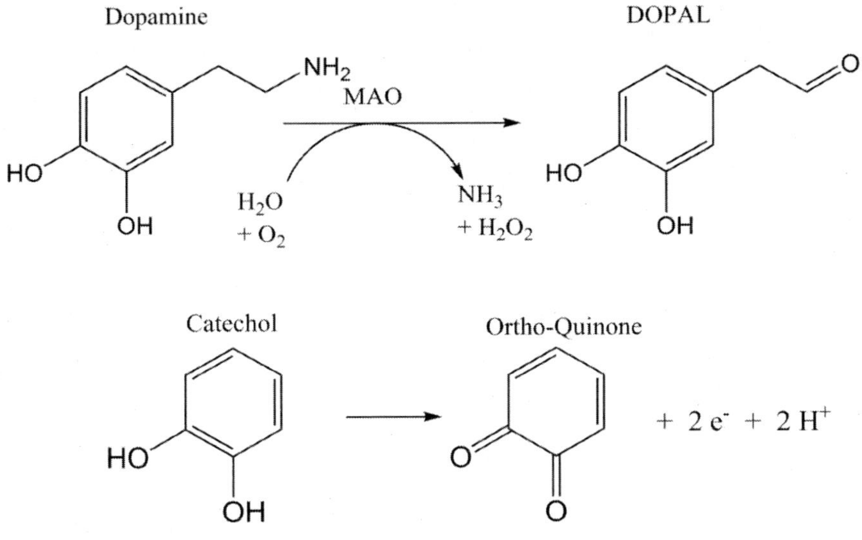

Figure 10. Oxidation of Dopamine to DOPAL and a Catechol to an Ortho-Quinone.

Dopaquinone has been reported to also cross-link proteins and has been shown to cross-link synaptosomal membrane proteins (Khan et al., 2001). These catechol derived quinones have also been shown to inhibit tyrosine hydroxylase (Xu et al., 1998; Kuhn et al., 1999) and more significantly, quinone formation has been linked to mitochondrial swelling (Berman & Hastings, 1999).

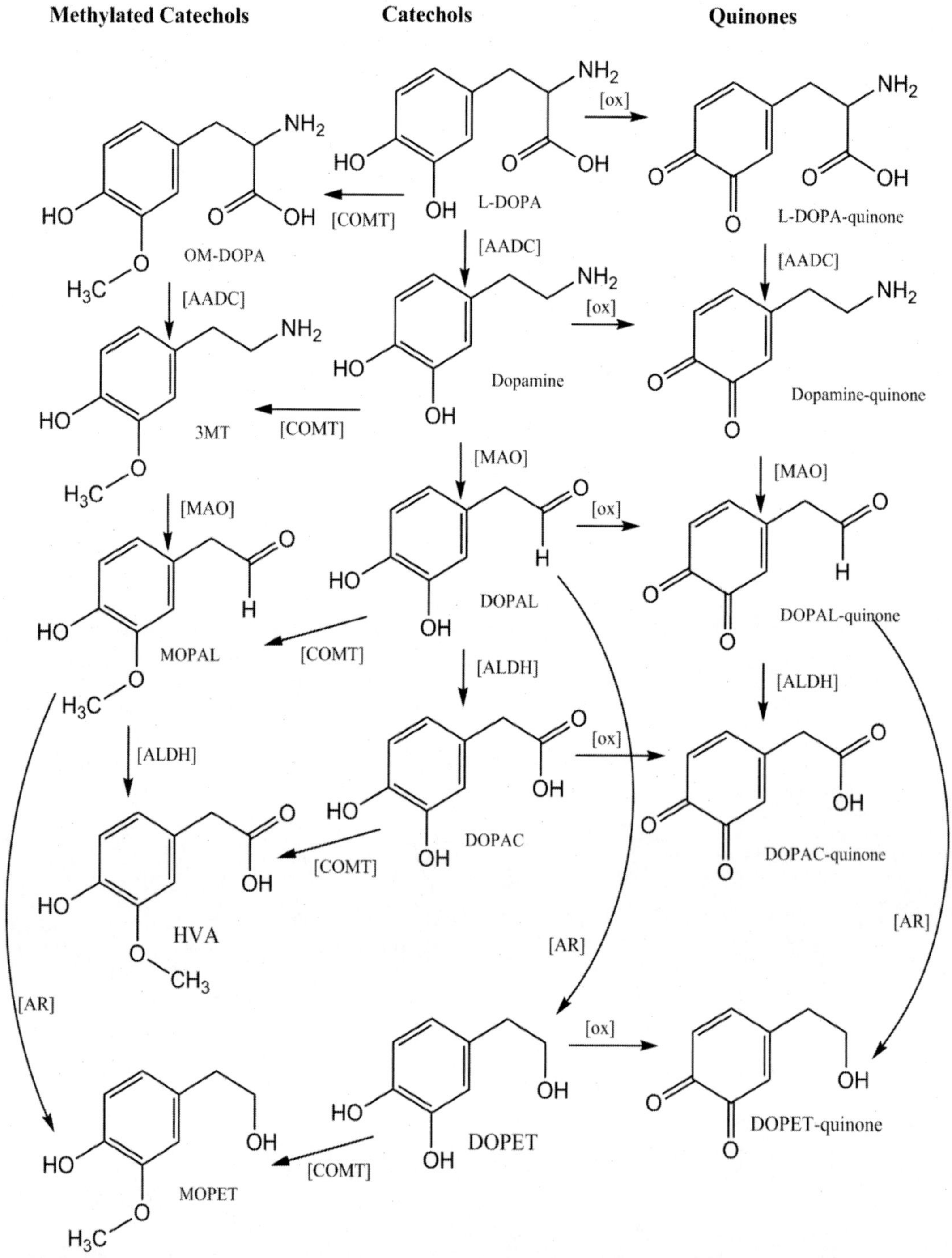

Figure 11. Metabolic pathway for dopamine that includes the oxidation to quinones and the alternative methylation to inhibit quinone formation. Reduction of the aldehyde by aldehyde reductase (AR) is also included in this scheme.

There are protective enzymes to decrease these quinone formations which include catechol-O-methyl transferase (COMT), which methylates one of the catechol hydroxyl groups to inhibit the oxidation to the quinone and also quinone oxidoreductase to reverse the reaction back to the catechol. The loss of this ability, due to the deletion of 29-base pair nucleotides in the promoter region of the dihydronicotinamide riboside (NRH):quinone oxidoreductase 2 (NQO2) gene, is associated with the development of Parkinson's disease (Harada et al., 2001). Under normal conditions, catecholamines and/or their quinones can upregulate the expression of quinone oxido-reductases (van Muiswinkel et al., 2000), implying a critical importance of this enzyme. It has also been suggested that drugs that could upregulate these enzymes would be neuroprotective (Drukarch & van Muiswinkel, 2000). And of course we would expect that toxins that interfere with these enzymes could be toxic.

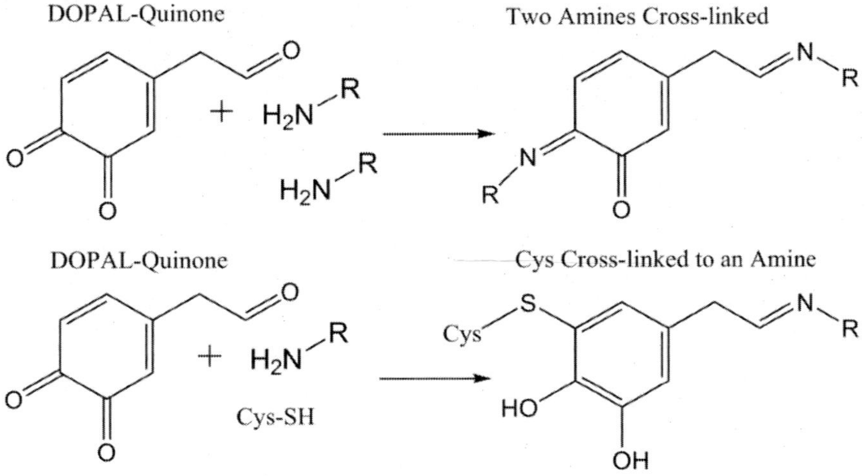

Figure 12. Cross-linking of proteins by DOPAL-quinone.

DOPAL and Quinones as Protein Cross-Linking Agents

One of the mechanisms by which quinones can be toxic is through the disruption of protein activity following adduct formation and cross-linking. Figure 12 shows the reaction of amine groups from a protein to the carbonyl groups and also the sulfhydryl of cysteine reacting with the quinone (Rees et al., 2009). The cross-linked amines can be either the N-terminal amine of the protein or the side group amine of lysine within a protein. This implies that DOPAL-quinone (Figure 12) is the most reactive and thus most toxic molecule.

DOPAL has been shown to be a cross-linking agent in proteins (Jinsmaa et al., 2011), and shown to specifically react with and inhibit tyrosine hydroxylase (Mexas et al., 2011). The inhibition of tyrosine hydroxylase was shown to be partially reversible. Doorn and coworkers have published compelling evidence that the most reactive cross-linker is the semi-quinone of DOPAL (Anderson et al., 2011). The oxidation of the catechol to the quinone takes place as a pair of one-electron transfers. The free radical intermediate between the catechol and the quinone is most reactive and thus these cross-links take place as the catechol is being oxidized.

THP and Other DOPAL Reaction Products

DOPAL's toxicity may also be due to other condensation product of DOPAL. DOPAL can react with dopamine to form a tetrahydroisoquinoline (TIQ) condensation product called Tetrahydropapaveroline (THP) (Tank & Weiner, 1977; Weiner, 1978; Tank et al., 1981) (Figure 13). However, DOPAL is still significantly more toxic than THP (Kristal et al., 2001).

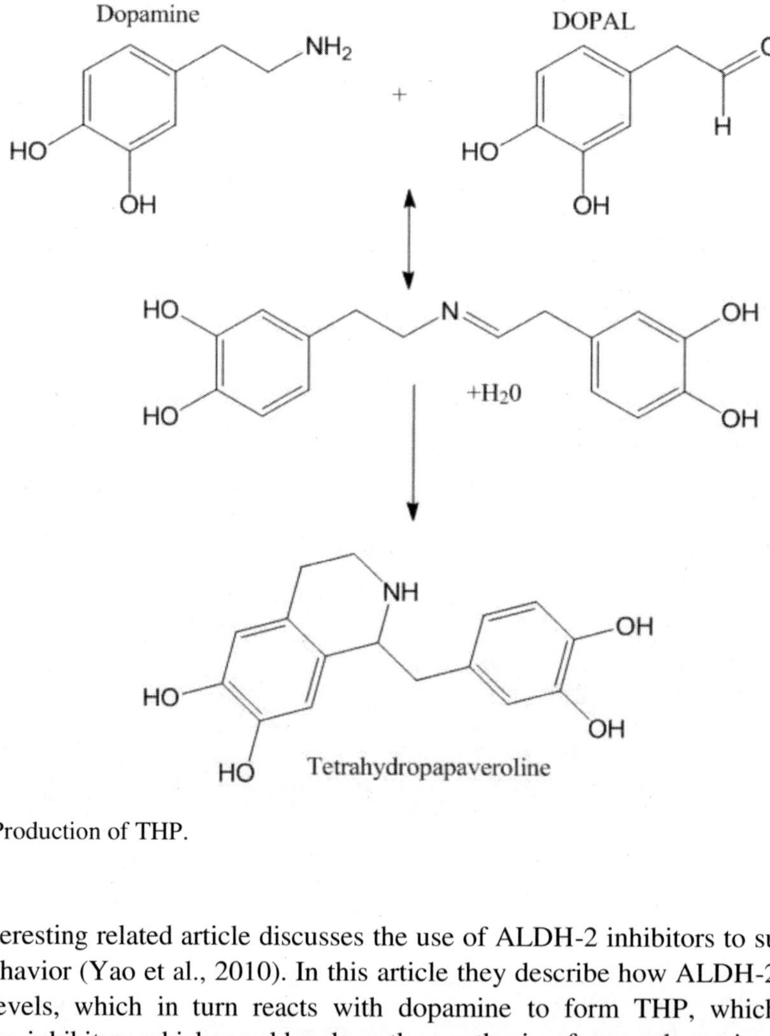

Figure 13. Production of THP.

An interesting related article discusses the use of ALDH-2 inhibitors to suppress cocaine seeking behavior (Yao et al., 2010). In this article they describe how ALDH-2i drugs elevate DOPAL levels, which in turn reacts with dopamine to form THP, which is a tyrosine hydroxylase inhibitor, which would reduce the synthesis of more dopamine. Although this article does not discuss Parkinson's directly, the implication could be that ALDH inactivation could also lead to increased DOPAL and THP, both of which inhibit tyrosine hydroxylase, thus resulting in eventual decreased dopamine output.

Additionally, it has been suggested that dopamine can be oxidized by prostaglandin H synthase into dopaminochrome, 2-(3,4-dihydroxyphenyl)-1-nitroethane and 2-(3,4,6-trihydroxyphenyl)-1-nitroethane (Mattammal et al., 1994) (Figure 14). The latter of which can be reduced by NADPH-cytochrome c reductase to 6-hydroxydopamine, another well documented dopaminergic neurotoxin. Further so, it has been shown that prostaglandin H syntheses levels were elevated in Parkinson's patients (Mattammal et al., 1995).

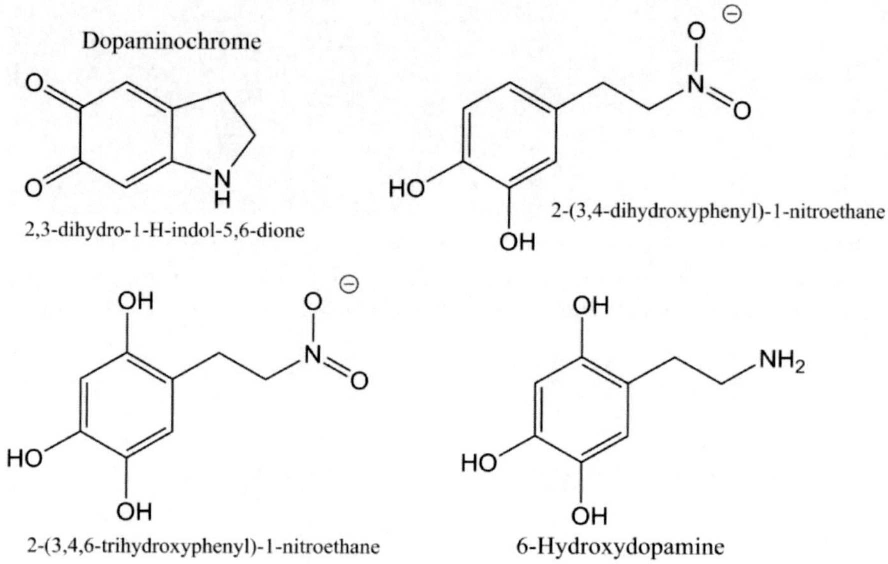

Figure 14. Other dopamine analog toxins.

Injections of DOPAL into Rat Brain Causes Loss of Cells

The injection of DOPAL directly into the brains of rats is problematic due to the fact that DOPAL is very unstable and must be synthesize a short time prior to use. This same fact is the reason that it is not a commercial product thus significantly reducing the amount of research on this molecule. DOPAL was injected into the substantia nigra and a loss of TH-immunopositive cells near the injection site (Figure 15A) was observed (Corso & Keller, 2000). Independent studies by Burke and co-workers complemented and confirmed these earlier findings with more convincing techniques. Stereological methods found a significant decrease of neutral red positive cells in the substantia nigra pars compacta (dopaminergic cells), and not in the pars reticulate (Panneton et al., 2010). This same group also found increased turning behavior in unilaterally injected rats similar to what has previously been shown following 6-OHDA or MPP^+ injections. Additional evidence of cell toxicity was the use of the cupric-silver stain for degenerating neurons showing the presence or argyrophilic cells in the substantia nigra pars compacta following injection of DOPAL (Corso & Keller, 2000) (Figure 15B).

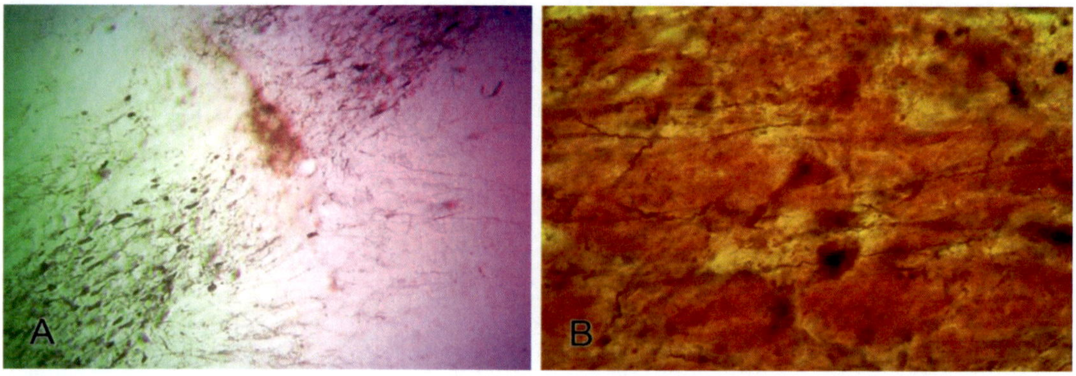

Figure 15. DOPAL injection in to the substantia nigra. (A) TH-immunostaining and (B) cupric silver staining. These photos were taken with an EDGE© 3-D white-light microscope using the red-green anaglyph option and can be observed in 3-D using red-green anaglyph glasses (Corso, 1998; Corso & Keller, 2000).

Summary and Conclusion

Starting with the MPTP story in the late 1970's and early 1980's, our understanding of the cell death associated with Parkinson's disease increased significantly. Combining our understanding of toxin-based studies and genetic studies indicates that there are several common features. The disorder is primarily the consequence of selective dopaminergic cell death. Lewy bodies consist of alpha-synuclein aggregates and aggregates are induced by DOPAL. Evidence shows that both mitochondrial inhibitors and products of oxidative stress inhibit aldehyde dehydrogenase either directly or indirectly and inhibitors of monoamine oxidase are shown to be protective. Therefore, all this evidence points at DOPAL being a central player in the mechanisms underlying many forms of neurodegeneration seen in Parkinson's disease.

References

Anderson, D. G., Mariappan, S. V., Buettner, G. R., & Doorn, J. A. (2011). Oxidation of 3,4-dihydroxyphenylacetaldehyde, a toxic dopaminergic metabolite, to a semiquinone radical and an ortho-quinone. *J.Biol.Chem., 286,* 26978-26986.

Ares-Santos, S., Granado, N., & Moratalla, R. (2013). The role of dopamine receptors in the neurotoxicity of methamphetamine. *J.Intern.Med., 273,* 437-453.

Asanuma, M., Miyazaki, I., & Ogawa, N. (2003). Dopamine- or L-DOPA-induced neurotoxicity: the role of dopamine quinone formation and tyrosinase in a model of Parkinson's disease. *Neurotox.Res., 5,* 165-176.

Berman, S. B. & Hastings, T. G. (1999). Dopamine oxidation alters mitochondrial respiration and induces permeability transition in brain mitochondria: implications for Parkinson's disease. *J Neurochem, 73,* 1127-37.

Bonnet, J. J., Legros, H., Janin, F., Dourmap, N., & Costentin, J. (2004). [Assessment of the in vitro and in vivo toxicity of 3,4-dihydroxyphenylacetaldehyde (DOPAL)]. *Ann.Pharm.Fr., 62,* 323-331.

Buervenich, S., Sydow, O., Carmine, A., Zhang, Z., Anvret, M., & Olson, L. (2000). Alcohol dehydrogenase alleles in Parkinson's disease. *Mov Disord, 15,* 813-8.

Burke, W. J., Kumar, V. B., Pandey, N., Panneton, W. M., Gan, Q., Franko, M. W. et al. (2008). Aggregation of alpha-synuclein by DOPAL, the monoamine oxidase metabolite of dopamine. *Acta Neuropathol., 115,* 193-203.

Burke, W. J., Li, S. W., Chung, H. D., Ruggiero, D. A., Kristal, B. S., Johnson, E. M. et al. (2004). Neurotoxicity of MAO metabolites of catecholamine neurotransmitters: role in neurodegenerative diseases. *Neurotoxicology, 25,* 101-115.

Burke, W. J., Schmitt, C. A., Gillespie, K. N., & Li, S. W. (1996). Norepinephrine transmitter metabolite is a selective cell death messenger in differentiated rat pheochromocytoma cells. *Brain Res., 722,* 232-235.

Buttner, S., Habernig, L., Broeskamp, F., Ruli, D., Vogtle, F. N., Vlachos, M. et al. (2013). Endonuclease G mediates alpha-synuclein cytotoxicity during Parkinson's disease. *EMBO J., 32,* 3041-3054.

Calne, D. B. & Langston, J. W. (1983). Aetiology of Parkinson's disease. *Lancet, 2,* 1457-9.

Cavalieri, E. L., Li, K. M., Balu, N., Saeed, M., Devanesan, P., Higginbotham, S. et al. (2002). Catechol ortho-quinones: the electrophilic compounds that form depurinating DNA adducts and could initiate cancer and other diseases. *Carcinogenesis, 23,* 1071-1077.

Choi, P., Golts, N., Snyder, H., Chong, M., Petrucelli, L., Hardy, J. et al. (2001). Co-association of parkin and alpha-synuclein. *Neuroreport, 12,* 2839-2843.

Corso, T. & Keller, G. (2000). Are the aldehyde products of monoamne oxidase significantly toxic? DOPAL as a possible neurotoxin contributing to Parkinson's disease. *Society for Neuroscience Abstracts, 26,* 92.9.

Corso, T. D. (1998). Real time 3-dimensional optical microscopy dramatically improves the interpretation and accuracy of silver and immuno-stained brain slices. In *Society for Neuroscience* (pp. 423.15).

Davis, G. C., Williams, A. C., Markey, S. P., Ebert, M. H., Caine, E. D., Reichert, C. M. et al. (1979). Chronic parkinsonism secondary to intravenous injection of meperidine analogues. *Psychiatry Research, 1,* 249-254.

Drukarch, B. & van Muiswinkel, F. L. (2000). Drug treatment of Parkinson's disease. Time for phase II. *Biochem Pharmacol, 59,* 1023-31.

Engelender, S. (2008). Ubiquitination of alpha-synuclein and autophagy in Parkinson's disease. *Autophagy., 4,* 372-374.

Florang, V. R., Rees, J. N., Brogden, N. K., Anderson, D. G., Hurley, T. D., & Doorn, J. A. (2007). Inhibition of the oxidative metabolism of 3,4-dihydroxyphenylacetaldehyde, a reactive intermediate of dopamine metabolism, by 4-hydroxy-2-nonenal. *Neurotoxicology, 28,* 76-82.

Fornai, F., Giorgi, F. S., Bassi, L., Ferrucci, M., Alessandri, M. G., & Corsini, G. U. (2000). Modulation of dihydroxyphenylacetaldehyde extracellular levels in vivo in the rat striatum after different kinds of pharmacological treatment. *Brain Research, 861,* 126-134.

Galvin, J. E. (2006). Interaction of alpha-synuclein and dopamine metabolites in the pathogenesis of Parkinson's disease: a case for the selective vulnerability of the substantia nigra. *Acta Neuropathol., 112,* 115-126.

Goldstein, D. S., Sullivan, P., Cooney, A., Jinsmaa, Y., Sullivan, R., Gross, D. J. et al. (2012). Vesicular uptake blockade generates the toxic dopamine metabolite 3,4-dihydroxyphenylacetaldehyde in PC12 cells: relevance to the pathogenesis of Parkinson's disease. *J.Neurochem., 123,* 932-943.

Goldstein, D. S., Sullivan, P., Holmes, C., Kopin, I. J., Basile, M. J., & Mash, D. C. (2011). Catechols in post-mortem brain of patients with Parkinson disease. *Eur.J.Neurol., 18,* 703-710.

Haque, N. S., LeBlanc, C. J., & Isacson, O. (1997). Differential dissection of the rat E16 ventral mesencephalon and survival and reinnervation of the 6-OHDA-lesioned striatum by a subset of aldehyde dehydrogenase-positive TH neurons. *Cell Transplant, 6,* 239-48.

Harada, S., Fujii, C., Hayashi, A., & Ohkoshi, N. (2001). An association between idiopathic Parkinson's disease and polymorphisms of phase II detoxification enzymes: glutathione S-transferase M1 and quinone oxidoreductase 1 and 2. *Biochem Biophys Res Commun, 288,* 887-92.

Holmes, C., Whittaker, N., Heredia-Moya, J., & Goldstein, D. S. (2010). Contamination of the norepinephrine prodrug droxidopa by dihydroxyphenylacetaldehyde. *Clin.Chem., 56,* 832-838.

Irwin, I., Langston, J. W., & DeLanney, L. E. (1987). 4-Phenylpyridine (4PP) and MPTP: the relationship between striatal MPP+ concentrations and neurotoxicity. *Life Sci, 40,* 731-40.

Jinsmaa, Y., Florang, V. R., Rees, J. N., Anderson, D. G., Strack, S., & Doorn, J. A. (2009). Products of oxidative stress inhibit aldehyde oxidation and reduction pathways in dopamine catabolism yielding elevated levels of a reactive intermediate. *Chem.Res.Toxicol., 22,* 835-841.

Jinsmaa, Y., Florang, V. R., Rees, J. N., Mexas, L. M., Eckert, L. L., Allen, E. M. et al. (2011). Dopamine-derived biological reactive intermediates and protein modifications: Implications for Parkinson's disease. *Chem.Biol.Interact., 192,* 118-121.

Kawahara, K., Hashimoto, M., Bar-On, P., Ho, G. J., Crews, L., Mizuno, H. et al. (2008). alpha-Synuclein aggregates interfere with Parkin solubility and distribution: role in the pathogenesis of Parkinson disease. *J.Biol.Chem., 283,* 6979-6987.

Kazmierczak, A., Adamczyk, A., & Benigna-Strosznajder, J. (2013). [The role of extracellular alpha-synuclein in molecular mechanisms of cell death]. *Postepy Hig.Med.Dosw.(Online.), 67,* 1047-1057.

Khan, F. H., Saha, M., & Chakrabarti, S. (2001). Dopamine induced protein damage in mitochondrial-synaptosomal fraction of rat brain. *Brain Res, 895,* 245-9.

Kim, H. J. (2013). Alpha-Synuclein Expression in Patients with Parkinson's Disease: A Clinician's Perspective. *Exp.Neurobiol., 22,* 77-83.

Kooncumchoo, P., Sharma, S., Porter, J., Govitrapong, P., & Ebadi, M. (2006). Coenzyme Q(10) provides neuroprotection in iron-induced apoptosis in dopaminergic neurons. *J.Mol.Neurosci., 28,* 125-141.

Kristal, B. S., Conway, A. D., Brown, A. M., Jain, J. C., Ulluci, P. A., Li, S. W. et al. (2001). Selective dopaminergic vulnerability: 3,4-dihydroxyphenylacetaldehyde targets mitochondria. *Free Radical Biology and Medicine, 30,* 924-931.

Kuhn, D. M., Arthur, R. E., Jr., Thomas, D. M., & Elferink, L. A. (1999). Tyrosine hydroxylase is inactivated by catechol-quinones and converted to a redox-cycling quinoprotein: possible relevance to Parkinson's disease. *J Neurochem, 73,* 1309-17.

Lamensdorf, I., Eisenhofer, G., Harvey-White, J., Hayakawa, Y., Kirk, K., & Kopin, I. J. (2000a). Metabolic stress in PC12 cells induces the formation of the endogenous dopaminergic neurotoxin, 3,4-dihydroxyphenylacetaldehyde. *J Neurosci Res, 60,* 552-8.

Lamensdorf, I., Eisenhofer, G., Harvey-White, J., Nechustan, A., Kirk, K., & Kopin, I. J. (2000b). 3,4-Dihydroxyphenylacetaldehyde potentiates the toxic effects of metabolic stress in PC12 cells. *Brain Research, 868,* 191-201.

Langston, J. W. & Ballard, P. (1984). Parkinsonism induced by 1-methyl-4-phenyl-1,2,3,6-tetrahydropyridine (MPTP): implications for treatment and the pathogenesis of Parkinson's disease. *Can J Neurol Sci, 11,* 160-5.

Langston, J. W., Ballard, P., Tetrud, J. W., & Irwin, I. (1983). Chronic Parkinsonism in humans due to a product of meperidine-analog synthesis. *Science, 219,* 979-80.

Langston, J. W. & Ballard, P. A., Jr. (1983). Parkinson's disease in a chemist working with 1-methyl-4-phenyl-1,2,5,6-tetrahydropyridine. *N Engl J Med, 309,* 310.

Langston, J. W., Forno, L. S., Rebert, C. S., & Irwin, I. (1984). Selective nigral toxicity after systemic administration of 1-methyl-4-phenyl-1,2,5,6-tetrahydropyrine (MPTP) in the squirrel monkey. *Brain Res, 292,* 390-4.

Langston, J. W., Irwin, I., Langston, E. B., & Forno, L. S. (1984a). 1-Methyl-4-phenylpyridinium ion (MPP+): identification of a metabolite of MPTP, a toxin selective to the substantia nigra. *Neurosci Lett, 48,* 87-92.

Langston, J. W., Irwin, I., Langston, E. B., & Forno, L. S. (1984b). Pargyline prevents MPTP-induced parkinsonism in primates. *Science, 225,* 1480-2.

Legros, H., Dingeval, M. G., Janin, F., Costentin, J., & Bonnet, J. J. (2004). Toxicity of a Treatment Associating Dopamine and Disulfiram for Catecholaminergic Neuroblastoma SH-SY5Y Cells: Relationships with 3,4-Dihydroxyphenylacetaldehyde Formation. *Neurotoxicology, 25,* 365-75.

Legros, H., Janin, F., Dourmap, N., Bonnet, J. J., & Costentin, J. (2004). Semi-chronic increase in striatal level of 3,4-dihydroxyphenylacetaldehyde does not result in alteration of nigrostriatal dopaminergic neurones. *J Neurosci Res, 75,* 429-35.

Li, H. & Dryhurst, G. (2001). Oxidative metabolites of 5-S-cysteinyldopamine inhibit the pyruvate dehydrogenase complex. *J Neural Transm, 108,* 1363-74.

Li, S. W., Lin, T. S., Minteer, S., & Burke, W. J. (2001). 3,4-Dihydroxyphenylacetaldehyde and hydrogen peroxide generate a hydroxyl radical: possible role in Parkinson's disease pathogenesis. *Brain Res.Mol.Brain Res., 93,* 1-7.

Lieberman, A., Lyons, K., Levine, J., & Myerburg, R. (2005). Statins, cholesterol, Co-enzyme Q10, and Parkinson's disease. *Parkinsonism.Relat Disord., 11,* 81-84.

Lipski, J., Nistico, R., Berretta, N., Guatteo, E., Bernardi, G., & Mercuri, N. B. (2011). L-DOPA: a scapegoat for accelerated neurodegeneration in Parkinson's disease? *Prog.Neurobiol., 94,* 389-407.

Mattammal, M. B., Chung, H. D., Strong, R., & Hsu, F. F. (1993). Confirmation of a dopamine metabolite in parkinsonian brain tissue by gas chromatography-mass spectrometry. *J Chromatogr, 614,* 205-12.

Mattammal, M. B., Haring, J. H., Chung, H. D., Raghu, G., & Strong, R. (1995). An endogenous dopaminergic neurotoxin: implication for Parkinson's disease. *Neurodegeneration, 4,* 271-81.

Mattammal, M. B., Strong, R., Lakshmi, V. M., Chung, H. D., & Stephenson, A. H. (1995). Prostaglandin H synthetase-mediated metabolism of dopamine: implication for Parkinson's disease. *J Neurochem, 64,* 1645-54.

Mattammal, M. B., Strong, R., White, E. t., & Hsu, F. F. (1994). Characterization of peroxidative oxidation products of dopamine by mass spectrometry. *J Chromatogr B Biomed Appl, 658,* 21-30.

McCaffery, P. & Drager, U. C. (1994). High levels of a retinoic acid-generating dehydrogenase in the meso-telencephalic dopamine system. *Proc Natl Acad Sci U S A, 91,* 7772-6.

McCormack, A. L., Thiruchelvam, M., Manning-Bog, A. B., Thiffault, C., Langston, J. W., Cory-Slechta, D. A. et al. (2002). Environmental risk factors and Parkinson's disease: selective degeneration of nigral dopaminergic neurons caused by the herbicide paraquat. *Neurobiol Dis, 10,* 119-27.

Mexas, L. M., Florang, V. R., & Doorn, J. A. (2011). Inhibition and covalent modification of tyrosine hydroxylase by 3,4-dihydroxyphenylacetaldehyde, a toxic dopamine metabolite. *Neurotoxicology, 32,* 471-477.

Mischley, L. K., Allen, J., & Bradley, R. (2012). Coenzyme Q10 deficiency in patients with Parkinson's disease. *J.Neurol.Sci., 318,* 72-75.

Mytilineou, C., Han, S. K., & Cohen, G. (1993). Toxic and protective effects of L-dopa on mesencephalic cell cultures. *J Neurochem, 61,* 1470-8.

Nelson, D. & Cox, M. (2000). Lehninger Principles of Biochemistry. *Worth Publishers.*

Olanow, C. W. (2004). Manganese-induced parkinsonism and Parkinson's disease. *Ann.N.Y.Acad.Sci., 1012,* 209-223.

Olney, J. W., Zorumski, C. F., Stewart, G. R., Price, M. T., Wang, G. J., & Labruyere, J. (1990). Excitotoxicity of L-dopa and 6-OH-dopa: implications for Parkinson's and Huntington's diseases. *Exp Neurol, 108,* 269-72.

Panneton, W. M., Kumar, V. B., Gan, Q., Burke, W. J., & Galvin, J. E. (2010). The neurotoxicity of DOPAL: behavioral and stereological evidence for its role in Parkinson disease pathogenesis. *PLoS.One., 5,* e15251.

Pardo, B., Mena, M. A., Fahn, S., & Garcia de Yebenes, J. (1993). Ascorbic acid protects against levodopa-induced neurotoxicity on a catecholamine-rich human neuroblastoma cell line. *Mov Disord, 8,* 278-84.

Ransom, B. R., Kunis, D. M., Irwin, I., & Langston, J. W. (1987). Astrocytes convert the parkinsonism inducing neurotoxin, MPTP, to its active metabolite, MPP+. *Neurosci Lett, 75,* 323-8.

Raphael Rubin & David S.Strayer (2012). *Rubin's Pathology, Clinicopathologic Foundations of Medicine*. (6th ed.) Wolters Kluwer/Lippincott Williams & Wilkins.

Rees, J. N., Florang, V. R., Anderson, D. G., & Doorn, J. A. (2007). Lipid peroxidation products inhibit dopamine catabolism yielding aberrant levels of a reactive intermediate. *Chem.Res.Toxicol., 20,* 1536-1542.

Rees, J. N., Florang, V. R., Eckert, L. L., & Doorn, J. A. (2009). Protein reactivity of 3,4-dihydroxyphenylacetaldehyde, a toxic dopamine metabolite, is dependent on both the aldehyde and the catechol. *Chem.Res.Toxicol., 22,* 1256-1263.

Seidl, S. E. & Potashkin, J. A. (2011). The promise of neuroprotective agents in Parkinson's disease. *Front Neurol., 2,* 68.

Sharma, S. K. & Ebadi, M. (2003). Metallothionein attenuates 3-morpholinosydnonimine (SIN-1)-induced oxidative stress in dopaminergic neurons. *Antioxid.Redox.Signal., 5,* 251-264.

Shoulson, I., Oakes, D., Fahn, S., Lang, A., Langston, J. W., LeWitt, P. et al. (2002). Impact of sustained deprenyl (selegiline) in levodopa-treated Parkinson's disease: a randomized placebo-controlled extension of the deprenyl and tocopherol antioxidative therapy of parkinsonism trial. *Ann Neurol, 51,* 604-12.

Siegle, G., Agranoff, B., Albers, R., Fisher, S., & Uhler, M. (1999). Basic Neurochemistry, Molecular, Cellular and Medical Aspects, 6th ed. *Lippincott Williams & Wilkins.*

Singleton, A. B., Farrer, M., Johnson, J., Singleton, A., Hague, S., Kachergus, J. et al. (2003). alpha-Synuclein locus triplication causes Parkinson's disease. *Science, 302,* 841.

Tanik, S. A., Schultheiss, C. E., Volpicelli-Daley, L. A., Brunden, K. R., & Lee, V. M. (2013). Lewy body-like alpha-synuclein aggregates resist degradation and impair macroautophagy. *J.Biol.Chem., 288,* 15194-15210.

Tank, A. W. & Weiner, H. (1977). The effects of ethanol on dopamine metabolism in rat liver and brain. *Adv Exp Med Biol, 85A,* 473-83.

Tank, A. W., Weiner, H., & Thurman, J. A. (1981). Enzymology and subcellular localization of aldehyde oxidation in rat liver : Oxidation of 3,4-dihydroxyphenylacetaldehyde derived from dopamine to 3,4-dihydroxyphenylacetic acid. *Biochemical Pharmacology, 30,* 3265-3275.

Tanner, C. M., Goldman, S. M., Aston, D. A., Ottman, R., Ellenberg, J., Mayeux, R. et al. (2002). Smoking and Parkinson's disease in twins. *Neurology, 58,* 581-8.

Tanner, C. M., Kamel, F., Ross, G. W., Hoppin, J. A., Goldman, S. M., Korell, M. et al. (2011). Rotenone, paraquat, and Parkinson's disease. *Environ.Health Perspect., 119,* 866-872.

Tetrud, J. W. & Langston, J. W. (1987). R-(-)-deprenyl as a possible protective agent in Parkinson's disease. *J Neural Transm Suppl, 25,* 69-79.

Tetrud, J. & Langston, J. (1989). The effect of deprenyl (selegiline) on the natural history of Parkinson's disease. *Science, 245,* 519-22.

Thiruchelvam, M., Brockel, B. J., Richfield, E. K., Baggs, R. B., & Cory-Slechta, D. A. (2000). Potentiated and preferential effects of combined paraquat and maneb on nigrostriatal dopamine systems: environmental risk factors for Parkinson's disease? *Brain Res, 873,* 225-34.

Thiruchelvam, M., Richfield, E. K., Baggs, R. B., Tank, A. W., & Cory-Slechta, D. A. (2000). The nigrostriatal dopaminergic system as a preferential target of repeated exposures to combined paraquat and maneb: implications for Parkinson's disease. *J Neurosci, 20,* 9207-14.

Thiruchelvam, M., Richfield, E. K., Goodman, B. M., Baggs, R. B., & Cory-Slechta, D. A. (2002). Developmental exposure to the pesticides paraquat and maneb and the Parkinson's disease phenotype. *Neurotoxicology, 23,* 621-33.

van Muiswinkel, F. L., Riemers, F. M., Peters, G. J., LaFleur, M. V., Siegel, D., Jongenelen, C. A. et al. (2000). L-Dopa stimulates expression of the antioxidant enzyme NAD(P)H:quinone oxidoreductase (NQO) in cultured astroglial cells. *Free Radic Biol Med, 29,* 442-53.

Vermeer, L. M., Florang, V. R., & Doorn, J. A. (2012). Catechol and aldehyde moieties of 3,4-dihydroxyphenylacetaldehyde contribute to tyrosine hydroxylase inhibition and neurotoxicity. *Brain Res., 1474,* 100-109.

Weiner, H. (1978). Relationship between 3,4-dihydroxyphenylacetaldehyde levels and tetrahydropapaveroline formation. *Alcohol Clin Exp Res, 2,* 127-31.

Wey, M. C., Fernandez, E., Martinez, P. A., Sullivan, P., Goldstein, D. S., & Strong, R. (2012). Neurodegeneration and motor dysfunction in mice lacking cytosolic and mitochondrial aldehyde dehydrogenases: implications for Parkinson's disease. *PLoS.One., 7,* e31522.

Xu, Y., Stokes, A. H., Roskoski, R., Jr., & Vrana, K. E. (1998). Dopamine, in the presence of tyrosinase, covalently modifies and inactivates tyrosine hydroxylase. *J Neurosci Res, 54,* 691-7.

Yao, L., Fan, P., Arolfo, M., Jiang, Z., Olive, M. F., Zablocki, J. et al. (2010). Inhibition of aldehyde dehydrogenase-2 suppresses cocaine seeking by generating THP, a cocaine use-dependent inhibitor of dopamine synthesis. *Nat.Med., 16,* 1024-1028.

Yasuda, T. & Mochizuki, H. (2010). The regulatory role of alpha-synuclein and parkin in neuronal cell apoptosis; possible implications for the pathogenesis of Parkinson's disease. *Apoptosis., 15,* 1312-1321.

Zhang, X., Li, L., Zhang, L., Borowitz, J. L., & Isom, G. E. (2009). Cyanide-induced death of dopaminergic cells is mediated by uncoupling protein-2 up-regulation and reduced Bcl-2 expression. *Toxicol.Appl.Pharmacol., 238,* 11-19.

In: The Central Catecholaminergic System
Editor: Bertalan Dudás
ISBN: 978-1-63117-937-2

Chapter 8

The Role of Fibroblast Growth Factor (FGF) Signaling on Dopaminergic Function in Parkinson's Disease

Aaron Kucinski, Ryan Curl, Robert S. Miletich, Thomas D. Corso, Ewa K. Stachowiak and Michal K. Stachowiak

Introduction

Parkinson's disease is a prevalent and debilitating neurodegenerative disease, which results in severe movement and cognitive deficits. About 1% to 2% of the population in North America will eventually develop this disorder, a prevalence which has essentially remained unchanged for the past 40 years (Rubin & Strayer, 2012). The trademark feature of this disorder is an impairment of dopamine transmission resulting from degeneration of dopamine neurons in the substantia nigra pars compacta and their projections to the dorsolateral striatum via the nigrostriatal pathway (Dauer & Przedborski, 2003). This progressive degeneration of these basal nuclei motor circuits results in bradykinesia, resting tremor and altered motor coordination (Rodriguez-Oroz et al., 2009). The previous chapter discussed evidence for selective dopaminergic degeneration resulting from exposure to environmental toxins such as MPTP (1-methyl-4-phenyl-1,2,3,6-tetrahydropyridine) or paraquat, but there are also genetically associated forms of Parkinson's disease as well as genetic susceptibilities to environmental and metabolic stresses. Particularly factors that involve elevated levels of reactive oxygen species (ROS) (Adams, Jr. et al., 2001; Jenner, 2003) and age related decline of protective mechanisms normally found in healthy neurons are of particular interest (Harman, 2006).

The maturation and protection of developing neurons as well as the maintenance and survival of adult neurons requires small proteins called neurotrophic factors (Connor & Dragunow, 1998; Harman, 2006). Many neurotrophic factors have antioxidant effects and have been shown to promote the survival of dopamine neurons, including fibroblast growth factor 2 (FGF-2, also known as basic FGF) (Grothe & Timmer, 2007), glial cell line-derived neurotrophic factor (GDNF) (Andereggen et al., 2009; Lin et al., 1993), epidermal growth factor (EGF) (Hadjiconstantinou et al., 1991), brain-derived neurotrophic factor (BDNF) (Hyman et al., 1991), conserved dopamine neurotrophic factor (CDNF) (Lindholm et al., 2007) and mesencephalic astrocyte-derived neurotrophic factor (MANF) (Petrova et al., 2003). These findings are important since there are reports that show decreased levels of FGF, DNF, NGF and GDNF in the nigrostriatal dopamine system and cerebrospinal fluid of Parkinson's disease patients (Howells et al., 2000; Mogi et al., 1999; Nagatsu et al., 2000; Parain et al., 1999; Tooyama et al., 1994). Also, genetic links between CDNF (Choi et al., 2011) BDNF (Chen et al., 2011) and FGF (Mizuta et al., 2008; Wang et al., 2008) and Parkinson's disease have been found. FGF distinguishes itself from other neurotrophic factors due to its critical role in supporting both developing and adult dopamine systems (Krejci et al., 2009; Mason, 2007). Important features of FGF-2 are that it promotes the growth and survival of cultured dopamine neurons (Giacobini et al., 1993; Krejci et al., 2009; Li et al., 2006; Mayer et al., 1993a), protects against neurotoxin-induced cell death (Casper & Blum, 1995; Date et al., 1993; Hsuan et al., 2006; Otto & Unsicker, 1993; Peng et al., 2008; Zawada et al., 1996) and increases in neuronal survival when co-grafted with dopamine neurons (Mayer et al., 1993b; Timmer et al., 2004; Timmer et al., 2007; Tooyama et al., 1994). It was also reported that FGF signaling increases dopamine levels in calbindin-negative substantia nigra neurons, those neurons that are at greatest risk in Parkinson's disease patients (Murase & McKay, 2006). In human Parkinson's disease patients, a reduction in the percentage of FGF- 2 immunoreactive dopamine neurons relative to healthy subjects was found (12.7% FGF-2 positive dopamine neurons versus 82% FGF-2 positive dopamine neurons in control brains) (Tooyama et al., 1994). Furthermore, Timmer and colleagues (2007) reported that in adult FGF-2 knockout mice with 6-hydroxydopamine (6-OHDA) lesions, there were significantly fewer surviving dopamine neurons compared to lesioned wild-type controls (Timmer et al., 2007). Thus, the FGF system merits considerable attention for investigation of Parkinson's disease prevention and therapy.

Although about 80% - 90% of patients suffering from Parkinson's disease acquire what is termed the "sporadic" or no known genetic origin of the disease, a diversity of genetic causes have been identified in recent years. These include defects of autosomal dominant genes affecting alpha-synuclein (Polymeropoulos et al., 1997), the leucine-rich repeat kinase 2 (LRRK2) (Zimprich et al., 2004), the autosomal recessive genes Parkin (encoded by the PARK2 gene) (Valente et al., 2004) and PARK7 (aka DJ-1) (Bonifati et al., 2003), and recently FGF20 (Wang et al., 2008). Given this diversity, it is likely that these genes influence common mechanisms affecting the development, maintenance and protection of dopamine neurons.

FGFR1 Signaling

FGF-2 has a high affinity for the fibroblast growth factor receptor 1 (FGFR1), which is present in the developing postnatal and adult substantia nigra (Andereggen et al., 2009; Tooyama et al., 1994) where it is localized to dopamine neurons and glial cells (Lin et al., 1993). Exogenous treatment with FGF-2 has neurotrophic effects on cultured dopamine neurons (Klejbor et al., 2006) and rat embryonic dopamine neurons after toxin exposure

(Giacobini et al., 1993). FGFR1 has been shown to be multifunctional depending on the location of the receptor during the cells development. On the cell surface, FGFR1 supports proliferation of neural progenitor cells and also activates cell survival related pathways in mature neurons. In the cell nucleus, FGFR1 stimulates differentiation as shown in the subventricular zone of mice *in vitro* and *in vivo* (Stachowiak et al., 2003; Stachowiak et al., 2007). It is postulated that such mechanisms involving signaling by FGF and related receptors act as intermediaries in diverse biological pathways as found in the recently established "Integrative Nuclear FGFR1 Signaling" (INFS) pathway (Fang et al., 2005; Stachowiak et al., 2007). Central to the INFS mechanism, which is activated by FGFs and other diverse stimuli, is the nuclear translocation of newly synthesized FGFR1 (along with its ligand) and its direct modulation of several homeostatic gene programs (Dunham-Ems et al., 2009; Maher, 1996; Myers et al., 2003; Reilly & Maher, 2001; Stachowiak et al., 1996). INFS may link signaling pathways in which Parkinson's disease-linked mutations have been reported and reconcile how genetic and non-genetic factors converge during degeneration of nigrostriatal dopamine neurons in Parkinson's disease.

Disrupted FGFR1 Signaling

An important role of FGF receptor signaling to the survival of dopamine neurons was shown using transfections of DNA coding dominant negative FGFR1(TK-) protein with deleted the tyrosine kinase domain directly into the substantia nigra in vivo and in cultured neurons (Stachowiak et al., 2003). In vivo transfection of FGFR1(TK-) into the adult rat midbrain using polyethylenimine resulted in a loss of TH-immunopositive neurons in the substantia nigra pars compacta and depletion of striatal dopamine (Corso et al., 2005). These findings agree with the report of profound reduction of FGF-2 immunoreactive dopamine neurons in the brains of Parkinson's disease patients (Tooyama et al., 1994). Together, this evidence substantiates a functional impact of FGF in the pathophysiology of Parkinson's disease (Zhang et al., 1988).

To further assess the role of substantia nigra-expressed fibroblast growth factor and its homologues in Parkinson's disease, a transgenic mouse model was engineered expressing FGFR1(TK-) from the tyrosine hydroxylase gene promoter (termed *th-fgfr1(tk-)*), thus restricting the mutation to dopaminergic neurons (Klejbor et al., 2006). Phenotypically, *th-fgfr1(tk-)* mice have smaller and less dense midbrain dopamine neurons, resembling the dopamine neuronal hypoplasia observed in adult Parkinson's disease patients (Ma et al., 1996; Moller, 1992). These mice display behavioral abnormalities associated with dysfunctional dopamine release such as impaired sensorimotor gating and cognitive dysfunction (Klejbor et al., 2006; Klejbor et al., 2009; Kucinski et al., 2012a).

Mice with Disrupted FGFR1 Signaling Are More Vulnerable to Dopaminergic Toxins

Unilateral injection of the dopamine toxin 6-hydroxydopamine (6-OHDA) to the medial forebrain bundle of *th-fgfr1(tk-)* mice generated a robust unilateral Parkinson's disease model

(Kucinski et al., 2012b). With the 6-OHDA lesions, *th-fgfr1(tk-)* mice made a higher percentage of contralateral rotations with apomorphine administration compared to lesioned wild type mice and showed an extensive unilateral reduction of tyrosine hydroxylase (TH) immunoreactivity in nigrostriatal dopamine neurons and loss of striatal dopamine and dopamine metabolites. Furthermore, unilaterally lesioned *th-fgfr1(tk-)* mice exhibited consistent spontaneous (drug free) motor impairments including ipsilateral rotation preference in the novel Cylinder Turning Test and a reduced latency to remain on the accelerating rotarod. These findings in *th-fgfr1(tk-)* mice, consistent with FGF-2 knockout mice (Timmer et al., 2007), indicate increased susceptibility of dopamine neurons with impaired FGFR1 signaling.

Paraquat, a widely used pesticide is considered an environmental neurotoxin which has been shown to increase the risk of Parkinson's disease (Ascherio et al., 2006; Liou et al., 1997; Tanner et al., 2011). Paraquat has a similar structure to MPTP and its metabolite MPP^+ (Figure 1).

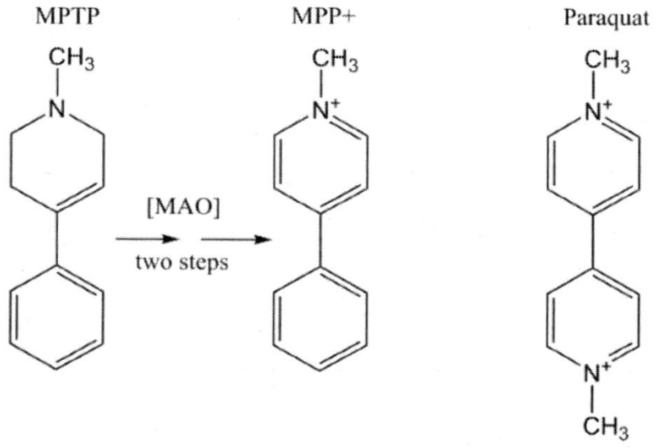

Figure 1. Comparison of the structure of paraquat to the structures of 1-methyl-4-phenyl-1,2,3,6-tetrahydropyridine (MPTP) and 1-methyl-4-phenylpyridine (MPP^+)

Exposure to the widely used manganese-based fungicide, maneb, has also been associated with Parkinson's disease development (Liu et al., 2003). Paraquat is thought to enter the brain via neutral amino acid transporters and enter cells via a sodium dependent process. Due to the fact that paraquat is a very efficient redox cycling compound, it is thought that it damages cells by inducing oxidative stress. It is unclear how maneb passes the blood brain barrier, however, it has been shown to inhibit mitochondrial complex III. Together, paraquat and maneb inhibit the Bak-dependent pathway while potentiating apoptosis via BAX protein (Fei et al., 2008). Paraquat and maneb target the substantia nigra and corpus striatum leading to increased oxidative stress, lipid peroxidation, drastically increased neuronal α-synuclein pathology and degeneration of dopaminergic neurons (Brooks et al., 1999; Cory-Slechta et al., 2005; Norris et al., 2007; Patel et al., 2006; Thiruchelvam et al., 2000).

Using the *th-fgfr1(tk-)* animal model, it was determined that systemic injections of paraquat and maneb caused a significant depletion of dopamine (Figure 2) and dihydroxyphenylacetic acid (DOPAC; Figure 3) in the striatum of male mice. Levo-dihydroxy phenylalanine (L- DOPA; Figure 4) and homovanyllic acid (HVA; Figure 5) were also reduced. Interestingly, no significant changes in any of the dopamine markers were observed in female mice. In addition to dopamine biomarkers, serotonin (Figure 6) and noradrenaline (Figure 7) levels were also significantly reduced in the striatum of male but not female animals. Administration of paraquat and maneb to *th-fgfr1(tk-)* mice replicates the findings in human Parkinson's patients that in addition to dopamine neurons, noradrenergic and serotoninergic neurons are also compromised in the striatum (Thiruchelvam et al., 2002).

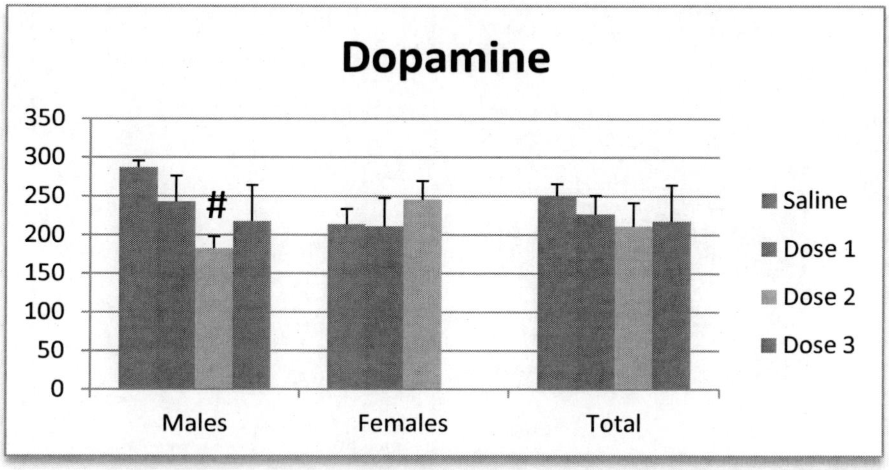

Figure 2. Dopamine concentrations in the striatum measured with high-pressure liquid chromatography (HPLC). Significant decrease has been found in dopamine following the treatment with medium doses of paraquat and maneb in male [*fgfr1 (tk-)*] mice when compared to the saline-treated ones ($p<0.05$). No significant differences were observed in the female animals. The animals were injected every other day with low, medium and high doses of paraquat and maneb for 7 weeks. Dose 1: low dose paraquat (5 mg/kg) and maneb (15 mg/kg); dose 2: medium dose of paraquat (10 mg/kg) and maneb (30 mg/kg); dose 3: high dose of paraquat (15 mg/kg) and maneb (45 mg/kg). Because of the extreme death (75%) in the group treated with high doses of toxins, these animals were given the medium dose after 2 weeks. Pound sign denotes significance.

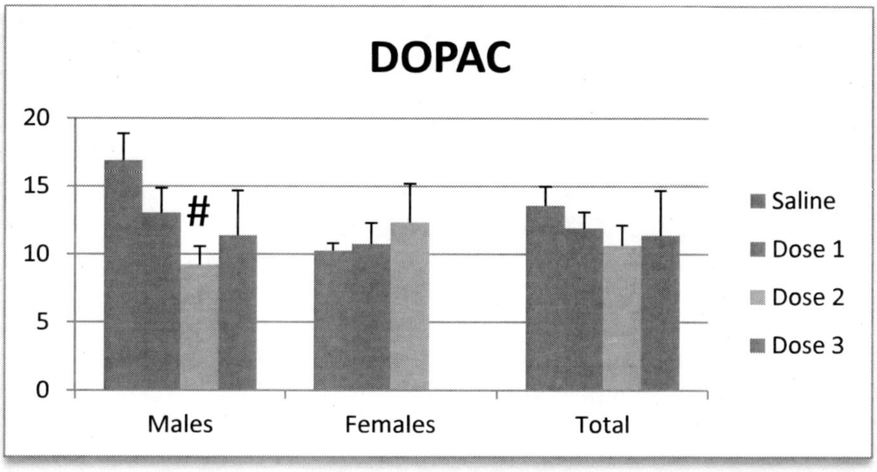

Figure 3. Dihydroxyphenylacetic acid (DOPAC) concentrations in the striatum measured with high-pressure liquid chromatography (HPLC). Significant decrease has been found in DOPAC following the treatment with medium doses of paraquat and maneb in male [*fgfr1 (tk-)*] mice when compared to the saline-treated ones ($p<0.05$). No significant differences were observed in the female animals. The animals were injected every other day with low, medium and high doses of paraquat and maneb for 7 weeks. Dose 1: low dose paraquat (5 mg/kg) and maneb (15 mg/kg); dose 2: medium dose of paraquat (10 mg/kg) and maneb (30 mg/kg); dose 3: high dose of paraquat (15 mg/kg) and maneb (45 mg/kg). Because of the extreme death (75%) in the group treated with high doses of toxins, these animals were given the medium dose after 2 weeks. Pound sign denotes significance.

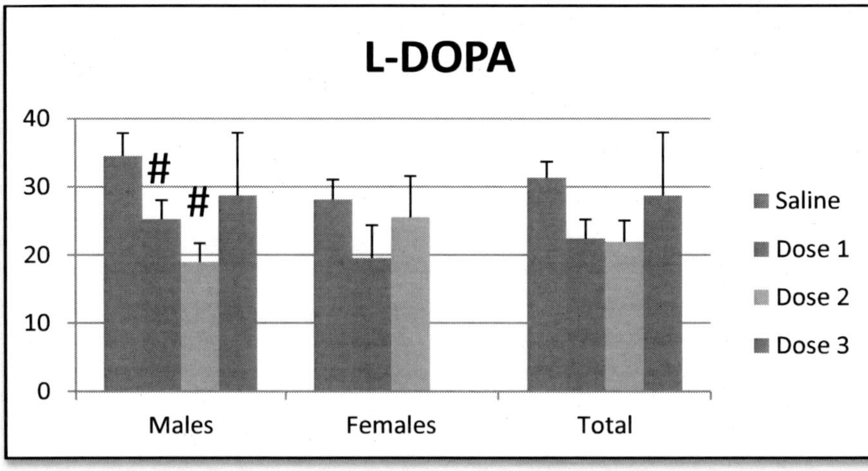

Figure 4. Levo-dihydroxy phenylalanine (L-DOPA) concentrations in the striatum measured with high-pressure liquid chromatography (HPLC). Significant decrease has been found in dopamine following the treatment with low and medium doses of paraquat and maneb in male [*fgfr1 (tk-)*] mice when compared to the saline-treated ones ($p<0.05$). No significant differences were observed in the female animals. The animals were injected every other day with low, medium and high doses of paraquat and maneb for 7 weeks. Dose 1: low dose paraquat (5 mg/kg) and maneb (15 mg/kg); dose 2: medium dose of paraquat (10 mg/kg) and maneb (30 mg/kg); dose 3: high dose of paraquat (15 mg/kg) and maneb (45 mg/kg). Because of the extreme death (75%) in the group treated with high doses of toxins, these animals were given the medium dose after 2 weeks. Pound signs denote significance.

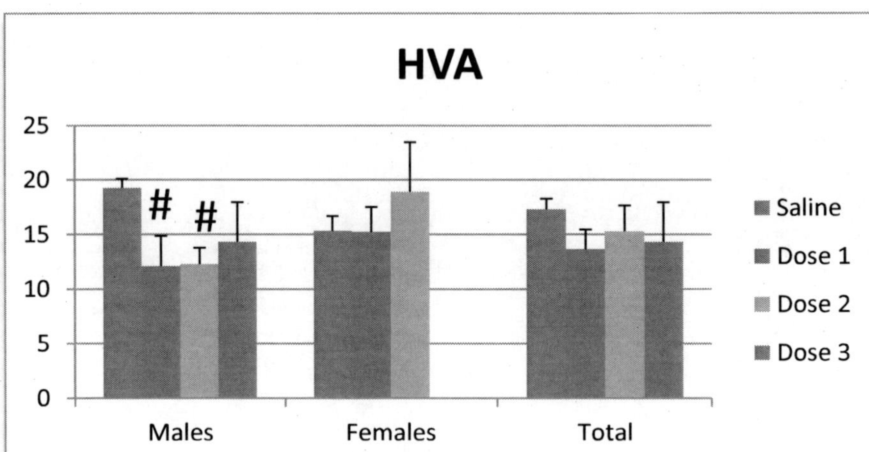

Figure 5. Homovanyllic acid (HVA) concentrations in the striatum measured with high-pressure liquid chromatography (HPLC). Significant decrease has been found in HVA following the treatment with low and medium doses of paraquat and maneb in male [*fgfr1 (tk-)*] mice when compared to the saline-treated ones ($p<0.05$). No significant differences were observed in the female animals. The animals were injected every other day with low, medium and high doses of paraquat and maneb for 7 weeks. Dose 1: low dose paraquat (5 mg/kg) and maneb (15 mg/kg); dose 2: medium dose of paraquat (10 mg/kg) and maneb (30 mg/kg); dose 3: high dose of paraquat (15 mg/kg) and maneb (45 mg/kg). Because of the extreme death (75%) in the group treated with high doses of toxins, these animals were given the medium dose after 2 weeks. Pound signs denote significance.

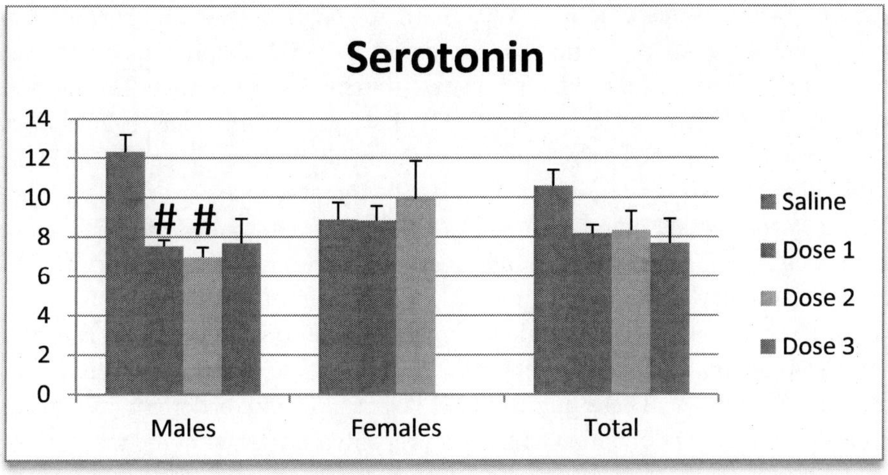

Figure 6. Serotonin concentrations in the striatum measured with high-pressure liquid chromatography (HPLC). Significant decrease has been found in serotonin following the treatment with low and medium doses of paraquat and maneb in male [*fgfr1 (tk-)*] mice when compared to the saline-treated ones ($p<0.05$). No significant differences were observed in the female animals. The animals were injected every other day with low, medium and high doses of paraquat and maneb for 7 weeks. Dose 1: low dose paraquat (5 mg/kg) and maneb (15 mg/kg); dose 2: medium dose of paraquat (10 mg/kg) and maneb (30 mg/kg); dose 3: high dose of paraquat (15 mg/kg) and maneb (45 mg/kg). Because of the extreme death (75%) in the group treated with high doses of toxins, these animals were given the medium dose after 2 weeks. Pound signs denote significance.

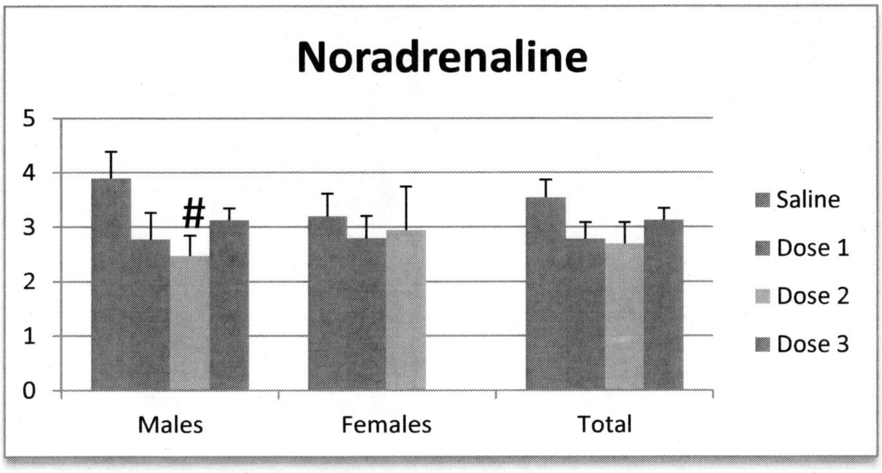

Figure 7. Noradrenaline concentrations in the striatum measured with high-pressure liquid chromatography (HPLC). Significant decrease has been found in serotonin following the treatment with medium doses of paraquat and maneb in male [*fgfr1 (tk-)*] mice when compared to the saline-treated ones ($p<0.05$). No significant differences were observed in the female animals. The animals were injected every other day with low, medium and high doses of paraquat and maneb for 7 weeks. Dose 1: low dose paraquat (5 mg/kg) and maneb (15 mg/kg); dose 2: medium dose of paraquat (10 mg/kg) and maneb (30 mg/kg); dose 3: high dose of paraquat (15 mg/kg) and maneb (45 mg/kg). Because of the extreme death (75%) in the group treated with high doses of toxins, these animals were given the medium dose after 2 weeks. Pound sign denotes significance.

The lack of change in the female animals reaffirms previous reports that females appear to be more resistant to paraquat and maneb (Barlow et al., 2004). Numerous studies have also reported a higher prevalence of Parkinson's disease in men than in women (Baldereschi et al., 2000; Bower et al., 1999; Mayeux et al., 1992). Estrogen therapy has been shown to be beneficial to women during the early stages of Parkinson's disease (Saunders-Pullman et al., 1999), but not the later stages (Strijks et al., 1999). Increased levels of estrogen could be neuroprotective in the female animals. Positron emission tomography (PET) scans on these same mice showed a significant paraquat and maneb-induced reduction of the [C11]d-threo-methylphenidate binding potential indicating reduced number of dopamine transporter (DAT) sites in the striatum and loss of dopamine terminals. This outcome is consistent with the depletion of dopamine and dopamine metabolites in the striatum of the paraquat and maneb treated male mice (Figure 8). These animals also display locomotor deficits in both the male and females even though the dopamine depletion was only significant in the males.

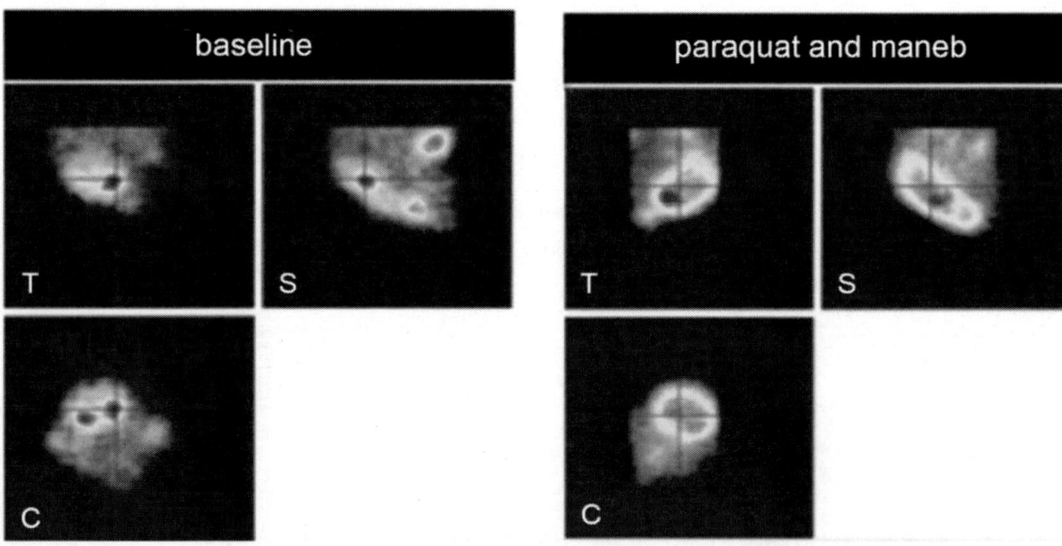

Binding Potential (BP): Receptor density and ligand affinity

Mice treatment (n)	BP Mean ± SEM
Baseline (6)	1.1183 ± .09228
Saline (2)	1.2150 ± .00500
paraquat + maneb (3)	0.6967 ± .03180#

Figure 8. Parametric, positron emission tomography (PET) images of *[C-11]* d-threo-*methylphenidate (MP)* binding potential from a baseline and animals treated with medium dose of paraquat (10 mg/kg) and maneb (30 mg/kg) for 4 weeks. MP is a ligand for the dopamine transporter, and provides an index of dopaminergic terminals. Orthogonal projections in the transverse (T), sagittal (S) and coronal (C) planes are demonstrated as examples from the dataset. Two mice are simultaneously imaged laying supine side by side, while the anesthesia was induced and maintained with isoflurane. Tracer was administered as a bolus penile injection. Average dose was 214 + 69 microCi. 24 scans were taken by increasing in duration from 15-600 seconds. Total acquisition time was 60 min. Images were reconstructed using filtered back projection. Concorde, Amide and SPM softwares were used for image analysis and modeling. Binding potential was derived from the Simplified Reference Tissue Model, using cerebellum as reference tissue. Pound sign denotes significance.

Conclusion

There is increasing evidence that Parkinson's disease may be elicited by a failure of endogenous neuroprotective mechanisms, such as impaired growth factor support of nigrostriatal dopamine neurons. FGF 2 and related growth factors protect dopamine neurons from cell death and promote dopamine neuronal growth and there are deficits of these growth factors in Parkinson's disease, highlighting the critical value of investigating these proteins for Parkinson's disease prevention and therapy. Multiple genes are associated with Parkinson's disease and there likely exists common intermediary signaling pathways, such as INFS, which integrate genetic and non-genetic risk factors for the disease. Transgenic *th-fgfr1(tk-)* mice with a deficiency of FGF signaling in nigrostriatal dopaminergic neurons are highly susceptible to damage from oxidative stress incurred by administration of neurotoxins 6-OHDA, paraquat and maneb.

Although the *fgfr1(tk-)* model replicates Parkinsonian features when neurotoxins target dopamine neurons that lack FGFR1 neurotrophic support, paradoxically, in young animals without neurotoxins there is elevated dopamine release in the striatum and a behavioral phenotype that resembles schizophrenia. The following chapter discusses that aspect of this model.

References

Adams, J. D., Jr., Chang, M. L., & Klaidman, L. (2001). Parkinson's disease--redox mechanisms. *Curr.Med.Chem., 8,* 809-814.

Andereggen, L., Meyer, M., Guzman, R., Ducray, A. D., & Widmer, H. R. (2009). Effects of GDNF pretreatment on function and survival of transplanted fetal ventral mesencephalic cells in the 6-OHDA rat model of Parkinson's disease. *Brain Res., 1276,* 39-49.

Ascherio, A., Chen, H., Weisskopf, M. G., O'Reilly, E., McCullough, M. L., Calle, E. E. et al. (2006). Pesticide exposure and risk for Parkinson's disease. *Ann Neurol, 60.*

Baldereschi, M., Di Carlo, A., Rocca, W. A., Vanni, P., Maggi, S., Perissinotto, E. et al. (2000). Parkinson's disease and parkinsonism in a longitudinal study: two-fold higher incidence in men. ILSA Working Group. Italian Longitudinal Study on Aging. *Neurology, 55.*

Barlow, B. K., Richfield, E. K., Cory-Slechta, D. A., & Thiruchelvam, M. (2004). A fetal risk factor for Parkinson's disease. *Dev Neurosci, 26.*

Bonifati, V., Rizzu, P., van Baren, M. J., Schaap, O., Breedveld, G. J., Krieger, E. et al. (2003). Mutations in the DJ-1 gene associated with autosomal recessive early-onset parkinsonism. *Science, 299.*

Bower, J. H., Maraganore, D. M., McDonnell, S. K., & Rocca, W. A. (1999). Incidence and distribution of parkinsonism in Olmsted County, Minnesota, 1976-1990. *Neurology, 52.*

Brooks, A. I., Chadwick, C. A., Gelbard, H. A., Cory-Slechta, D. A., & Federoff, H. J. (1999). Paraquat elicited neurobehavioral syndrome caused by dopaminergic neuron loss. *Brain Res, 823.*

Casper, D. & Blum, M. (1995). Epidermal growth factor and basic fibroblast growth factor protect dopaminergic neurons from glutamate toxicity in culture. *J Neurochem, 65.*

Chen, L., Wang, Y., Xiao, H., Wang, L., Wang, C., Guo, S. et al. (2011). The 712A/G polymorphism of Brain-derived neurotrophic factor is associated with Parkinson's disease but not Major Depressive Disorder in a Chinese Han population. *Biochem.Biophys.Res.Commun., 408,* 318-321.

Choi, J. M., Hong, J. H., Chae, M. J., Ngyuen, P. H., Kang, H. S., Ma, H. I. et al. (2011). Analysis of mutations and the association between polymorphisms in the cerebral dopamine neurotrophic factor (CDNF) gene and Parkinson disease. *Neurosci.Lett., 493,* 97-101.

Connor, B. & Dragunow, M. (1998). The role of neuronal growth factors in neurodegenerative disorders of the human brain. *Brain Res.Brain Res.Rev., 27,* 1-39.

Corso, T. D., Torres, G., Goulah, C., Roy, I., Gambino, A. S., Nayda, J. et al. (2005). Transfection of tyrosine kinase deleted FGF receptor-1 into rat brain substantia nigra reduces the number of tyrosine hydroxylase expressing neurons and decreases concentration levels of striatal dopamine. *Brain Res Mol Brain Res, 139.*

Cory-Slechta, D. A., Thiruchelvam, M., Richfield, E. K., Barlow, B. K., & Brooks, A. I. (2005). Developmental pesticide exposures and the Parkinson's disease phenotype. *Birth Defects Res A Clin Mol Teratol, 73.*

Date, I., Yoshimoto, Y., Imaoka, T., Miyoshi, Y., Gohda, Y., Furuta, T. et al. (1993). Enhanced recovery of the nigrostriatal dopaminergic system in MPTP-treated mice following intrastriatal injection of basic fibroblast growth factor in relation to aging. *Brain Res, 621.*

Dauer, W. & Przedborski, S. (2003). Parkinson's disease: mechanisms and models. *Neuron, 39,* 889-909.

Dunham-Ems, S. M., Lee, Y. W., Stachowiak, E. K., Pudavar, H., Claus, P., Prasad, P. N. et al. (2009). Fibroblast growth factor receptor-1 (FGFR1) nuclear dynamics reveal a novel mechanism in transcription control. *Mol Biol Cell, 20.*

Fang, X., Stachowiak, E. K., Dunham-Ems, S. M., Klejbor, I., & Stachowiak, M. K. (2005). Control of CREB-binding protein signaling by nuclear fibroblast growth factor receptor-1: a novel mechanism of gene regulation. *J Biol Chem, 280.*

Fei, Q., McCormack, A. L., Di Monte, D. A., & Ethell, D. W. (2008). Paraquat neurotoxicity is mediated by a Bak-dependent mechanism. *J Biol Chem, 283.*

Giacobini, M. M., Stromberg, I., Almstrom, S., Cao, Y., & Olson, L. (1993). Fibroblast growth factors enhance dopamine fiber formation from nigral grafts. *Brain Res.Dev.Brain Res., 75,* 65-73.

Grothe, C. & Timmer, M. (2007). The physiological and pharmacological role of basic fibroblast growth factor in the dopaminergic nigrostriatal system. *Brain Res.Rev., 54,* 80-91.

Hadjiconstantinou, M., Fitkin, J. G., Dalia, A., & Neff, N. H. (1991). Epidermal growth factor enhances striatal dopaminergic parameters in the 1-methyl-4-phenyl-1,2,3,6-tetrahydropyridine-treated mouse. *J.Neurochem., 57,* 479-482.

Harman, D. (2006). Free radical theory of aging: an update: increasing the functional life span. *Ann.N.Y.Acad.Sci., 1067,* 10-21.

Howells, D. W., Porritt, M. J., Wong, J. Y., Batchelor, P. E., Kalnins, R., Hughes, A. J. et al. (2000). Reduced BDNF mRNA expression in the Parkinson's disease substantia nigra. *Exp.Neurol., 166,* 127-135.

Hsuan, S. L., Klintworth, H. M., & Xia, Z. (2006). Basic fibroblast growth factor protects against rotenone-induced dopaminergic cell death through activation of extracellular signal-regulated kinases 1/2 and phosphatidylinositol-3 kinase pathways. *J Neurosci, 26.*

Hyman, C., Hofer, M., Barde, Y. A., Juhasz, M., Yancopoulos, G. D., Squinto, S. P. et al. (1991). BDNF is a neurotrophic factor for dopaminergic neurons of the substantia nigra. *Nature, 350,* 230-232.

Jenner, P. (2003). Oxidative stress in Parkinson's disease. *Ann.Neurol., 53 Suppl 3,* S26-S36.

Klejbor, I., Kucinski, A., Wersinger, S. R., Corso, T., Spodnik, J. H., Dziewiatkowski, J. et al. (2009). Serotonergic hyperinnervation and effective serotonin blockade in an FGF receptor developmental model of psychosis. *Schizophr Res, 113.*

Klejbor, I., Myers, J. M., Hausknecht, K., Corso, T. D., Gambino, A. S., Morys, J. et al. (2006). Fibroblast growth factor receptor signaling affects development and function of dopamine neurons - inhibition results in a schizophrenia-like syndrome in transgenic mice. *J Neurochem, 97.*

Krejci, P., Prochazkova, J., Bryja, V., Kozubik, A., & Wilcox, W. R. (2009). Molecular pathology of the fibroblast growth factor family. *Hum.Mutat., 30,* 1245-1255.

Kucinski, A., Syposs, C., Wersinger, S., Bencherif, M., Stachowiak, M. K., & Stachowiak, E. K. (2012a). alpha7 neuronal nicotinic receptor agonist (TC-7020) reverses increased striatal dopamine release during acoustic PPI testing in a transgenic mouse model of schizophrenia. *Schizophr Res, 136.*

Kucinski, A., Wersinger, S., Stachowiak, E., Radell, M., Hesse, R., Corso, T. et al. (2012b). Unilateral 6-OHDA th-fgfr1(tk-) mouse model supports the role of FGFs in Parkinson's disease and the effects of nicotine and L-DOPA on spontaneous motor impairments. *Health, 4,* 1178-1190.

Li, A., Guo, H., Luo, X., Sheng, J., Yang, S., Yin, Y. et al. (2006). Apomorphine-induced activation of dopamine receptors modulates FGF-2 expression in astrocytic cultures and promotes survival of dopaminergic neurons. *FASEB J., 20,* 1263-1265.

Lin, L. F., Doherty, D. H., Lile, J. D., Bektesh, S., & Collins, F. (1993). GDNF: a glial cell line-derived neurotrophic factor for midbrain dopaminergic neurons. *Science, 260,* 1130-1132.

Lindholm, P., Voutilainen, M. H., Lauren, J., Peranen, J., Leppanen, V. M., Andressoo, J. O. et al. (2007). Novel neurotrophic factor CDNF protects and rescues midbrain dopamine neurons in vivo. *Nature, 448,* 73-77.

Liou, H. H., Tsai, M. C., Chen, C. J., Jeng, J. S., Chang, Y. C., Chen, S. Y. et al. (1997). Environmental risk factors and Parkinson's disease: a case-control study in Taiwan. *Neurology, 48.*

Liu, K. H., Kim, C. S., & Kim, J. H. (2003). Human exposure assessment to mancozeb during treatment of mandarin fields. *Bull Environ Contam Toxicol, 70.*

Ma, S. Y., Rinne, J. O., Collan, Y., Roytta, M., & Rinne, U. K. (1996). A quantitative morphometrical study of neuron degeneration in the substantia nigra in Parkinson's disease. *J Neurol Sci, 140.*

Maher, P. A. (1996). Nuclear Translocation of fibroblast growth factor (FGF) receptors in response to FGF-2. *J Cell Biol, 134.*

Mason, I. (2007). Initiation to end point: the multiple roles of fibroblast growth factors in neural development. *Nat.Rev.Neurosci., 8,* 583-596.

Mayer, E., Dunnett, S. B., Pellitteri, R., & Fawcett, J. W. (1993a). Basic fibroblast growth factor promotes the survival of embryonic ventral mesencephalic dopaminergic neurons--I. Effects in vitro. *Neuroscience, 56,* 379-388.

Mayer, E., Fawcett, J. W., & Dunnett, S. B. (1993b). Basic fibroblast growth factor promotes the survival of embryonic ventral mesencephalic dopaminergic neurons--II. Effects on nigral transplants in vivo. *Neuroscience, 56.*

Mayeux, R., Denaro, J., Hemenegildo, N., Marder, K., Tang, M. X., Cote, L. J. et al. (1992). A population-based investigation of Parkinson's disease with and without dementia. Relationship to age and gender. *Arch Neurol, 49.*

Mizuta, I., Tsunoda, T., Satake, W., Nakabayashi, Y., Watanabe, M., Takeda, A. et al. (2008). Calbindin 1, fibroblast growth factor 20, and alpha-synuclein in sporadic Parkinson's disease. *Hum.Genet., 124,* 89-94.

Mogi, M., Togari, A., Kondo, T., Mizuno, Y., Komure, O., Kuno, S. et al. (1999). Brain-derived growth factor and nerve growth factor concentrations are decreased in the substantia nigra in Parkinson's disease. *Neurosci.Lett., 270,* 45-48.

Moller, A. (1992). Mean volume of pigmented neurons in the substantia nigra in Parkinson's disease. *Acta Neurol Scand Suppl, 137.*

Murase, S. & McKay, R. D. (2006). A specific survival response in dopamine neurons at most risk in Parkinson's disease. *J Neurosci, 26.*

Myers, J. M., Martins, G. G., Ostrowski, J., & Stachowiak, M. K. (2003). Nuclear trafficking of FGFR1: a role for the transmembrane domain. *J Cell Biochem, 88.*

Nagatsu, T., Mogi, M., Ichinose, H., & Togari, A. (2000). Changes in cytokines and neurotrophins in Parkinson's disease. *J.Neural Transm.Suppl,* 277-290.

Norris, E. H., Uryu, K., Leight, S., Giasson, B. I., Trojanowski, J. Q., & Lee, V. M. (2007). Pesticide exposure exacerbates alpha-synucleinopathy in an A53T transgenic mouse model. *Am J Pathol, 170.*

Otto, D. & Unsicker, K. (1993). FGF-2-mediated protection of cultured mesencephalic dopaminergic neurons against MPTP and MPP+: specificity and impact of culture conditions, non-dopaminergic neurons, and astroglial cells. *J Neurosci Res, 34.*

Parain, K., Murer, M. G., Yan, Q., Faucheux, B., Agid, Y., Hirsch, E. et al. (1999). Reduced expression of brain-derived neurotrophic factor protein in Parkinson's disease substantia nigra. *Neuroreport, 10,* 557-561.

Patel, S., Singh, V., Kumar, A., Gupta, Y. K., & Singh, M. P. (2006). Status of antioxidant defense system and expression of toxicant responsive genes in striatum of maneb- and paraquat-induced Parkinson's disease phenotype in mouse: mechanism of neurodegeneration. *Brain Res, 1081.*

Peng, J., Xie, L., Jin, K., Greenberg, D. A., & Andersen, J. K. (2008). Fibroblast growth factor 2 enhances striatal and nigral neurogenesis in the acute 1-methyl-4-phenyl-1,2,3,6-tetrahydropyridine model of Parkinson's disease. *Neuroscience, 153.*

Petrova, P., Raibekas, A., Pevsner, J., Vigo, N., Anafi, M., Moore, M. K. et al. (2003). MANF: a new mesencephalic, astrocyte-derived neurotrophic factor with selectivity for dopaminergic neurons. *J.Mol.Neurosci., 20,* 173-188.

Polymeropoulos, M. H., Lavedan, C., Leroy, E., Ide, S. E., Dehejia, A., Dutra, A. et al. (1997). Mutation in the alpha-synuclein gene identified in families with Parkinson's disease. *Science, 276.*

Reilly, J. F. & Maher, P. A. (2001). Importin beta-mediated nuclear import of fibroblast growth factor receptor: role in cell proliferation. *J Cell Biol, 152.*

Rodriguez-Oroz, M. C., Jahanshahi, M., Krack, P., Litvan, I., Macias, R., Bezard, E. et al. (2009). Initial clinical manifestations of Parkinson's disease: features and pathophysiological mechanisms. *Lancet Neurol., 8,* 1128-1139.

Rubin, R. & Strayer, D. S. (2012). *Rubin's Pathology: Clinicopathologic Foundations of Medicine.* (6 ed.) Baltimore, MD: Lippincott Williams & Wilkins.

Saunders-Pullman, R., Gordon-Elliott, J., Parides, M., Fahn, S., Saunders, H. R., & Bressman, S. (1999). The effect of estrogen replacement on early Parkinson's disease. *Neurology, 52.*

Stachowiak, E. K., Fang, X., Myers, J., Dunham, S., & Stachowiak, M. K. (2003). cAMP-induced differentiation of human neuronal progenitor cells is mediated by nuclear fibroblast growth factor receptor-1 (FGFR1). *J Neurochem, 84.*

Stachowiak, M. K., Maher, P. A., Joy, A., Mordechai, E., & Stachowiak, E. K. (1996). Nuclear accumulation of fibroblast growth factor receptors is regulated by multiple signals in adrenal medullary cells. *Mol Biol Cell, 7.*

Stachowiak, M. K., Maher, P. A., & Stachowiak, E. K. (2007). Integrative nuclear signaling in cell development--a role for FGF receptor-1. *DNA Cell Biol, 26.*

Strijks, E., Kremer, J. A., & Horstink, M. W. (1999). Effects of female sex steroids on Parkinson's disease in postmenopausal women. *Clin Neuropharmacol, 22.*

Tanner, C. M., Kamel, F., Ross, G. W., Hoppin, J. A., Goldman, S. M., Korell, M. et al. (2011). Rotenone, paraquat, and Parkinson's disease. *Environ.Health Perspect., 119,* 866-872.

Thiruchelvam, M., Richfield, E. K., Baggs, R. B., Tank, A. W., & Cory-Slechta, D. A. (2000). The nigrostriatal dopaminergic system as a preferential target of repeated exposures to combined paraquat and maneb: implications for Parkinson's disease. *J Neurosci, 20.*

Thiruchelvam, M., Richfield, E. K., Goodman, B. M., Baggs, R. B., & Cory-Slechta, D. A. (2002). Developmental exposure to the pesticides paraquat and maneb and the Parkinson's disease phenotype. *Neurotoxicology, 23,* 621-633.

Timmer, M., Cesnulevicius, K., Winkler, C., Kolb, J., Lipokatic-Takacs, E., Jungnickel, J. et al. (2007). Fibroblast growth factor (FGF)-2 and FGF receptor 3 are required for the development of the substantia nigra, and FGF-2 plays a crucial role for the rescue of dopaminergic neurons after 6-hydroxydopamine lesion. *J Neurosci, 27.*

Timmer, M., Muller-Ostermeyer, F., Kloth, V., Winkler, C., Grothe, C., & Nikkhah, G. (2004). Enhanced survival, reinnervation, and functional recovery of intrastriatal dopamine grafts co-transplanted with Schwann cells overexpressing high molecular weight FGF-2 isoforms. *Exp Neurol, 187.*

Tooyama, I., McGeer, E. G., Kawamata, T., Kimura, H., & McGeer, P. L. (1994). Retention of basic fibroblast growth factor immunoreactivity in dopaminergic neurons of the substantia nigra during normal aging in humans contrasts with loss in Parkinson's disease. *Brain Res., 656,* 165-168.

Valente, E. M., Abou-Sleiman, P. M., Caputo, V., Muqit, M. M., Harvey, K., Gispert, S. et al. (2004). Hereditary early-onset Parkinson's disease caused by mutations in PINK1. *Science, 304.*

Wang, G., van der Walt, J. M., Mayhew, G., Li, Y. J., Zuchner, S., Scott, W. K. et al. (2008). Variation in the miRNA-433 binding site of FGF20 confers risk for Parkinson disease by overexpression of alpha-synuclein. *Am.J.Hum.Genet., 82,* 283-289.

Zawada, W. M., Kirschman, D. L., Cohen, J. J., Heidenreich, K. A., & Freed, C. R. (1996). Growth factors rescue embryonic dopamine neurons from programmed cell death. *Exp Neurol, 140.*

Zhang, W. Q., Tilson, H. A., Nanry, K. P., Hudson, P. M., Hong, J. S., & Stachowiak, M. K. (1988). Increased dopamine release from striata of rats after unilateral nigrostriatal bundle damage. *Brain Res., 461,* 335-342.

Zimprich, A., Biskup, S., Leitner, P., Lichtner, P., Farrer, M., Lincoln, S. et al. (2004). Mutations in LRRK2 cause autosomal-dominant parkinsonism with pleomorphic pathology. *Neuron, 44.*

In: The Central Catecholaminergic System
Editor: Bertalan Dudás
ISBN: 978-1-63117-937-2

Chapter 9

Schizophrenia and the Dopaminergic System

Robert S. Miletich, Aaron Kucinski, Sridhar Narla, Courtney Benson, Scott Wersinger, Thomas D. Corso, Merouane Bencherif, Ewa K. Stachowiak and Michal K. Stachowiak

Introduction

Schizophrenia has been a scourge on all human societies in all locations on the planet. It affects approximately 1% of the population and it is characterized by three clusters of symptoms: positive, negative and cognitive (Kuepper et al., 2012; van Os & Kapur, 2009). Positive symptoms are those of psychosis, which includes hallucinations and delusions. Negative symptoms include emotional blunting, flattened affect, anhedonia, loss of motivation. Cognitive symptoms include deficits in working memory and executive function. Functional prognosis seems to be most related to the severity of these cognitive symptoms. These cognitive problems have been long recognized and are crystallized in Kraepelin's 1893 characterization of schizophrenia as "dementia praecox". Their probable relation to frontal lobe dysfunction was also recognized by Kraepelin. This "hypofrontality" has been characterized in multiple ways over the years, most recently with functional neuroimaging, where diminished frontal lobe activation has been associated with performance deficits in working memory, problem solving, shifting sets and executive cognitive processes (Meyer-Lindenberg et al., 2002; Simpson et al., 2010).

The dopamine hypothesis of schizophrenia stands as the predominant explanation of the disease's etiology and pathophysiology (Davis et al., 1991; Howes & Kapur, 2009; Kuepper et al., 2012; Simpson et al., 2010; Tost et al., 2010). Although its form has evolved since it was first proposed in the 1970's, the basic tenet that dopamine plays a central role in this disorder has remained valid. It was originally formed from the serendipitous discovery that chlorpromazine and other related compounds, called neuroleptics, had antipsychotic properties. It was at this same time epoch of the mid-20th century that dopamine was found in the brain and that it possessed neurotransmitter action. The dopamine hypothesis was strengthened with the observation that stimulant drugs, like amphetamine, acting through releasing catecholamines, especially dopamine, were capable of causing psychosis. The dopamine hypothesis of schizophrenia was firmly established in the 1970s when the newly developed receptor binding assay revealed that neuroleptic clinical efficacy directly correlated with dopamine receptor subtype D_2 affinity (Beaulieu & Gainetdinov, 2011; Howes & Kapur, 2009). This chapter will provide an overview of our current understandings of dopamine in schizophrenia. This is not a comprehensive review, as this is a very active literature. Over 3000 articles have been published on dopamine and schizophrenia in the past five years. Over 10 times that number have been published since the dopamine hypothesis was originally formulated in the mid-20th century.

The role of dopamine in schizophrenia has been elaborated by assays in both animal models and humans (Davis et al., 1991; Howes & Kapur, 2009; Tost et al., 2010). These have included histologic, anatomic, biochemical, electrophysiologic and behavioral investigations. In vivo functional neuroimaging studies have been particular fruitful as they allow study of the brain in living patients with schizophrenia. They also allow for the effect of antipsychotic drugs on brain activity to be quantified. It was initially posited that there was near uniform change in the dopamine systems of patients with schizophrenia. This specifically centered on dopamine receptors, in particular, the D_2 subtype. A number of groups found increased expression of D_2 receptors in schizophrenia.

Five subtypes of dopamine receptors have been identified. These subtypes can be categorizes into the D_1-like (D_1, D_5) and the D_2-like (D_2, D_3, D_4) families. The members of each family have similar pharmacology. These have different distributions in the brain. The highest concentrations are in the striatum where both D_1 and D_2 receptors are present. There are far fewer D_2 receptors in the cerebral cortex, where there is a predominance of D_1 receptors, highest in the frontal cortex. The number of D_3, D_4 and D_5 subtypes are low and no unequivocal role in the pathophysiology of schizophrenia has been identified (Beaulieu & Gainetdinov, 2011).

The presence of increased D_2 receptors in patients with schizophrenia was controversial for many years. Opposing camps using different tracers found either increases or no change of D_2 receptors (Davis et al., 1991; Howes & Kapur, 2009; D. F. Wong et al., 1986). A historical confound has been that D_2 receptor blockade, the main therapy of schizophrenia, results in a compensatory D_2 receptor upregulation. This indicates the need to study drug-naive and drug-withdrawn subjects if the native state of schizophrenia is to be characterized. With metanalytic pooling of all findings and control of experimental conditions, the weight of the evidence supports increased striatal D_2 receptor expression in patients with schizophrenia. The presence of D_1 receptor changes in the frontal cortices remains controversial and awaits more selective D_1 receptor probe development.

The dopamine hypothesis originally focused on the dopamine receptor. As more data accumulated, it was apparent that there are abnormalities of the dopaminergic neuron itself (Heinz & Schlagenhauf, 2010; Meyer-Lindenberg et al., 2002; Patel et al., 2010) (Figure 1). There is an enhancement of dopamine presynaptic activity, resulting in increased dopamine synthesis and increased baseline and stimulus-induced release of dopamine into the synaptic cleft. This results in increased dopamine receptor occupancy in both baseline and dopamine release-stimulated conditions. Functional neuroimaging has played a paramount role in these discoveries.

Functional neuroimaging and postmortem studies have not consistently revealed changes in the dopamine transporter (DAT) (Kuepper et al., 2012). Besides the increased dynamics of the striatal dopaminergic synapse, reflected in increased baseline and evoked dopamine release and D_2 receptor occupancy, there are abnormalities of other aspects of the dopaminergic neuron. There is a decreased size of dopaminergic neurons which is associated with decreased volumes of both the substantia nigra and ventral tegmental area. In patients with schizophrenia and Asperger's syndrome not subjected to neuroleptic treatments, there is a significant decrease in the volume of the substantia nigra (−21%) and reduction of mean nerve cell volume in the substantia nigra pars compacta (SNc) (−15%) and ventral tegmental area (VTA) (−17%) (Bogerts et al., 1983). Altered dendritic morphology (Ikemoto et al., 2009) and synaptic contacts (Kolomeets & Uranova, 1999) of dopaminergic neurons have also been reported in the brain of patients with schizophrenia.

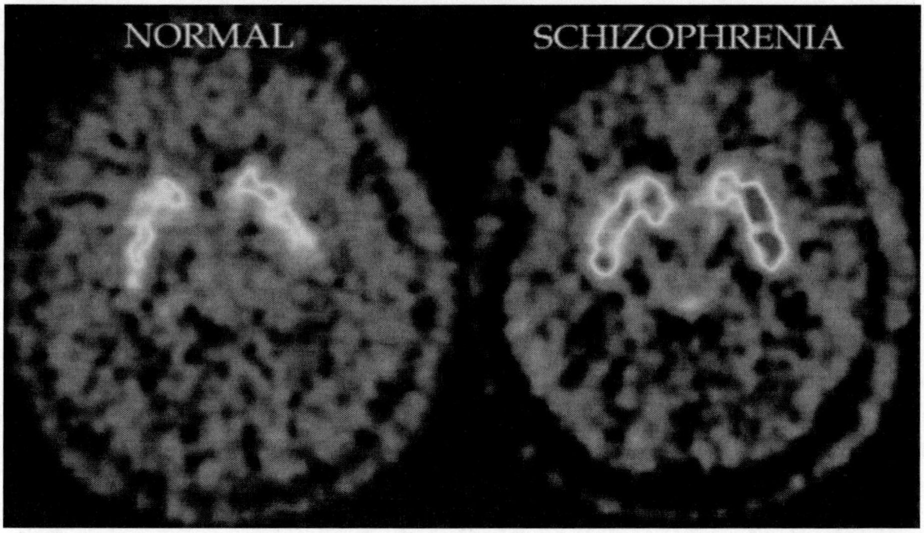

Figure 1. Human 6-[^{18}F]fluoro-L-dopa positron emission tomography of a normal volunteer (author RSM) on the left and a drug-withdrawn schizophrenic patient on the right. Images shown are brain uptake from 90 to 120 minutes after bolus IV administration. The greatest activity is present in the striatum, with lesser amounts of specific signal in the mesencephalon/diencephalon. There is greater 6-[^{18}F]fluoro-L-dopa striatal sequestration in schizophrenia, indicating increased presynaptic dopamine synthesis.

It also became apparent that the aberrant dopamine physiology was not homogenous across all dopaminergic neurons within the brain (Davis et al., 1991; Kuepper et al., 2012). There are different dopaminergic systems in the brain, identified by their cells of origin and their projections sites. The largest of these are the nigrostriatal, mesolimbic and mesocortical systems. Although there is some overlap between these dopaminergic systems, they are distinct by having different connections. The nigrostriatal system arises from cell bodies in the substantia nigra and innervates the dorsal striatum. The mesolimbic and mesocortical systems arise from cell bodies in the ventral tegmental area and innervate the ventral striatum with other limbic structures and cerebral cortex, respectively. An aged version of the dopamine hypothesis supported the mesolimbic dopaminergic system as having exclusive importance in schizophrenia. It is now apparent that there is pathophysiologic involvement of all three dopaminergic systems. The changes are not uniform in all dopaminergic systems. There is evidence of a frontal hypodopaminergia concomitant with the striatal hyperdopaminergia. The evidence has been stronger and more consistent for the striatal changes than for the frontal changes. Animal models have also shown an inverse relation between the striatal and cortical targeting dopaminergic systems (Meyer-Lindenberg et al., 2002; Simpson et al., 2010). This remains an area with uncertainties as to how this inverse relation develops and is maintained.

Not only are there disparate abnormalities of the different dopaminergic systems, there are also important interactions with other neurotransmitter systems, as well (Carlsson et al., 2001; Coyle et al., 2010; I. Klejbor et al., 2009; Patel et al., 2010; Shin et al., 2011). These interactions occur in both heterosynaptic loci, resulting in alterations of neurotransmitter release, but also in summed, sequential homosynaptic loci. The complexity of these neurotransmitter interactions stems from the fact that the significance of any neurotransmitter system resides within the neuronal connectivity network of which it is an element. In simpler words, the various neurotransmitter systems "talk" to one another. Thus, an abnormality in one necessarily affects the functions of others.

The second longstanding theory of schizophrenia is the serotonin hypothesis (5-HT) (Shin et al., 2011). This concept was initiated by the structural resemblance of hallucinogenic drugs to 5-HT, drugs which were capable of inducing psychosis. Much work has revealed that a significant component of the unique action of the newer atypical antipsychotics arises from their antagonist action at 5-HT receptors, in particular the 5-HT_{2A} subtype. The atypical antipsychotics, while useful for ameliorating the positive symptoms of schizophrenia, showed fewer motor side effects than the typical antipsychotics. They were also initially thought to have some efficacy in decreasing the negative schizophrenia symptoms, again unlike the typical antipsychotics. However, metanalysis has not borne this out (Coyle et al., 2010). Their therapeutic spectrum likely is due to this combined action on both 5-HT and D_2 receptors. The anatomic locus of this action is currently unknown. Some have supported a cortical site, while we, using a transgenic mouse schizophrenia model, have implicated brainstem 5-HT_{2A} receptors of importance (I. Klejbor et al., 2009). Using the known cellular connectivities of the substantia nigra and ventral tegmental area, we have proposed a model which readily explains the frontal hypodopaminergia and striatal hyperdopaminergia of schizophrenia and their therapeutic correction with blockade of both 5-HT_{2A} and D_2 receptors (I. Klejbor et al., 2009). Despite these more recent findings, it remains true that all antipsychotic drugs currently employed clinically have D_2 receptor antagonism as the major vehicle for their clinical efficacy.

It is clear that dopamine is involved in schizophrenia clinical expression. It is accepted that the striatal hyperdopaminergia is a key component for the expression of the positive symptoms of schizophrenia. The negative and cognitive schizophrenia symptoms are thought to result from limbic and frontal cortical dysfunction in schizophrenia (Kuepper et al., 2012). The negative and cognitive symptoms have been resistant to antipsychotic drug therapy. The cognitive symptoms of Kraepelin's dementia praecox have been refractory to intervention. However, all three symptom clusters are related to the underlying disease process. We have shown using positron emission tomography that the hypofrontality in shifting set executive cognitive function was directly correlated with the striatal hyperdopaminergia in the individual patient (Meyer-Lindenberg et al., 2002). This remains a very active field of investigation to this day as the need for effective pharmacologic therapy to address the negative and cognitive symptoms remains great. It has also been suggested that dopamine may play slightly different role in different phases of the disease (Patel et al., 2010).

A more recent formulation of the dopamine hypothesis acknowledges the separate scientific findings that dopamine is of importance for both reward mechanisms and for sensory salience. It is now thought that since dopamine mediates reward and salience assessment of sensory phenomena normally, that its primary importance with regard to mediation of the positive schizophrenia symptoms is related to abnormal sensory processing, resulting in hallucinations and in assigning inappropriate importance or aberrant salience to these abnormal sensations, fueling delusional thought processes (Heinz & Schlagenhauf, 2010; Kapur, 2004; Lau et al., 2013).

Abundant clinical data supports a neurodevelopment origin to schizophrenia (Bertolino & Blasi, 2009; Howes & Kapur, 2009; Lau et al., 2013; MacDonald & Schulz, 2009; Tost et al., 2010). This idea states that schizophrenia is an emergent illness whose etiology likely involves a multi-hit process wherein susceptibility genes interact with internal and external environmental factors, the interacting constellation of which ultimately results in the clinical syndrome. Environmental stress in multiple forms, including obstetrical, nurturing, physical and emotional deprivations, appears necessary for schizophrenia to emerge. We (I. Klejbor et al., 2006b; Stachowiak et al., 2013) and others (Terwisscha van Scheltinga et al., 2010) have strongly implicated disrupted FGF function in this process. The histologic alterations in human schizophrenia, including altered size of dopamine cells and their respective brain nuclei support the notion that this neurodevelopmental pathology affects dopaminergic systems. But how can changes in dopamine result in schizophrenia? What is the developmental mechanism? It may be that altered dopamine during neurodevelopment is actually related to the emergence of schizophrenia (Simpson et al., 2010). In support of this possibility, our recent work in a transgenic mouse model, th(tk-)/th(tk-), has replicated many of the structural and functional changes seen in human schizophrenia. This model produces aberrant functioning of the Integrative Nuclear FGF Signaling pathway (INFS) in developing dopaminergic neurons. As such, this work supports key roles for both dopaminergic systems and INFS in the origin of schizophrenia (I. Klejbor et al., 2006b; Stachowiak et al., 2013).

Although much progress has been made in understanding the role of dopamine in schizophrenia, many controversies and uncertainties remain. Primary among these remain the documentation of frontal lobe hypodopaminergia. The data which exists has been inconsistent, controversial and/or indirect. The presence of striatal hyperdopaminergia is well-established. Whether this plays an etiologic role is the development of schizophrenia is supported by indirect evidence and needs to be more firmly established. Dopamine alone is not responsible for this pathology and undoubtedly the interactions of regionally specific dopaminergic subsystems with other neurotransmitter systems are of importance as well. How alterations of dopamine function during development result in the altered anatomy needs to be elaborated. Many questions have been answered, but many questions remain. The fact remains though, that treatment based on dopamine has proven efficacious and useful, especially for the positive symptoms of schizophrenia. More selective target or cocktail approach addressing multiple neurotransmitter systems may further improve therapeutics.

It has been stated that the dopamine hypothesis does explain the pathophysiology of schizophrenia, but not necessarily the cause *per se* (Lau et al., 2013). We submit that the more proximate factors to the disease etiology is related to aberrant neurodevelopment which creates altered physiology for the dopaminergic system as well as other neurotransmitter systems, including 5-HT and nicotinic systems.

Modeling Schizophrenia in Transgenic Mice by Attenuation of Dopamine Neurons Development

In this context of dopamine hypothesis we developed a transgenic mouse model (Ilona Klejbor et al., 2006a), called th(tk-)/th(tk-) or *th-fgfr1(tk-)*, which results from hypoplastic development of dopaminergic neurons induced by a dominant negative mutant of FGFR1, tyrosine kinase-deleted FGFR1(TK-)(Ilona Klejbor et al., 2006a). Restriction of mutant expression to catecholamine-neurons containing brain regions (Ilona Klejbor et al., 2006a) is achieved by fusion with the tyrosine hydroxylase (TH) promoter. Similar to human schizophrenia, where histologic alterations, include altered size of dopaminergic cells and their respective brain nuclei (Bogerts et al., 1983) there was a reduction of size and density of SNc and VTA TH-immunoreactive neurons(Ilona Klejbor et al., 2006a). Paradoxically, there were increases of dopamine and its metabolites in terminal regions of the nigrostriatal dopaminergic system, consistent with increased dopamine transmission. In contrast, there appeared to be a reduction of these measures present in the prefrontal cortex. These findings are consistent with human PET studies(Meyer-Lindenberg et al., 2002) and postmortem evidence of increased subcortical dopamine synthesis in schizophrenia (Mueller et al., 2004; Toru et al., 1982).

How dopaminergic neuronal hypoplasia could paradoxically lead to dopamine hypertransmission in the subcortical basal ganglia with concurrent DA hypotransmission in the frontal cortex? In the developing brain, 5-HT and dopaminergic systems compete for neuronal target sites and a dynamic relationship between the two systems persists into adulthood (Bruno et al., 1987; Rodriguez-Pallares et al., 2003; Stachowiak et al., 1984). In FGFR1 knockout embryos and adult mice there was a caudal shift in embryonic and adult midbrain dopaminergic neurons and an increase in 5-HT neurons in that region (Jukkola et al., 2006). Quantitative immunohistology of adult *th-fgfr1(tk-)* mice revealed hyperinnervation of hypoplastic midbrain dopaminergic neurons by serotonergic terminals (Fig.2). This was corroborated by increased tissue levels of 5-HT and 5-HT metabolite 5-hydroxyindoleacetic acid (5-HIAA) in the SN and VTA of adult transgenic mice. Evidence suggests an overactive 5-HT system in schizophrenia (Bartfai et al., 1983; Hansson et al., 1994) (for discussion see also (I. Klejbor et al., 2009)) and drugs that target 5-HT receptors, including atypical antipsychotics (AAP), are efficacious against positive schizophrenia symptoms attributable to dopaminergic hypertransmission (Abel et al., 1996; Bartfai et al., 1983; Harrison, 1999; Lieberman et al., 1998; Schmidt et al., 1993). In *th-fgfr1(tk-)* mice, the hyperinnervation of substantia nigra pars reticulata (SNr) by 5-HT terminals may also contribute to dopamine hypertransmission while direct hyperinnervation of VTA dopaminergic neurons by serotonergic terminals could lead to dopamine hypotransmission in prefrontal cortex.(I. Klejbor et al., 2009) (Figure 2).

In *th-fgfr1(tk-)* mice, developmental targeting of midbrain dopaminergic neurons with the FGFR(TK-) mutation not only impairs midbrain dopaminergic neuronal morphology and dopamine transmission in the striatum but also causes abnormal neuronal layering and morphology in the frontal cortex. Stereological analysis of the anterior cingulate area of the brain cortex verified reduced densities of NeuN positive neurons in *th-fgfr1(tk-)* mice versus control C57bl/6J animals, which were confined to the first three layers - molecular, granular and outer pyramidal of the cortex. Moreover, cells with granular neuronal morphology were displaced into the superficial molecular layer and cortical stratification was less pronounced in transgenic mice. Thus, the hyperactivity of the nigrostriatal pathway might also perturb cortical development. Importantly, myelinated cortical fibers in *th-fgfr1(tk-)* mice were also disorganized. Neurons in these superficial layers integrate function of cortical columns and control the activities of glutamatergic projection neurons, which arise in deeper cortical layers and innervate to control striatal dopaminergic terminals and midbrain dopaminergic neurons.

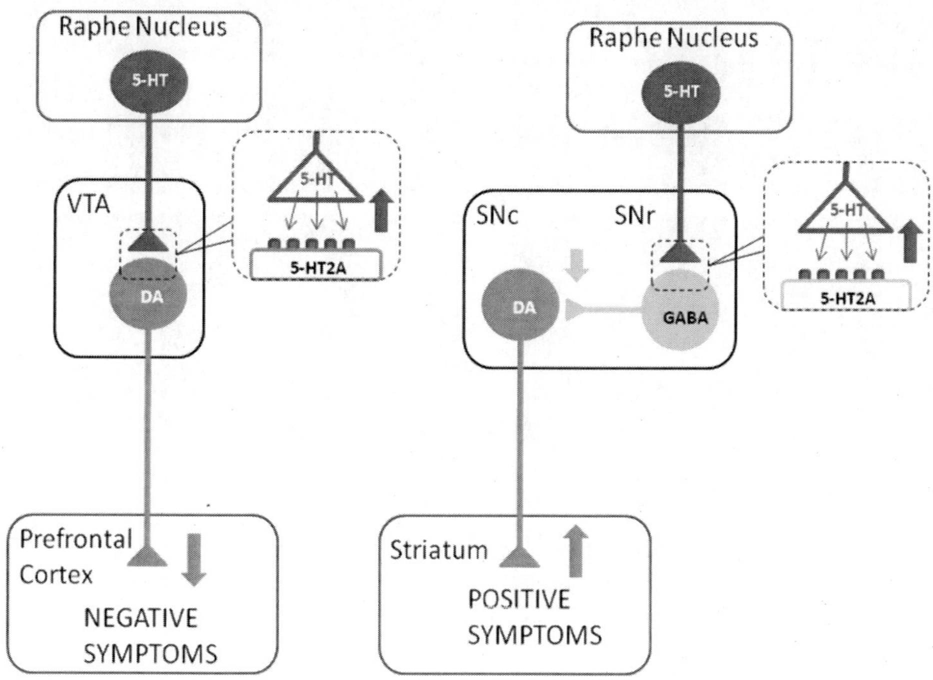

Figure 2. Correction of positive and negative symptoms in an FGF/dopamine developmental model of psychosis – why 5-HT_{2A} antagonists are effective therapeutic agents. Serotonergic hyperinnervation results in overstimulation of 5-HT_{2A} receptors in parabrachial pigmentosus and paranigral nuclei of the VTA and in the SNr. In VTA stimulation of 5-HT_{2A} reduces the activity of dopaminergic hypoplastic mesocortical neurons leading to hypofrontality and negative symptoms *(social disconnection)*. In contrast, overstimulation of 5-HT_{2A} in SNr may increase the activity of dopaminergic SNc neurons causing an excessive dopamine output by the hypoplastic nigro-striatal system and impaired sensory gating. Activation of the SNc dopaminergic neurons may be mediated by GABAergic SNr interneurons. Abbreviations: FGF-fibroblast growth factor, 5-HT – 5-Hydroxytryptamine, VTA – ventral tegmental area, SNr – substantia nigra pars reticulata, SNc – subtantia nigra pars compacta, DA - Dopamine, from: (I. Klejbor et al., 2009).

In summary, impaired development of dopaminergic neurons affects neuronal systems which are innervated by dopaminergic neurons or receive dopaminergic input indicating that developmental hypoplasia of dopaminergic neurons can lead to widespread structural brain disorganization as observed in schizophrenia (Figure 3).

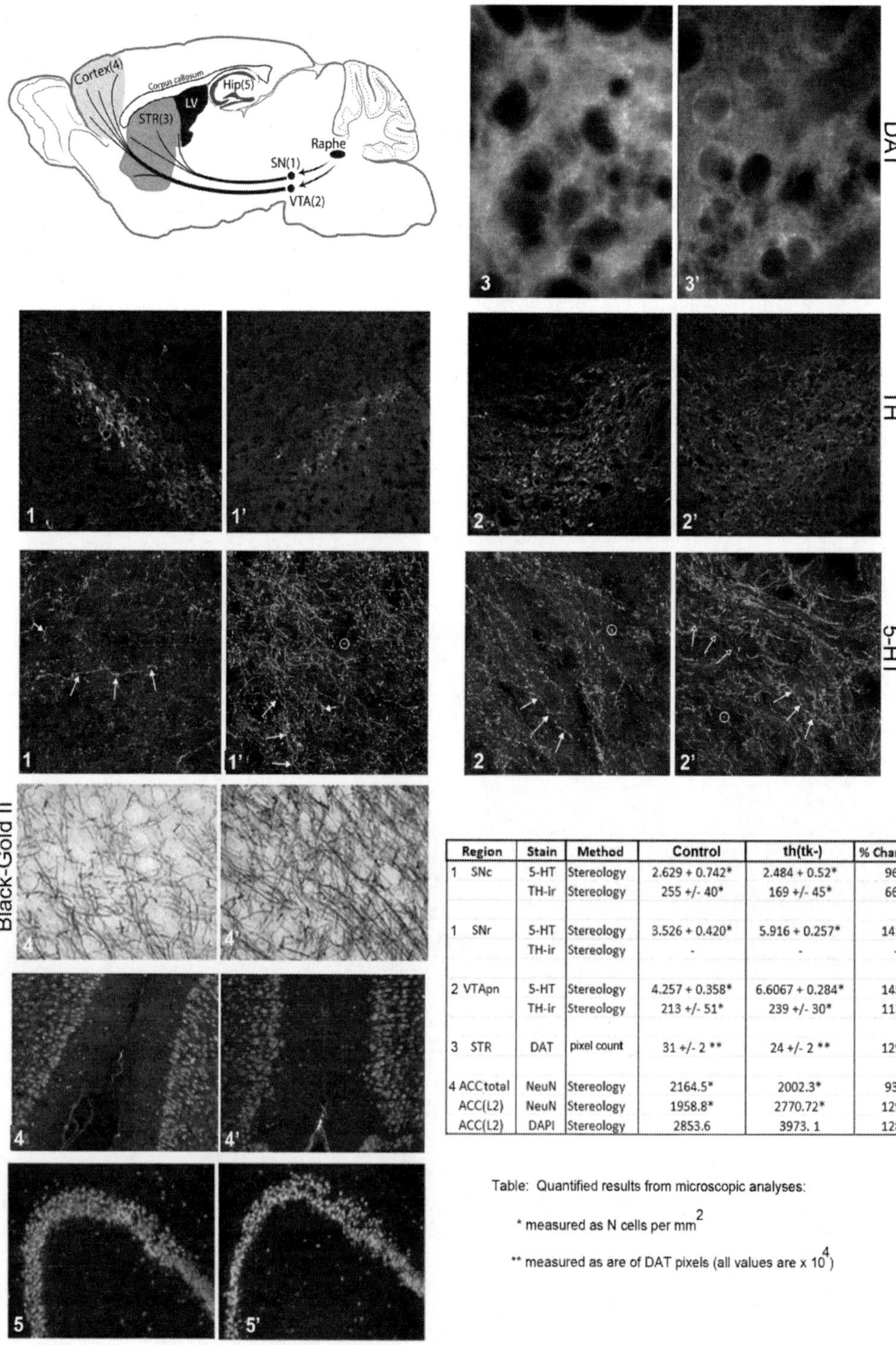

Region	Stain	Method	Control	th(tk-)	% Change
1 SNc	5-HT	Stereology	2.629 + 0.742*	2.484 + 0.52*	96%
	TH-ir	Stereology	255 +/- 40*	169 +/- 45*	66%
1 SNr	5-HT	Stereology	3.526 + 0.420*	5.916 + 0.257*	141%
	TH-ir	Stereology	-	-	-
2 VTApn	5-HT	Stereology	4.257 + 0.358*	6.6067 + 0.284*	145%
	TH-ir	Stereology	213 +/- 51*	239 +/- 30*	112%
3 STR	DAT	pixel count	31 +/- 2 **	24 +/- 2 **	129%
4 ACCtotal	NeuN	Stereology	2164.5*	2002.3*	93%
ACC(L2)	NeuN	Stereology	1958.8*	2770.72*	129%
ACC(L2)	DAPI	Stereology	2853.6	3973. 1	128%

Table: Quantified results from microscopic analyses:

* measured as N cells per mm^2

** measured as are of DAT pixels (all values are x 10^4)

Figure 3. Brain malformations in *th-fgfr1(tk-)* mice. Brain structures: 1–SN, 2–VTA, 3–striatum, 4–Anterior Cingulate Cortex, 5–hippocampus, pyramidal layer (from Stachowiak et al., 2013, Schizophrenia Research)

Dopaminergic systems: Examples of tyrosine hydroxylase (TH) immunoreactive (IR) fluorescent dopaminergic neurons in midbrain nuclei at postnatal day (PD) 360 of control and *th-fgfr1(tk-)* mice are shown. Stereological counting and measurements revealed reduced size of dopaminergic neurons at PD 0 (SNc -27%, VTA -21%) and at PD 360 (SNc -15%, VTA -10%). Density of dopaminergic neurons was reduced at PD 0 (SNc -26%, VTA -34%) and at PD 360 (SNc -34%). Density of terminals in striatum (3) expressing dopamine transporter protein (DAT) was reduced by 23% in *th-fgfr1(tk-)* mice (all differences are statistically significant) (I. Klejbor et al., 2006b).
5-HT systems: 5-HT-IR fluorescent cellular element neurons in midbrain nuclei of 6 months (PD 180) old mice. Brain sections were stained with anti-5-HT polyclonal Ab and Cy3 conjugated secondary Ab. Examples of 5-HT immunostaining in the VTA paranigral nucleus and substantia nigra pars reticulate (SNr) are shown. The 5-HT-IR fibers innervating the VTA or SN are predominantly smooth with small varicosities and thus similar to the D-type produced by the dorsal raphe nucleus (Fibiger & Miller, 1977; van der Kooy & Hattori, 1980). The PN has a dense network of long 5-HT-IR fibers with small varicosities, numerous puncta and smooth fibers without varicosities. In *th-fgfr1(tk-)* mice stereological counts revealed an increased number of incoming **5-HT fibers** in the paranigral nucleus (1) and the parabrachial pigmentosus nucleus of the VTA, as well as in the SNr (2) when compared to controls. These axons formed dense networks of 5-HT-IR fibers with numerous varicosities. Also, using HPLC analysis we found increased levels of 5-HT in the SN and increased 5-HT metabolite 5-Hydroxyindoleacetic acid (5-HIAA) in the VTA of adult *th-fgfr1(tk-)* mice (from: (I. Klejbor et al., 2009).
Cortical system (PD180): Gray matter staining cortical neurons with anti-NeuN antibody and stereological counting revealed -7.5% reduction of neuronal density in the Anterior Cingulate region. Subregional analysis of cortical layers revealed a 35% increase of NeuN+ cells and a 22% increase in DAPI+ cells in superficial cortical layers (Layers 1 and 2 sampled). Black-Gold II staining displayed more myelinated, disorganized fibers in *th-fgfr1(tk-)* mice compared to nontransgenic controls (S. Narla, C. Syposs, E.K. Stachowiak – previously unpublished observations).
Hippocampal pyramidal layer: Neurons stained with anti-NeuN. Preliminary analyses suggest reduced densities of pyramidal neurons in *th-fgfr1(tk-)* mice.

Behavioral Deficits and Reversal by Anti-Dopamine Drugs

The striatum, a center of convergence of input from descending cortical and lower brain regions, mediates goal-directed behavior and motor output by computing information related to cognition, motivation, sensory motor integration, and motor learning (Chudasama & Robbins, 2006; Gruber & McDonald, 2012). Hyperactive striatal dopaminergic transmission is an important feature of schizophrenia (Brunelin et al., 2013). One particular symptom of schizophrenia attributable to hyperactive striatal dopamine release is impaired sensorimotor gating, defined as a reduced ability to sort and filter sensory input and control motor reflex responses (Swerdlow & Geyer, 1998). Prepulse inhibition (PPI) of the startle response, a measure of sensorimotor gating, is determined by the extent that a subject's systematic bodily response to a moderately intense sensory stimulus is attenuated when immediately preceded by a ‘prepulse’ stimulus of a lower intensity. With normal gating circuitry, an organism learns to filter extraneous sensory input in order to focus attention and react appropriately to relevant sensory information. Reduced PPI in human patients often co-occurs with other cognitive impairments such as attention deficits and disorganized thought as well as positive symptoms such as hallucinations and delusions (Braff et al., 1999). Thus, impaired PPI potentially lies at the interface of cognitive dysfunction and positive symptoms and is widely considered a reliable endophenotypic marker of the disease (Braff, 2010; Koch, 2013; Takahashi et al., 2011). Systemic administration of dopamine releasing agent amphetamine and dopamine agonist apomorphine (Powell et al., 2009; Swerdlow & Geyer, 1998) as well as local application of apomorphine into the striatum (Wan et al., 1995) disrupts PPI in rodents. Furthermore, typical antipsychotics that block D_2 receptors attenuate PPI deficits (Mansbach et al., 1988).

In the *th-fgfr1(tk-)* mouse model, which features a developmental disruption of midbrain dopaminergic neurons and elevated striatal dopamine transmission, acoustic PPI of the startle response is severely reduced in adult animals (Hauser et al., 2009; I. Klejbor et al., 2009; I. Klejbor et al., 2006b; Kucinski et al., 2012). Similar PPI deficits have been observed in other genetic models of schizophrenia and in mice with hyper-dopaminergic tone such as dopamine transporter protein (DAT) knockout mice (Geyer et al., 2002; Powell et al., 2009; Ralph et al., 2001). In schizophrenia, behavioral symptoms often follow a predictable time course with cognitive impairments typically appearing in childhood, and positive symptoms and negative symptoms, such as social and motivational deficits, manifesting in late adolescence or early adulthood, despite the presence of genetic and anatomical abnormalities at birth (Thompson et al., 2004; A. H. Wong & Van Tol, 2003). In *th-fgfr1(tk-)* mice, reduced PPI does not appear until approximately 4 months of age relative to controls. This delayed onset coincides with evolving neurochemical changes in transgenic mice. For example, increased tissue levels of dopamine in the striatum and 5-HT in the midbrain relative to controls are not observed until adulthood (I. Klejbor et al., 2009; I. Klejbor et al., 2006b). Thus, the developmental dopamine *-th-fgfr1(tk-)* model uniquely recreates a temporal aspect of the human disease. The reduced PPI in adult *th-fgfr1(tk-)* mice is normalized with systemic administration of the D_2 receptor antagonist (typical antipsychotic) flupentixol (I. Klejbor et al., 2006b).

Schizophrenia patients often simultaneously display symptoms attributable to cortical reduction of dopamine transmission (negative symptoms and cognitive dysfunction) and elevated subcortical (striatal) dopamine activity (positive symptoms), perhaps reflecting the interconnectedness of cortical and subcortical brain regions. Disruption of cortical layering and connections were also found in *th-fgfr1(tk-)* mice (Figure 3), and may play a role in sensory gating, cognitive and social behavior deficits.

Mirroring human schizophrenia patients that exhibit reduced social interactions and an inability to form new contacts, *th-fgfr1(tk-)* mice displayed reduced social interaction in a resident-intruder paradigm, not attributable to anxiety-related behavior(Hauser et al., 2009; I. Klejbor et al., 2009). Another feature of schizophrenia associated with reduced cortical dopamine is working memory impairments (Davis et al., 1991; Goldman-Rakic et al., 2004). Using a behavioral paradigm that tests for temporal (recent versus old) components of working memory (DeVito et al., 2009), *th-fgfr1(tk-)* mice were found to be unable to distinguish between old and recently investigated objects, a distinction that was successfully made by control mice, indicating working memory dysfunction.

In addition to developmental abnormalities of the nigrostriatal dopaminergic system in *th-fgfr1(tk-)* mice, the co-developing serotonergic system also develops abnormally, evident by 5-HT axonal hyperplasia and elevated 5-HT release in adult mice (as discussed above and on Figure 2) In recent years, atypical antipsychotics (AAP) have often shown efficacy in treating both the positive and negative symptoms of schizophrenia and are effective in autism (Rausch et al., 2005) through strong 5-HT_{2A} and weaker D_2 receptor antagonism (Gray & Roth, 2007; Meltzer et al., 2003). Increased levels of 5-HT metabolite 5-hydroxyindoleacetic acid (5-HIAA) have been reported (Hansson et al., 1994) in human schizophrenia patients and the observed increase in ratio of 5-HT to dopamine metabolites predicts a favorable response to clozapine treatment (Pickar et al., 1994). It has been suggested that in the first episode, since they respond very well to selective 5-HT_{2A} antagonism, subjects with schizophrenia have an enhanced central serotonin tone, as supported by the increased fenfluramine-induced prolactin response (Abel et al., 1996). There is a general consensus that 5-HT_{2A} antagonistic therapeutic action of atypical antipsychotic drugs is through an influence on dopamine function (Gray & Roth, 2007; Lieberman et al., 1998; Meltzer et al., 2003). Serotonin neurons originating in the dorsal and main raphe nuclei innervate dopaminergic terminal regions (e.g. prefrontal cortex and striatum). The strongest 5-HT innervation is in the ventral midbrain structures, including the VTA and SN (Moukhles et al., 1997), suggesting that observed changes in CSF 5-HIAA levels in schizophrenia could reflect alterations that occur in 5-HT terminals in this brain region.

Blocking 5-HT_{2A} receptors in *th-fgfr1(tk-)* mice with specific antagonist M100907 normalized PPI and startle impairments (I. Klejbor et al., 2009). The atypical antipsychotics clozapine and quetiapine also normalized PPI while quetiapine and M100907, but not clozapine, improved social withdrawal, mimicking findings in human patients (Zhong et al., 2006). We hypothesized that 5-HT_{2A} antagonism improved PPI deficits in *th-fgfr1(tk-)* mice by attenuating the inhibitory influence of hyperinnervating 5-HT fibers onto GABAergic interneurons of the SNr, thus increasing inhibition of SNc midbrain neurons and subsequently decreasing dopamine release into the striatum. Simultaneously, blockade of 5-HT_{2A} receptors directly on the somatodendritic regions of VTA neurons may increase 5-HT-mediated dopamine release in the frontal cortex and improve social withdrawal (I. Klejbor et al., 2009).

Recently, the nicotinic acetylcholine system has emerged as potential target for supplemental or alternative therapies to common neuroleptic treatments for schizophrenia therapy. Schizophrenia patients smoke at a remarkably high rate and volume relative to the general population (Dome et al., 2010; Tidey et al., 2005; Williams et al., 2010). Numerous studies confirm that the primary psychoactive chemical in cigarette smoke, nicotine, improves cognitive function and enhances emotionality and motivation (Adan et al., 2004; Harris et al., 2004; Levin et al., 2006; Newhouse et al., 2004; Stolerman et al., 2000). Smoking and nicotine administration improve impaired PPI in schizophrenic patients (Kumari et al., 2001; Postma et al., 2006; Woznica et al., 2009), an effect mediated by central neuronal nicotinic receptors (NNRs) (George et al., 2006). NNRs have a widespread and dense localization on multiple neuronal systems, including dopaminergic, GABAegic and glutamatergic neurons (Albuquerque et al., 2009; Wonnacott, 1997). The α7 NNR subtype in particular (NNRs are comprised of pentameric combinations of α and β subunits; α7 receptors have five α subunits) has a close association with dopaminergic systems in the midbrain, striatum and cortex (Kaiser & Wonnacott, 2000; Livingstone et al., 2009; Mameli-Engvall et al., 2006; Wonnacott et al., 2000), thus in position to mediate abnormal dopamine release in multiple brain regions affected in schizophrenia.

In *th-fgfr1(tk-)* mice, selective α7 NNR agonists TC-5619 and TC-7020 (Marrero et al., 2010) improved PPI deficits (Hauser et al., 2009; Kucinski et al., 2012) consistent with the effects of α7 NNR agonists on PPI in other mouse models of schizophrenia (Acker et al., 2008; Hajos et al., 2005; Kohnomi et al., 2010; Tietje et al., 2008; Wallace et al., 2011). Interestingly, low doses of AAP clozapine and TC-5619 that alone had no effect additively enhanced PPI (Hauser et al., 2009), consistent with previous studies showing that nicotine enhanced clozapine's alleviating effects on PPI and other cognitive impairments (Levin et al., 2005; Levin & Rezvani, 2007). α7 NNRs are found on 5-HT neurons in the dorsal raphe and may influence 5-HT release (Aznar et al., 2005). Furthermore, 5-HT is an antagonist of α7-wild-type NNR through interactions at, or near the acetylcholine-binding sites (Fucile et al., 2002). Hence, α7 NNR agonists could function to overcome the potential suppression of α7 NNR activity by excessive 5-HT released from the hyperplastic 5-HT terminals. In addition to the therapeutic effects on PPI, α7 NNRs agonists were found to improve behavioral impairments associated with hypofrontality in *th-fgfr1(tk-)* mice. TC-5619 improved social interaction deficits, an effect that was augmented by clozapine (Hauser et al., 2009) TC-7020 increased investigation preference for old objects in transgenic animals, suggesting an improvement in working memory. The improvement of working memory by TC-7020 in *th-fgfr1(tk-)* mice may be associated with the normalization of hyperactive dopamine release in the dorsal striatum by α7 NNR agonism as previously demonstrated (Kucinski et al., 2012). Recent reports have suggested that the dorsal striatum plays an important role in cognitive function mediated by dopamine activity (Cools, 2011; Simpson et al., 2010). It was also shown that α7 NNR agonism and an α7 allosteric potentiator increased dopamine release in the PFC of rats (Livingstone et al., 2009), an effect that could potentially mediate and enhance executive functions such as working memory and attention (Floresco & Magyar, 2006; Schultz, 2002). Thus, agonism of α7 NNRs may facilitate the normalization of impaired dopamine transmission in multiple brain regions and offer the possibility that α7 nicotinic-targeting compounds improve cognitive function in human patients.

Dopamine Hyper-Release and Normalization with Drugs

To further investigate potential hypertransmission of dopamine in the striatum of *th-fgfr1(tk−)* mice and its role in the manifestation of schizophrenia-like symptoms in these mice, *in vivo* microdialysis was performed while mice simultaneously underwent PPI testing (Kucinski et al., 2012)(Figure 4). Although no differences in dopamine release between *th-fgfr1(tk−)* mice and controls were observed during baseline activity, the transgenic mice showed a robust elevation of dopamine in the dorsal striatum during the acoustic PPI test session. An elevation of dopamine during phasic activity is consistent with evidence from human schizophrenia patients that striatal dopamine transmission is most pronounced during periods when psychotic episodes are likely to manifest (Laruelle et al., 1999). Furthermore, the dopamine hypertransmission provides experimental support for the human schizophrenia hypothesis that excessive striatal dopamine release disrupts normal inhibitory gating circuitry and contributes to reduced cognitive control over sensory filtering and motor reflex responses. The elevation of dopamine release in the dorsal striatum is consistent with recent PET evidence that increases in amphetamine-induced dopamine release in schizophrenia patients is more pronounced in the caudate nucleus of the dorsal striatum than the ventral striatum (Kegeles et al., 2010). The ventral tier of the striatum (nucleus accumbens) is known to be a center of integration for computation of information related to motivation, reward and emotion (Sesack & Grace, 2010). The dorsal striatum, on the other hand, is comprised of the putamen, which has strong connections with primary motor cortical areas that control basic movement, and the caudate, which forms close associations with cognitive regions of the frontal cortex that are involved in higher level processing of sensory information (Grahn et al., 2009). The elevated tissue levels of dopamine and dopamine metabolites in the dorsal striatum of *th-fgfr(tk−)* mice together with elevated dopamine release during PPI testing together provide strong evidence that hypertransmission in this region is a primary culprit of a cognitive/ positive schizophrenia-like symptom.

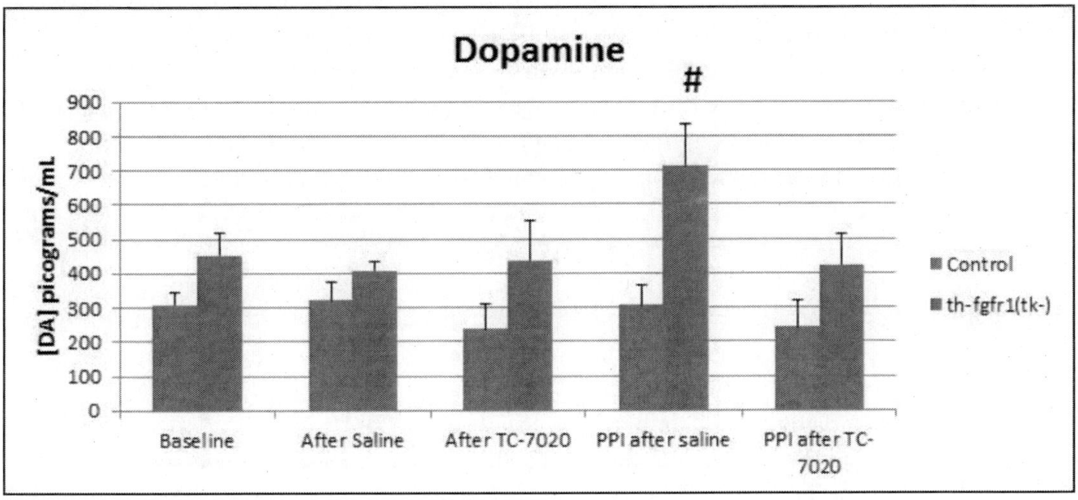

Figure 4. Dopamine release in the striatum during an acoustic PPI test session *th-fgfr1(tk-)* and control mice. The levels of dopamine (picograms/mL) collected under various conditions. Data from both treatment groups were combined for the baseline data (n = 10 control and 10 *th-fgfr1(tk-)* mice). The values are the means of single values derived for each mouse from the average amount of dopamine in two (for post injection) or three (baseline and post PPI) successive fractions per condition. # Significant difference between control and *th-fgfr1(tk-)* ($p<0.05$ post hoc after main effect of genotype, from: (Kucinski et al., 2012).

Administration of α7 NNR agonist during PPI testing TC-7020 normalized excessive striatal dopamine release in *th-fgfr(tk−)* mice, directly demonstrating an α7 NNR-mediated suppression of schizophrenia-associated hyperdopaminergic innervations (Kucinski et al., 2012)(Figure 4). α7 NNRs are selectively localized on midbrain dopaminergic neurons in the SNc and VTA as well as on glutamate terminals in the midbrain and striatum, which are in close contact with dopaminergic neurons (Champtiaux et al., 2003; Gotti et al., 2009; Jones & Wonnacott, 2004; Salminen et al., 2004). This places α7 NNRs in a position to mediate dopaminergic neuronal firing and excessive striatal dopamine release. Furthermore, it was also shown in rats that α7 NNR agonists increased dopamine release in the PFC (Livingstone et al., 2009). Dopamine release in the PFC was shown to be mediated in part by the α7 NNRs in a manner that is regulated by "cross-talk" with glutamate terminals (Livingstone et al., 2009). Thus, α7 NNR agonism could improve cognitive and negative symptoms by enhancing impaired dopamine transmission in the PFC. In total, systemic activation of nicotinic receptors appears to have the potential to simultaneously mediate cortical and subcortical impairments of dopamine transmission as well as the activity of other transmitter systems impaired in schizophrenia.

New Models to Understand Schizophrenia

While new drug targets help treat more symptoms of schizophrenia they do not alter the fundamental pathology of the impaired dopamine system. While the role of impaired development of dopaminergic system has been known for decades it is only recently that the progress has been made in understanding the underlying genetic cause of this impaired dopamine system. A network of some 160 genes selected from linkage, association, and gene expression literature reports have been proposed to contribute to the etiology of the disease (Rodriguez-Murillo et al., 2012; Sun). These genes mediate a wide range of neurodevelopmental events including progenitor cell proliferation and differentiation, migration, cytoskeleton reorganization, axonal connectivity and patterning of brain structures (Ayalew et al., 2012; Jaaro-Peled et al., 2009; Moskvina et al., 2009; Potkin et al., 2010; Sun et al., 2010).

How does altered expression of such a variety of genes lead to the complex set of abnormalities observed in the schizophrenic brain? It has been hypothesized that the protein products of these genes converge on common neurodevelopmental pathways that affect the development of multiple neural circuits and neurotransmitter systems. One such neurodevelopmental pathway is Integrative Nuclear FGFR1 Signaling (INFS). INFS integrates diverse neurogenic signals that direct the postmitotic development of embryonic stem cells, neural progenitors and immature neurons, by direct gene reprogramming. Additionally, FGFR1 and its partner proteins link multiple upstream pathways in which schizophrenia-linked genes are known to function and interact directly with those genes. To test such a hypothesis a new model system is required.

One promising model is human induced pluripotent stem cells (hiPSCs) reprogrammed from fibroblasts. Using skin cells from patients with schizophrenia provides a non-invasive *in vitro* model to study disease states from individual patients. Fibroblasts from control and schizophrenia patients were reprogrammed into human induced pluripotent stem cells (hiPSCs) using transcription factors OCT4, SOX2, KLF4, cMYC, and LIN28 (Brennand et al., 2011). The hiPSCs were differentiated into neural progenitor cells (NPCs), which were further developed into mature neurons for one to three months. When hiPSC neurons were co-cultured with astrocytes, robust synapse maturation and neuronal connectivity occurred.

Most hiPSC-derived neurons were glutamatergic and expressed VGLUT1, approximately 30% of the neurons were GABAergic, expressing GAD65/67, and less than 10% of the neurons were dopaminergic, testing positive for tyrosine-hydroxylase. When derived from patients with schizophrenia, hiPSC neurons displayed a marked decrease in neuronal connectivity as compared to hiPSC neurons derived from controls. Schizophrenia patients' hiPSC neurons displayed a decrease in the number of neurites, suggesting a decrease in synaptic maturation. A total of 596 unique genes were found significantly up- or down-regulated in hiPSC neurons derived from patients with schizophrenia as compared to hiPSC neurons derived from controls. Expression of genes encoding glutamate receptors, dopamine receptors, cAMP, and WNT were impaired in hiPSC neurons derived from patients with schizophrenia, which are required for refining synaptic connections and long-term potentiation. This data supports the model of schizophrenia whereby combinations of different gene disruptions disturb the key pathways affected in schizophrenia. Further investigation of hiPSC derived from schizophrenic patients may reveal specific developmental and functional impairments of dopaminergic neurons, and the role INFS plays in it.

References

Abel, K. M., O'Keane, V., & Murray, R. M. (1996). Enhancement of the prolactin response to d-fenfluramine in drug-naive schizophrenic patients. *Br J Psychiatry, 168*(1), 57-60.

Acker, B. A., Jacobsen, E. J., Rogers, B. N., Wishka, D. G., Reitz, S. C., Piotrowski, D. W., et al. (2008). Discovery of N-[(3R,5R)-1-azabicyclo[3.2.1]oct-3-yl]furo[2,3-c]pyridine-5-carboxamide as an agonist of the alpha7 nicotinic acetylcholine receptor: in vitro and in vivo activity. *Bioorg Med Chem Lett, 18*(12), 3611-3615.

Adan, A., Prat, G., & Sanchez-Turet, M. (2004). Effects of nicotine dependence on diurnal variations of subjective activation and mood. *Addiction, 99*(12), 1599-1607.

Albuquerque, E. X., Pereira, E. F., Alkondon, M., & Rogers, S. W. (2009). Mammalian nicotinic acetylcholine receptors: from structure to function. *Physiol Rev, 89*(1), 73-120.

Ayalew, M., Le-Niculescu, H., Levey, D. F., Jain, N., Changala, B., Patel, S. D., et al. (2012). Convergent functional genomics of schizophrenia: from comprehensive understanding to genetic risk prediction. *Mol Psychiatry.*

Aznar, S., Kostova, V., Christiansen, S. H., & Knudsen, G. M. (2005). Alpha 7 nicotinic receptor subunit is present on serotonin neurons projecting to hippocampus and septum. *Synapse, 55*(3), 196-200.

Bartfai, A., Levander, S. E., & Sedvall, G. (1983). Smooth pursuit eye movements, clinical symptoms, CSF metabolites, and skin conductance habituation in schizophrenic patients. *Biol Psychiatry, 18*(9), 971-987.

Beaulieu, J. M., & Gainetdinov, R. R. (2011). The physiology, signaling, and pharmacology of dopamine receptors. *Pharmacol Rev, 63*(1), 182-217.

Bertolino, A., & Blasi, G. (2009). The genetics of schizophrenia. *Neuroscience, 164*(1), 288-299.

Bogerts, B., Hantsch, J., & Herzer, M. (1983). A morphometric study of the dopamine-containing cell groups in the mesencephalon of normals, Parkinson patients, and schizophrenics. *Biol Psychiatry, 18*(9), 951-969.

Braff, D. L. (2010). Prepulse inhibition of the startle reflex: a window on the brain in schizophrenia. *Curr Top Behav Neurosci, 4*, 349-371.

Braff, D. L., Swerdlow, N. R., & Geyer, M. A. (1999). Symptom correlates of prepulse inhibition deficits in male schizophrenic patients. *Am J Psychiatry, 156*(4), 596-602.

Brennand, K. J., Simone, A., Jou, J., Gelboin-Burkhart, C., Tran, N., Sangar, S., et al. (2011). Modelling schizophrenia using human induced pluripotent stem cells. *Nature, 473*(7346), 221-225.

Brunelin, J., Fecteau, S., & Suaud-Chagny, M. F. (2013). Abnormal striatal dopamine transmission in schizophrenia. *Curr Med Chem, 20*(3), 397-404.

Bruno, J. P., Jackson, D., Zigmond, M. J., & Stricker, E. M. (1987). Effect of dopamine-depleting brain lesions in rat pups: role of striatal serotonergic neurons in behavior. *Behav Neurosci, 101*(6), 806-811.

Carlsson, A., Waters, N., Holm-Waters, S., Tedroff, J., Nilsson, M., & Carlsson, M. L. (2001). Interactions between monoamines, glutamate, and GABA in schizophrenia: new evidence. *Annu Rev Pharmacol Toxicol, 41*, 237-260.

Champtiaux, N., Gotti, C., Cordero-Erausquin, M., David, D. J., Przybylski, C., Lena, C., et al. (2003). Subunit composition of functional nicotinic receptors in dopaminergic neurons investigated with knock-out mice. *Journal of Neuroscience, 23*(21), 7820-7829.

Chudasama, Y., & Robbins, T. W. (2006). Functions of frontostriatal systems in cognition: comparative neuropsychopharmacological studies in rats, monkeys and humans. *Biol Psychol, 73*(1), 19-38.

Cools, R. (2011). Dopaminergic control of the striatum for high-level cognition. *Curr Opin Neurobiol, 21*(3), 402-407.

Coyle, J. T., Balu, D., Benneyworth, M., Basu, A., & Roseman, A. (2010). Beyond the dopamine receptor: novel therapeutic targets for treating schizophrenia. *Dialogues Clin Neurosci, 12*(3), 359-382.

Davis, K. L., Kahn, R. S., Ko, G., & Davidson, M. (1991). Dopamine in schizophrenia: a review and reconceptualization. *Am J Psychiatry, 148*(11), 1474-1486.

DeVito, L. M., Konigsberg, R., Lykken, C., Sauvage, M., Young, W. S., 3rd, & Eichenbaum, H. (2009). Vasopressin 1b receptor knock-out impairs memory for temporal order. *J Neurosci, 29*(9), 2676-2683.

Dome, P., Lazary, J., Kalapos, M. P., & Rihmer, Z. (2010). Smoking, nicotine and neuropsychiatric disorders. *Neurosci Biobehav Rev, 34*(3), 295-342.

Fibiger, H. C., & Miller, J. J. (1977). An anatomical and electrophysiological investigation of the serotonergic projection from the dorsal raphenucleus to the substantia nigra in the rat. *Neuroscience, 2*, 975-987.

Floresco, S. B., & Magyar, O. (2006). Mesocortical dopamine modulation of executive functions: beyond working memory. *Psychopharmacology (Berl), 188*(4), 567-585.

Fucile, S., Palma, E., Eusebi, F., & Miledi, R. (2002). Serotonin antagonizes the human neuronal alpha7 nicotinic acetylcholine receptor and becomes an agonist after L248T alpha7 mutation. *Neuroscience, 110*(1), 169-179.

George, T. P., Termine, A., Sacco, K. A., Allen, T. M., Reutenauer, E., Vessicchio, J. C., et al. (2006). A preliminary study of the effects of cigarette smoking on prepulse inhibition in schizophrenia: involvement of nicotinic receptor mechanisms. *Schizophr Res, 87*(1-3), 307-315.

Geyer, M. A., McIlwain, K. L., & Paylor, R. (2002). Mouse genetic models for prepulse inhibition: an early review. *Mol Psychiatry, 7*(10), 1039-1053.

Goldman-Rakic, P. S., Castner, S. A., Svensson, T. H., Siever, L. J., & Williams, G. V. (2004). Targeting the dopamine D1 receptor in schizophrenia: insights for cognitive dysfunction. *Psychopharmacology (Berl), 174*(1), 3-16.

Gotti, C., Clementi, F., Fornari, A., Gaimarri, A., Guiducci, S., Manfredi, I., et al. (2009). Structural and functional diversity of native brain neuronal nicotinic receptors. *Biochem Pharmacol, 78*(7), 703-711.

Grahn, J. A., Parkinson, J. A., & Owen, A. M. (2009). The role of the basal ganglia in learning and memory: neuropsychological studies. *Behav Brain Res, 199*(1), 53-60.

Gray, J. A., & Roth, B. L. (2007). The pipeline and future of drug development in schizophrenia. *Mol Psychiatry, 12*(10), 904-922.

Gruber, A. J., & McDonald, R. J. (2012). Context, emotion, and the strategic pursuit of goals: interactions among multiple brain systems controlling motivated behavior. *Front Behav Neurosci, 6*, 50.

Hajos, M., Hurst, R. S., Hoffmann, W. E., Krause, M., Wall, T. M., Higdon, N. R., et al. (2005). The selective alpha7 nicotinic acetylcholine receptor agonist PNU-282987 [N-[(3R)-1-Azabicyclo[2.2.2]oct-3-yl]-4-chlorobenzamide hydrochloride] enhances GABAergic synaptic activity in brain slices and restores auditory gating deficits in anesthetized rats. *J Pharmacol Exp Ther, 312*(3), 1213-1222.

Hansson, L. O., Waters, N., Winblad, B., Gottfries, C. G., & Carlsson, A. (1994). Evidence for biochemical heterogeneity in schizophrenia: a multivariate study of monoaminergic indices in human post-mortal brain tissue. *J Neural Transm Gen Sect, 98*(3), 217-235.

Harris, J. G., Kongs, S., Allensworth, D., Martin, L., Tregellas, J., Sullivan, B., et al. (2004). Effects of nicotine on cognitive deficits in schizophrenia. *Neuropsychopharmacology, 29*(7), 1378-1385.

Harrison, P. J. (1999). The neuropathology of schizophrenia. A critical review of the data and their interpretation. *Brain, 122 (Pt 4)*, 593-624.

Hauser, T. A., Kucinski, A., Jordan, K. G., Gatto, G. J., Wersinger, S. R., Hesse, R. A., et al. (2009). TC-5619: an alpha7 neuronal nicotinic receptor-selective agonist that demonstrates efficacy in animal models of the positive and negative symptoms and cognitive dysfunction of schizophrenia. *Biochem Pharmacol, 78*(7), 803-812.

Heinz, A., & Schlagenhauf, F. (2010). Dopaminergic dysfunction in schizophrenia: salience attribution revisited. *Schizophr Bull, 36*(3), 472-485.

Howes, O. D., & Kapur, S. (2009). The dopamine hypothesis of schizophrenia: version III--the final common pathway. *Schizophr Bull, 35*(3), 549-562.

Ikemoto, K., Nishi, K., Kunii, Y., Wada, A., Yang, Q., Takase, I., et al. (2009). A study of monoamine neuronal systems of schizophrenic patients: using forensic autopsy brains. *Leg Med (Tokyo), 11 Suppl 1*, S165-167.

Jaaro-Peled, H., Hayashi-Takagi, A., Seshadri, S., Kamiya, A., Brandon, N. J., & Sawa, A. (2009). Neurodevelopmental mechanisms of schizophrenia: understanding disturbed postnatal brain maturation through neuregulin-1-ErbB4 and DISC1. *Trends Neurosci, 32*(9), 485-495.

Jones, I. W., & Wonnacott, S. (2004). Precise localization of alpha7 nicotinic acetylcholine receptors on glutamatergic axon terminals in the rat ventral tegmental area. *Journal of Neuroscience, 24*(50), 11244-11252.

Jukkola, T., Lahti, L., Naserke, T., Wurst, W., & Partanen, J. (2006). FGF regulated gene-expression and neuronal differentiation in the developing midbrain-hindbrain region. *Dev Biol, 297*(1), 141-157.

Kaiser, S., & Wonnacott, S. (2000). alpha-bungarotoxin-sensitive nicotinic receptors indirectly modulate [(3)H]dopamine release in rat striatal slices via glutamate release. *Mol Pharmacol, 58*(2), 312-318.

Kapur, S. (2004). How antipsychotics become anti-"psychotic"--from dopamine to salience to psychosis. *Trends Pharmacol Sci, 25*(8), 402-406.

Kegeles, L. S., Abi-Dargham, A., Frankle, W. G., Gil, R., Cooper, T. B., Slifstein, M., et al. (2010). Increased synaptic dopamine function in associative regions of the striatum in schizophrenia. *Arch Gen Psychiatry, 67*(3), 231-239.

Klejbor, I., Kucinski, A., Wersinger, S. R., Corso, T., Spodnik, J. H., Dziewiatkowski, J., et al. (2009). Serotonergic hyperinnervation and effective serotonin blockade in an FGF receptor developmental model of psychosis. *Schizophr Res, 113*(2-3), 308-321.

Klejbor, I., Myers, J. M., Hausknecht, K., Corso, T. D., Gambino, A. S., Morys, J., et al. (2006a). Fibroblast growth factor receptor signaling affects development and function of dopamine neurons - inhibition results in a schizophrenia-like syndrome in transgenic mice. *Journal of Neurochemistry, 97*(5), 1243-1258.

Klejbor, I., Myers, J. M., Hausknecht, K., Corso, T. D., Gambino, A. S., Morys, J., et al. (2006b). Fibroblast growth factor receptor signaling affects development and function of dopamine neurons - inhibition results in a schizophrenia-like syndrome in transgenic mice. [Research Support, Non-U.S. Gov't]. *J Neurochem, 97*(5), 1243-1258.

Koch, M. (2013). Clinical relevance of animal models of schizophrenia. *Suppl Clin Neurophysiol, 62*, 113-120.

Kohnomi, S., Suemaru, K., Goda, M., Choshi, T., Hibino, S., Kawasaki, H., et al. (2010). Ameliorating effects of tropisetron on dopaminergic disruption of prepulse inhibition via the alpha(7) nicotinic acetylcholine receptor in Wistar rats. *Brain Res, 1353*, 152-158.

Kolomeets, N. S., & Uranova, N. A. (1999). Synaptic contacts in schizophrenia: studies using immunocytochemical identification of dopaminergic neurons. *Neurosci Behav Physiol, 29*(2), 217-221.

Kucinski, A., Syposs, C., Wersinger, S., Bencherif, M., Stachowiak, M. K., & Stachowiak, E. K. (2012). alpha7 neuronal nicotinic receptor agonist (TC-7020) reverses increased striatal dopamine release during acoustic PPI testing in a transgenic mouse model of schizophrenia. *Schizophr Res, 136*(1-3), 82-87.

Kuepper, R., Skinbjerg, M., & Abi-Dargham, A. (2012). The dopamine dysfunction in schizophrenia revisited: new insights into topography and course. *Handb Exp Pharmacol*(212), 1-26.

Kumari, V., Soni, W., & Sharma, T. (2001). Influence of cigarette smoking on prepulse inhibition of the acoustic startle response in schizophrenia. *Hum Psychopharmacol, 16*(4), 321-326.

Laruelle, M., Abi-Dargham, A., Gil, R., Kegeles, L., & Innis, R. (1999). Increased dopamine transmission in schizophrenia: relationship to illness phases. *Biol Psychiatry, 46*(1), 56-72.

Lau, C. I., Wang, H. C., Hsu, J. L., & Liu, M. E. (2013). Does the dopamine hypothesis explain schizophrenia? *Rev Neurosci, 24*(4), 389-400.

Levin, E. D., McClernon, F. J., & Rezvani, A. H. (2006). Nicotinic effects on cognitive function: behavioral characterization, pharmacological specification, and anatomic localization. *Psychopharmacology (Berl), 184*(3-4), 523-539.

Levin, E. D., Petro, A., & Caldwell, D. P. (2005). Nicotine and clozapine actions on pre-pulse inhibition deficits caused by N-methyl-D-aspartate (NMDA) glutamatergic receptor blockade. *Prog Neuropsychopharmacol Biol Psychiatry, 29*(4), 581-586.

Levin, E. D., & Rezvani, A. H. (2007). Nicotinic interactions with antipsychotic drugs, models of schizophrenia and impacts on cognitive function. *Biochem Pharmacol, 74*(8), 1182-1191.

Lieberman, J. A., Mailman, R. B., Duncan, G., Sikich, L., Chakos, M., Nichols, D. E., et al. (1998). Serotonergic basis of antipsychotic drug effects in schizophrenia. *Biological Psychiatry, 44*(11), 1099-1117.

Livingstone, P. D., Srinivasan, J., Kew, J. N., Dawson, L. A., Gotti, C., Moretti, M., et al. (2009). alpha7 and non-alpha7 nicotinic acetylcholine receptors modulate dopamine release in vitro and in vivo in the rat prefrontal cortex. *Eur J Neurosci, 29*(3), 539-550.

MacDonald, A. W., & Schulz, S. C. (2009). What we know: findings that every theory of schizophrenia should explain. *Schizophr Bull, 35*(3), 493-508.

Mameli-Engvall, M., Evrard, A., Pons, S., Maskos, U., Svensson, T. H., Changeux, J. P., et al. (2006). Hierarchical control of dopamine neuron-firing patterns by nicotinic receptors. *Neuron, 50*(6), 911-921.

Mansbach, R. S., Geyer, M. A., & Braff, D. L. (1988). Dopaminergic stimulation disrupts sensorimotor gating in the rat. *Psychopharmacology (Berl), 94*(4), 507-514.

Marrero, M. B., Lucas, R., Salet, C., Hauser, T. A., Mazurov, A., Lippiello, P. M., et al. (2010). An alpha7 nicotinic acetylcholine receptor-selective agonist reduces weight gain and metabolic changes in a mouse model of diabetes. [Research Support, Non-U.S. Gov't]. *J Pharmacol Exp Ther, 332*(1), 173-180.

Meltzer, H. Y., Li, Z., Kaneda, Y., & Ichikawa, J. (2003). Serotonin receptors: their key role in drugs to treat schizophrenia. *Progress in Neuro-Psychopharmacology & Biological Psychiatry, 27*(7), 1159-1172.

Meyer-Lindenberg, A., Miletich, R. S., Kohn, P. D., Esposito, G., Carson, R. E., Quarantelli, M., et al. (2002). Reduced prefrontal activity predicts exaggerated striatal dopaminergic function in schizophrenia. *Nature Neuroscience, 5*(3), 267-271.

Moskvina, V., Craddock, N., Holmans, P., Nikolov, I., Pahwa, J. S., Green, E., et al. (2009). Gene-wide analyses of genome-wide association data sets: evidence for multiple common risk alleles for schizophrenia and bipolar disorder and for overlap in genetic risk. *Mol Psychiatry, 14*(3), 252-260.

Moukhles, H., Bosler, O., Bolam, J. P., Vallee, A., Umbriaco, D., Geffard, M., et al. (1997). Quantitative and morphometric data indicate precise cellular interactions between serotonin terminals and postsynaptic targets in rat substantia nigra. *Neuroscience, 76*(4), 1159-1171.

Mueller, H. T., Haroutunian, V., Davis, K. L., & Meador-Woodruff, J. H. (2004). Expression of the ionotropic glutamate receptor subunits and NMDA receptor-associated intracellular proteins in the substantia nigra in schizophrenia. *Brain Res Mol Brain Res, 121*(1-2), 60-69.

Newhouse, P., Singh, A., & Potter, A. (2004). Nicotine and nicotinic receptor involvement in neuropsychiatric disorders. *Curr Top Med Chem, 4*(3), 267-282.

Patel, N. H., Vyas, N. S., Puri, B. K., Nijran, K. S., & Al-Nahhas, A. (2010). Positron emission tomography in schizophrenia: a new perspective. *J Nucl Med, 51*(4), 511-520.

Pickar, D., Owen, R. R., Jr., Litman, R. E., Hsiao, J. K., & Su, T. P. (1994). Predictors of clozapine response in schizophrenia. *J Clin Psychiatry, 55 Suppl B*, 129-132.

Postma, P., Gray, J. A., Sharma, T., Geyer, M., Mehrotra, R., Das, M., et al. (2006). A behavioural and functional neuroimaging investigation into the effects of nicotine on sensorimotor gating in healthy subjects and persons with schizophrenia. *Psychopharmacology (Berl), 184*(3-4), 589-599.

Potkin, S. G., Macciardi, F., Guffanti, G., Fallon, J. H., Wang, Q., Turner, J. A., et al. (2010). Identifying gene regulatory networks in schizophrenia. *Neuroimage, 53*(3), 839-847.

Powell, S. B., Zhou, X., & Geyer, M. A. (2009). Prepulse inhibition and genetic mouse models of schizophrenia. *Behav Brain Res, 204*(2), 282-294.

Ralph, R. J., Paulus, M. P., Fumagalli, F., Caron, M. G., & Geyer, M. A. (2001). Prepulse inhibition deficits and perseverative motor patterns in dopamine transporter knock-out mice: differential effects of D1 and D2 receptor antagonists. *J Neurosci, 21*(1), 305-313.

Rausch, J. L., Sirota, E. L., Londino, D. L., Johnson, M. E., Carr, B. M., Bhatia, R., et al. (2005). Open-label risperidone for Asperger's disorder: negative symptom spectrum response. *J Clin Psychiatry, 66*(12), 1592-1597.

Rodriguez-Murillo, L., Gogos, J. A., & Karayiorgou, M. (2012). The genetic architecture of schizophrenia: new mutations and emerging paradigms. *Annu Rev Med, 63*, 63-80.

Rodriguez-Pallares, J., Guerra, M. J., & Labandeira-Garcia, J. L. (2003). Elimination of serotonergic cells induces a marked increase in generation of dopaminergic neurons from mesencephalic precursors. *European Journal of Neuroscience, 18*(8), 2166-2174.

Salminen, O., Murphy, K. L., McIntosh, J. M., Drago, J., Marks, M. J., Collins, A. C., et al. (2004). Subunit composition and pharmacology of two classes of striatal presynaptic nicotinic acetylcholine receptors mediating dopamine release in mice. *Mol Pharmacol, 65*(6), 1526-1535.

Schmidt, C. J., Kehne, J. H., Carr, A. A., Fadayel, G. M., Humphreys, T. M., Kettler, H. J., et al. (1993). Contribution of serotonin neurotoxins to understanding psychiatric disorders: the role of 5-HT2 receptors in schizophrenia and antipsychotic activity. *Int Clin Psychopharmacol, 8 Suppl 2*, 25-32.

Schultz, W. (2002). Getting formal with dopamine and reward. *Neuron, 36*(2), 241-263.

Sesack, S. R., & Grace, A. A. (2010). Cortico-Basal Ganglia reward network: microcircuitry. *Neuropsychopharmacology, 35*(1), 27-47.

Shin, J. K., Malone, D. T., Crosby, I. T., & Capuano, B. (2011). Schizophrenia: a systematic review of the disease state, current therapeutics and their molecular mechanisms of action. *Curr Med Chem, 18*(9), 1380-1404.

Simpson, E. H., Kellendonk, C., & Kandel, E. (2010). A possible role for the striatum in the pathogenesis of the cognitive symptoms of schizophrenia. *Neuron, 65*(5), 585-596.

Stachowiak, M. K., Bruno, J. P., Snyder, A. M., Stricker, E. M., & Zigmond, M. J. (1984). Apparent sprouting of striatal serotonergic terminals after dopamine-depleting brain lesions in neonatal rats. *Brain Res, 291*(1), 164-167.

Stachowiak, M. K., Kucinski, A., Curl, R., Syposs, C., Yang, Y., Narla, S., et al. (2013). Schizophrenia: a neurodevelopmental disorder--integrative genomic hypothesis and therapeutic implications from a transgenic mouse model. *Schizophr Res, 143*(2-3), 367-376.

Stolerman, I. P., Mirza, N. R., Hahn, B., & Shoaib, M. (2000). Nicotine in an animal model of attention. *Eur J Pharmacol, 393*(1-3), 147-154.

Sun, J., Jia, P., Fanous, A. H., van den Oord, E., Chen, X., Riley, B. P., et al. (2010). Schizophrenia gene networks and pathways and their applications for novel candidate gene selection. *PLoS One, 5*(6), e11351.

Swerdlow, N. R., & Geyer, M. A. (1998). Using an animal model of deficient sensorimotor gating to study the pathophysiology and new treatments of schizophrenia. *Schizophr Bull, 24*(2), 285-301.

Takahashi, H., Hashimoto, R., Iwase, M., Ishii, R., Kamio, Y., & Takeda, M. (2011). Prepulse inhibition of startle response: recent advances in human studies of psychiatric disease. *Clin Psychopharmacol Neurosci, 9*(3), 102-110.

Terwisscha van Scheltinga, A. F., Bakker, S. C., & Kahn, R. S. (2010). Fibroblast growth factors in schizophrenia. *Schizophr Bull, 36*(6), 1157-1166.

Thompson, J. L., Pogue-Geile, M. F., & Grace, A. A. (2004). Developmental pathology, dopamine, and stress: a model for the age of onset of schizophrenia symptoms. *Schizophr Bull, 30*(4), 875-900.

Tidey, J. W., Rohsenow, D. J., Kaplan, G. B., & Swift, R. M. (2005). Cigarette smoking topography in smokers with schizophrenia and matched non-psychiatric controls. *Drug Alcohol Depend, 80*(2), 259-265.

Tietje, K. R., Anderson, D. J., Bitner, R. S., Blomme, E. A., Brackemeyer, P. J., Briggs, C. A., et al. (2008). Preclinical characterization of A-582941: a novel alpha7 neuronal nicotinic receptor agonist with broad spectrum cognition-enhancing properties. *CNS Neurosci Ther, 14*(1), 65-82.

Toru, M., Nishikawa, T., Mataga, N., & Takashima, M. (1982). Dopamine metabolism increases in post-mortem schizophrenic basal ganglia. *J Neural Transm, 54*(3-4), 181-191.

Tost, H., Alam, T., & Meyer-Lindenberg, A. (2010). Dopamine and psychosis: theory, pathomechanisms and intermediate phenotypes. *Neurosci Biobehav Rev, 34*(5), 689-700.

van der Kooy, D., & Hattori, T. (1980). Dorsal raphe cells with collateral projections to the caudate-putamen and substantia nigra: a fluorescent retrograde double labeling study in the rat. *Brain Research, 186*(1), 1-7.

van Os, J., & Kapur, S. (2009). Schizophrenia. *Lancet, 374*(9690), 635-645.

Wallace, T. L., Callahan, P. M., Tehim, A., Bertrand, D., Tombaugh, G., Wang, S., et al. (2011). RG3487, a novel nicotinic alpha7 receptor partial agonist, improves cognition and sensorimotor gating in rodents. *J Pharmacol Exp Ther, 336*(1), 242-253.

Wan, F. J., Geyer, M. A., & Swerdlow, N. R. (1995). Presynaptic dopamine-glutamate interactions in the nucleus accumbens regulate sensorimotor gating. *Psychopharmacology (Berl), 120*(4), 433-441.

Williams, J. M., Gandhi, K. K., Lu, S. E., Kumar, S., Shen, J., Foulds, J., et al. (2010). Higher nicotine levels in schizophrenia compared with controls after smoking a single cigarette. *Nicotine Tob Res, 12*(8), 855-859.

Wong, A. H., & Van Tol, H. H. (2003). Schizophrenia: from phenomenology to neurobiology. *Neurosci Biobehav Rev, 27*(3), 269-306.

Wong, D. F., Wagner, H. N., Jr., Tune, L. E., Dannals, R. F., Pearlson, G. D., Links, J. M., et al. (1986). Positron emission tomography reveals elevated D_2 dopamine receptors in drug-naive schizophrenics. *Science, 234*, 1558-1563.

Wonnacott, S. (1997). Presynaptic nicotinic ACh receptors. *Trends Neurosci, 20*(2), 92-98.

Wonnacott, S., Kaiser, S., Mogg, A., Soliakov, L., & Jones, I. W. (2000). Presynaptic nicotinic receptors modulating dopamine release in the rat striatum. *Eur J Pharmacol, 393*(1-3), 51-58.

Woznica, A. A., Sacco, K. A., & George, T. P. (2009). Prepulse inhibition deficits in schizophrenia are modified by smoking status. *Schizophr Res, 112*(1-3), 86-90.

Zhong, K. X., Sweitzer, D. E., Hamer, R. M., & Lieberman, J. A. (2006). Comparison of quetiapine and risperidone in the treatment of schizophrenia: A randomized, double-blind, flexible-dose, 8-week study. *J Clin Psychiatry, 67*(7), 1093-1103.

In: The Central Catecholaminergic System
Editor: Bertalan Dudás

ISBN: 978-1-63117-937-2

Chapter 10

Catecholamines and Bipolar Disorder

Moritz Mühlbacher and Irene Lehner-Adam

Introduction

Definition

Bipolar affective disorder, also known as manic depression, is a spectrum of mental disorders characterized by cyclic mood swings. Episodes of elevated mood known as mania and episodes of lowered mood known as depression typically alternate with euthymic periods of complete or incomplete remission.

Depressive Episodes

Depressive episodes, clinically diagnosed not only by presence of depressed mood but also by anhedonia and loss of energy, are a major cause of morbidity worldwide. Lifetime prevalence ranges from 8 – 12 percent in most countries, and a considerable proportion of all patients may suffer from chronically recurring, unipolar depressive episodes (Andrade et al., 2003). Bipolar depressive episodes are not generally different from unipolar depressive episodes, but the rate of "atypical" depression, characterized by increased sleep, increased appetite and undiminished affective reactivity, may be elevated in comparison to unipolar depression (Mitchell et al., 2001).

Conversion from Unipolar Depression to Bipolar Disorder and Switch

Patients diagnosed with (unipolar) depression are at considerable risk of developing hypomanic or manic episodes in later life. Large cohort studies reported a conversion rate of up to 39 percent in patients diagnosed with unipolar depression followed up prospectively for an average of 20 years from the onset of the disorder (Angst et al., 2005). The risk seems to be particularly high if psychotic symptoms like hallucinations and delusions are present during the initial depressive episode (Beesdo et al., 2009). A "switch" to mania or hypomania may occur at any given point of time during the course of the disorder. In many cases, switch phenomena are preceded by stressful events, although such well-known triggers may also be absent in other cases. Of interest, many drugs enhancing catecholaminergic transmission can either mimic manic symptoms in healthy patients or catalyze manic episodes in bipolar patients, a phenomenon named treatment emergent affective switch (TEAS). The same is true for a number of psychotropic drugs with a negative impact on catecholaminergic function which can elicit depressive symptoms in vulnerable individuals.

Manic and Hypomanic Episodes

Bipolar disorder is typified by mood swings toward the pathologically elevated, manic end of the affective spectrum. Approximately one percent of the population is affected by the classic, Type I bipolar disorder with full-blown manic episodes. During these manic episodes, mood is elevated out of keeping with the individual's circumstances and may vary from carefree joviality to almost uncontrollable excitement or irritability (Figure 1). Typically, manic patients also experience inflated self-esteem or ideas of grandiosity, decreased need for sleep, flight of ideas, distractibility, increase in goal-directed activity, and excessive involvement in pleasurable activities with high risk for negative and painful consequences. Some manic patients also suffer from psychotic symptoms like hallucinations and delusions. An additional two to five percent of the general population may suffer from Type II bipolar disorder with frequent and long depressive episodes followed by hypomanic states of attenuated severity (Figure 2). Hypomania typically lacks immediate negative consequences and therefore tends to remain underdiagnosed with a high estimated number of unreported cases (Ferrari et al., 2011).

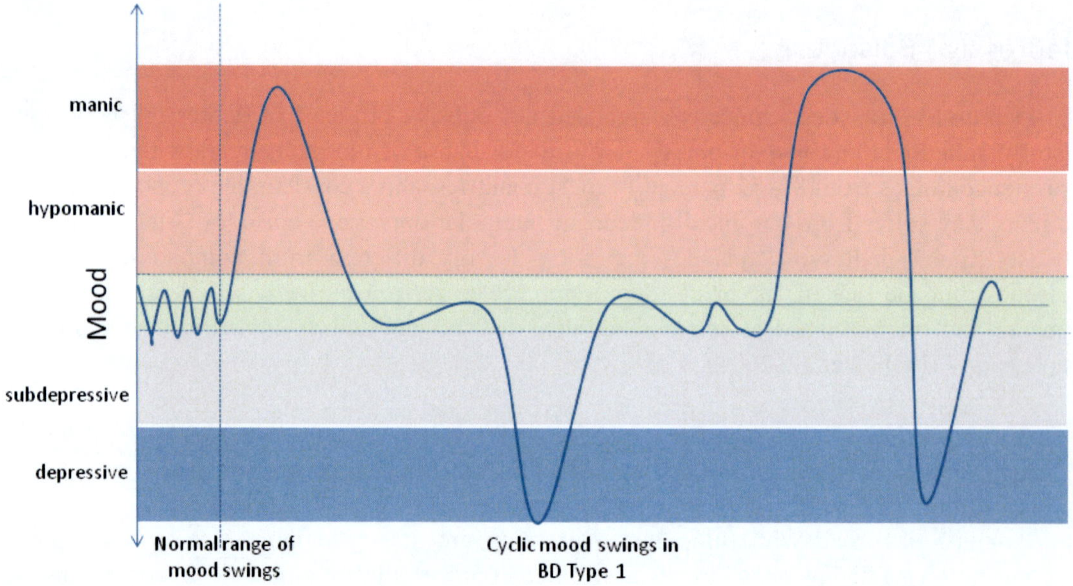

Figure 1. Bipolar Disorder Type I. Cycling mood swings with full blown mania and depression.

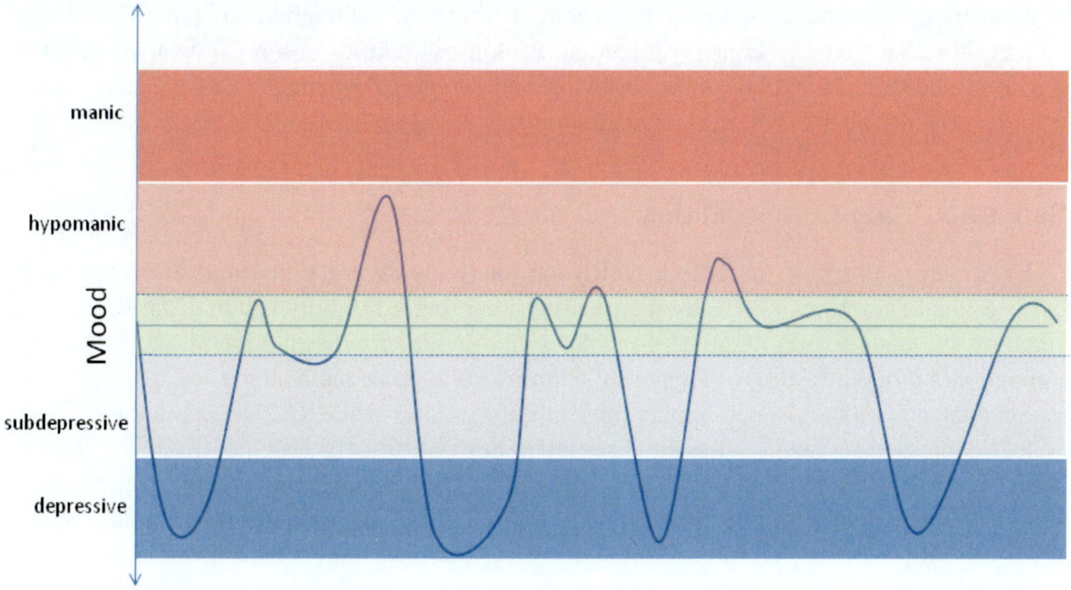

Figure 2. Bipolar Disorder Type II. Cyclic mood swings of depressive phases alternating with hypomanic states.

Mixed Episodes

A considerable number of bipolar patients also experience mixed episodes, when several manic and depressive symptoms (Table 1) are present at the same time or alternate very rapidly. In their extreme form, mania and depression can supersede one another with minimal intervals of hours or even minutes, referred to as "ultra-rapid cycling". These precarious conditions count among the most difficult to treat challenges in psychiatry.

Table 1. Typical psychopathological symptoms of manic and depressive episodes

Manic Episode	Depressive Episode
Elevated or irritated mood	Lowered (depressed or irritable) mood
Inflated self-esteem or grandiosity	Feelings of worthlessness and excessive or inappropriate guilt
Decreased need for sleep	Insomnia
More talkative than usual or pressure to keep talking Psychomotor acceleration	Slow speech Psychomotor retardation
Flight of ideas or subjective experience that thoughts are racing	Diminished ability to think or concentrate, or more indecisiveness
Increase in goal-directed activity	Fatigue or Loss of energy
Excessive involvement in pleasurable activities with high risk for painful consequences	Decreased interest or pleasure, Anhedonia, Anergia

In many regards, mania seems to be the direct "opposite" of depression, with clinical core features altered in the exact contrary direction. Biological theories of bipolar disorder needs to be able to address and explain the underlying neurochemical changes responsible for those cycling bidirectional changes in psychopathology.

"Remission" and Comorbidities

Even during times of remission, which may individually vary in length from weeks to years, residual symptoms may often be present, comprising not only residual sub-depressive symptoms but also a wide range of possible cognitive deficits. During the last few decades, thorough and diligent testing of supposedly "remitted" bipolar patients has led to the finding that attenuated symptoms often remain present during times when the patients themselves do not feel depressed or manic. Bipolar disorder is now commonly accepted to be of chronic nature and not simply caused by episodic 1 disturbances of brain functioning. Neuroanatomical and neurochemical changes are thought to be present throughout the whole course of the disorder. During remission, these changes may result in minor clinical symptoms, often not immediately noticeable and without greater functional impairment. However, when a new phase is triggered, the central nervous system seems to lack important safeguards and appears to be more vulnerable to derailment. In addition, there is a statistically significant increased risk for severe comorbidities which have a negative impact on the overall outcome (Young & Grunze, 2013).

"Neuroprogression"

There is now strong evidence for progressive neuropathological changes in bipolar disorder, including a shortening of interval-episode with each reoccurrence, gradual deterioration of underlying aberrant regulatory systems in various neurotransmitter systems and even a subtle loss of brain mass in different regions of the central nervous system (Berk et al., 2011). Although recent research about possible causes of neuroprogression have by and large focused on inflammation, oxidative stress, neuroprotective factors or glutamatergic mechanisms, catecholamines are inextricably intertwined with each of these factors and may well be involved in the pathophysiology of bipolar disorder itself (Gama et al., 2013).

Global Burden and Impact

Bipolar disorder has been deemed the most expensive behavioral health care diagnosis in the United States (Peele et al., 2003). Working life may be reduced by up to 14 years and life expectancy by up to 9 years (Coryell et al., 1993). Furthermore, bipolar disorder is associated with a high rate of severe comorbidities like addictive disorders, cardiovascular disease and diabetes, adding to their overall significance. Interestingly, both types of bipolar disorder, with their typical symptoms during manic and depressive episodes, cognitive deficits during times of remission and a considerable proportion of comorbidities have been linked to a possible imbalance or dysregulation of catecholaminergic transmission (Fitzgerald, 2013a; Fitzgerald, 2013b). With regard to these facts, bipolar disorder can serve as an epitome to investigate the role of catecholamines in the pathogenesis of complex medical conditions.

The Catecholamine Theory of Affective Disorders

Scientific attempts to comprehend the brain's role in mania and depression from a neurobiological point of view began in the second half of the twentieth century and coincided with the arrival of the first effective mood-altering drugs and the discovery of their mechanism of action. One of the first scientific concepts was the catecholaminergic theory of affective disorders (Schildkraut, 1995; Schildkraut, 1965). Reduced and simplified to its central assumption, the catecholamine theory linked depressive states to a relative lack of catecholaminergic neurotransmission, and mania to a relative hyperfunction of the same system. While it is obvious from today's point of view that this theory falls short of explaining all of the essential aspects of affective disorders, imbalances in catecholaminergic transmission still remain one of the backbones of scientific research interests in this field. Developing medications targeting the catecholaminergic system continues to be the primary goal of the vast majority of all currently licensed drugs in psychiatry and certainly merits further investigation with special focus on their interrelations with other transmitter systems.

Evidence from Animal and Behavioral Studies

Dopamine and noradrenaline are known to regulate core aspects of psychopathology related to bipolar disorder. These include general arousal, anxiety, psychomotor regulation, aspects of cognitive functioning, novelty seeking and motivation towards pleasurable activities (Table 2).

By way of example, lower motor activity and hypophagia is observed in dopamine-deficient transgenic mice (Zhou & Palmiter, 1995) and animal models of depression have shown that dopamine agonists reduce depression-like behavior in experimental animals (Basso et al., 2005). In humans, ventral tegmental area dopamine neuron degeneration has been associated with depression (Torack & Morris, 1988).

The central dopaminergic system can be subdivided into three distinct parts. Of these, the mesolimbic system has arguably the largest impact on the human psyche. The mesolimbic dopamine system is mostly responsible for facilitating purposeful behavior directed towards new stimuli and goals. Dopamine supports motivation. A stimulus followed by a positive response elicits a release of dopamine in the brain, linking the original stimulus to positive feelings and conferring to it incentive salience and reinforcement. In the field of personality psychology, dopamine is associated with the desire for diversification and extraversion. Changes in serotonin (5-hydroxytryptamin) levels show similar effects on human behavior: high serotonin levels lead to shy and withdrawn behavior by suppressing dopamine action, while high dopamine or low serotonin levels induce curiosity and explorative behavior (Baarendse, Winstanley, & Vanderschuren, 2013). A marked increase in brain dopamine levels, induced by some drugs, can temporarily lead to high degrees of psychological elation because of their effects on reward behavior and can even induce psychotic symptoms (Lieberman et al., 1990). A higher general arousal level as well as better decision-making abilities are also functions dependent on dopamine and noradrenaline levels and result in redundant and complementary functions of both of these transmitters. It is well established that catecholamines exert an inverted U dose response on working memory performance, whereby too much or too little dopamine or noradrenaline impairs spatial working memory and delay-related neuron firing (Arnsten, 2007; Ramos & Arnsten, 2007). High levels of dopamine and noradrenaline will block input to the prefrontal cortex. A low level of these two transmitters will also cause dysfunction of the prefrontal cortex network and lead to a general decrease in its activity. Low dopamine and high noradrenaline levels will cause increased susceptibility to failures of working memory (Avery et al., 2013). It is generally assumed that clinical symptoms related to attention deficit are caused by functional disorders of catecholamines. Attention regulation occurs through an anterior system, mainly via dopamine as the corresponding neurotransmitter, and a posterior system (posterior and parietal cortex), with noradrenaline acting as neurotransmitter.

Catecholamines also play an important role in the regulation of aggression in mammals and humans because they modulate vulnerability and/or initiation of aggressive behavior in social situations (Yanowitch & Coccaro, 2011).

In the light of these findings, excess and deficiency of catecholaminergic transmission seem to serve well as a theory to explain the typical symptoms of depressive and manic episodes.

Table 2. Behavioral effects regulated by dopamine and noradrenaline

Dopamine	Noradrenaline
• Motivation towards pleasurable activities • Novelty seeking, curiosity, exploratory behavior • Psychomotor regulation • Cognitive function • Impulsivity	• General arousal as part of the "fight or flight" response to stressors • Attention and responding actions • Anxiety and aggression • Cognitive function

Pharmacological Evidence

The first antidepressants widely available and still in use today, tricyclic antidepressants, act by blocking noradrenaline transporters and serotonin transporters. Thus, they inhibit the reuptake of noradrenaline and serotonin at the synaptic cleft and increase the intrasynaptic concentration of both neurotransmitters. As the human prefrontal cortex largely lacks dopamine transporters, the reuptake of dopamine in the prefrontal cortex is managed by noradrenaline transporters (Valentini et al., 2004). Summing up, tricyclic antidepressants enhance serotoninergic and noradrenergic transmission in general, and dopaminergic transmission in the human prefrontal cortex. These properties are also the very mechanisms that are generally considered to be the first necessary step in a cascade of neurochemical or intracellular neuronal sequelae contributing to the antidepressant effect of the tricyclic antidepressants. On the other hand, psychotropics like reserpine – a formerly widely used blood pressure medication – lead to a depletion of catecholamines. Reserpine is also infamous for its high frequency of unwanted side effects, mainly severe depression, making a strong argument for catecholamine deficiency being a cause of depression.

These effects of various drugs on mood are correctly predicted by the catecholaminergic theory of affective disorders and seem to fit seamlessly into a simplified model, with depression and mania interpreted as catecholamine deficiency and excess, respectively. Additional exemplary evidence is summarized in Table 3.

Table 3. Pharmacological evidence for the catecholaminergic theory of affective disorders. Abbreviations: 5HT: serotonin; BD: bipolar disorder; DOPAC: 3,4 dihydroxyphenylacetic acid; DA: dopamine; NA: noradrenaline; MAO: monoaminooxydase

Substance	Mechanism of action	Clinical Effect
Tricyclic Antidepressants	Inhibition of NA and 5HT-reuptake	Mood↑ Manic switch in BD patients possible
MAO-Inhibitors	Inhibition of breakdown of NA, 5HT and DA	Mood↑ Manic switch in BD patients possible
A-Methyl tyrosine	Inhibits Tyrosine - Hydroxylase: DA, NA↓	Mood↓
Reserpine	NA, DA depletion	Mood↓
Methyldopa	Blocks DOPAC: DA, NA↓	Mood ↓
Amphetamines	Increase DA, NA functioning	Euphoria (healthy subjects) Manic switch in BD patients possible
L-DOPA, Dopamine Agonists	DA↑	Euphoria (healthy subjects) Manic switch in BD patients possible
Dopamine receptor D2R-Blockers (e.g. Haloperidol)	DA↓	Effective control of manic symptoms

Points to ponder

- If depression were a mere state of catecholamine deficiency, antidepressant drugs boosting catecholaminergic transmission should work immediately within the time frame of onset of their purported mechanism of action – a matter of minutes. This usually does not occur. It takes a minimum of 10 to 14 days on average for the first clinically relevant antidepressant effects to occur.
- Drugs like reserpine, which reduce catecholaminergic transmission in all patients, should also elicit depressive symptoms in all patients. However, only some of these patients – albeit a significantly large proportion – seem to be affected.

  A possible explanation of these discrepancies may be that (1) catecholamine deficiency may only be a secondary adaption to superordinate changes which take more time to remedy than catecholaminergic drugs necessitate for their first step of action, or (2) some individuals may be equipped with considerable safeguarding mechanisms for assaults against severe derailment in catecholaminergic transmission.

Genetic and Epigenetic Evidence

Affective disorders like unipolar depression and – to an even greater extent – bipolar disorder tends to run in families. The genetic load of bipolar disorder Type 1 is particularly high and there is a considerable overlap with other psychiatric disorders, including schizophrenia, schizoaffective disorders, anxiety disorders and autistic spectrum disorder, as well as various severe somatic comorbidities like metabolic syndrome (Schulze et al., 2012). If catecholamines were to play a pivotal role in the pathogenesis of these illnesses, a shared genetic background might be expected. However, the genetics of psychiatric disorders have proven to be particularly elusive and bipolar disorder is no exception in this regard. If anything, research efforts over the past few decades have painted a dotted picture of impressionistic quality with a wide variety of minor risk loci, each possibly contributing to certain aspects of the disorder. Not one single genetic marker nor even a typical combination of genetic polymorphisms related to a single transmitter tested to this day has been shown to contribute unequivocally and exclusively to the etiology of bipolar disorder. The majority of all genetic risk factors identified appear to be more closely related to serotonin, gamma amino butyric acid (GABA), glutamate or genes regulating circadian rhythms. Some of the identified loci even lie within regions of the genome whose exact functions still remain to be elucidated. That said, there is some evidence that genes related directly or indirectly to catecholaminergic transmission may be determinants of different aspects or subtypes of bipolar disorder (compare Table 4). Earlier studies focused on genes coding for enzymes involved in the metabolism of catecholamines or their receptors on cell membranes. In spite of some encouraging initial evidence for the involvement of subtypes of dopamine or noradrenaline receptors, transporters and related enzymes, many findings could not be replicated in larger samples or did not prove to be relevant risk factors in more recent genome-wide association studies (GWAS). Today, it seems more likely that a wide variety of genetic polymorphisms for unspecific factors involved in second messenger signaling, the cytoskeleton or maintenance of neuron-to-neuron and neuron-to-glia crosstalk, which ultimately affect catecholaminergic function and other neurotransmitters, are part of the pathophysiological background of bipolar disorder. Interestingly, though, there is relatively good evidence for epigenetic changes of the catecholaminergic system in bipolar disorder. Hypomethylation of the membrane-bound catecholamine-O-methyl transferase promoter, especially in the left frontal lobe, has been shown to be a significant risk factor in the development of bipolar disorder. This epigenetic change could increase gene expression and consequently contribute to an imbalance in dopamine and noradrenaline metabolism (Abdolmaleky et al., 2006). Genetic polymorphisms within dopamine receptor genes appear to be associated with gender differences, type of bipolar disorder and related comorbidities. There is also some evidence that different variants of the catecholamine-O-methyl transferase gene have an impact on the course of the disorder, like age of onset and number or polarity of episodes. Polymorphisms of the monoamine oxidase-A gene might account for ethnic differences and a special variant of the monoamine oxidase-A gene seems to be associated with increased risk of elevated impulsivity, especially when combined with a history of severe childhood trauma, across a wide range of psychiatric disorders (Buckholtz & Meyer-Lindenberg, 2012). Other catecholamine related genes (tyrosine hydroxylase-gene, dopamine beta hydroxylase-gene and dopa decarboxylase-gene) seem to have little or no impact on bipolar disorder. However, due to a dearth of gene-gene interaction studies, a possible role of particular genetic constellations cannot entirely be excluded. Table 4 provides exemplary genetic findings about the above-mentioned catecholamine-related genes in bipolar disorder.

Table 4. Genetic findings of catecholamine-related genes in bipolar disorder. Abbreviations: BD: bipolar disorder; COMT: catecholamine-O-methyl transferase, DBH: dopamine beta hydroxylase, DDC: DOPA decarboxylase, MAO-A: monoamino oxidase A; TH: tyrosine hydroxylase

Gene	Possible Relation to Bipolar Disorders	Source
COMT low-activity allele (MET158;COMTL)	Minor risk factor for BD	(Rotondo et al., 2002; Lee & Kim, 2010)
	Increased in patients with ultra-rapid cycling	(Kirov et al., 1998)
	Association of velocardiofacial syndrome and ultra-rapid cycling	(Lachman et al., 1996)
	Decrease of facial emotional recognition	(Soeiro-de-Souza et al., 2012; Lelli-Chiesa et al., 2011)
	Early age at onset of BD	(Massat et al., 2011)
	Fewer manic episodes	(Massat et al., 2011)
COMT-MB gene promoter hypomethylation	(Epigenetic) Risk factor for BD	(Abdolmaleky et al., 2006)
Dopamine D_2 receptor A1/A1 variant	Risk factor for BD in males, not females	(Wang et al., 2013)
Dopamine D_3 receptor Ser9gly	Risk factor in BD Type II and comorbid anxiety	(Chang et al., 2013)
	Interaction with COMT low activity allele in BD Type 1	(Lee et al., 2011)
TH	No significant association in meta-analysis	(Turecki, Rouleau, Mari, Joober, & Morgan, 1997)
DBH	No evidence for linkage	(Ewald, Mors, Flint, Eiberg, & Kruse, 1994)
DDC	No evidence for linkage	(Ewald, Mors, Eiberg, Flint, & Kruse, 1995)
MAO-A	Association with BD in Caucasians in meta-analysis (CA subtype)	(Fan et al., 2010)
	Increased Impulsivity and association with childhood trauma in male patients with mood disorder (uVNTR subtype)	(Huang et al., 2004; Buckholtz & Meyer-Lindenberg, 2008)

Points to ponder

- GWAS of almost all psychiatric disorders, especially within the affective and schizophrenic spectrums, have failed to yield consistent results pointing towards the involvement of only a handful responsible genetic polymorphisms and their related functions within the central nervous system. From today's point of view, it seems likely that hundreds or even thousands of genetic and epigenetic variables play a role to different aspects of psychiatric disorders.
- Some shared genetic and epigenetic changes might be relevant to the overlap in clinical psychopathology of psychiatric disorders which are considered separate entities in the current psychiatric classification. Such an overlap is well known for bipolar disorders and schizophrenia, anxiety disorders, impulse control disorders, attention deficit hyperactivity disorders and autism spectrum disorders (Schulze et al., 2012; Lee et al., 2013).
- With special regard to catecholamines, a partially shared genetic background might account for some common psychopathological symptoms like cognitive deficits, psychomotor disturbance, control of impulse and mood, novelty seeking, anxiety, delusions and hallucinations.
- While most catecholamine related genes may not confer a significant risk for the whole group of BD, some could still be of importance for familial variants or special phenotypes.

The Noradrenergic System

Peripheral Levels of Noradrenaline and Metabolites

Bipolar patients appear to have reduced to average resting output of plasma noradrenaline with a highly exaggerated noradrenaline response in standing during orthostatic challenge compared to healthy controls (Rudorfer et al., 1985). The plasma level of the main neuronal metabolite, 3-methoxy-4-hydroxy-phenylglycol (MHG), seems to be higher during manic episodes when compared to depression or remission (Maj et al., 1984). Consistent with the theory of an overall activation of the noradrenergic system, manic patients also tend to exhibit higher urinary concentrations of noradrenaline compared to depressed bipolar patients or healthy controls (Swann et al., 1987). Moreover, urinary excretion of the main extraneuronal noradrenaline metabolite, normetadrenaline, appears to be particularly high during depressive episodes (Maas et al., 1987). Clinical studies of noradrenergic receptors tend to rely on findings from receptors on easily accessible blood platelets and lymphocytes. It is not entirely clear whether results from such studies can be translated and used to formulate theories about corresponding changes in the central nervous system. Although results are often conflicting and prone to confounding factors, they are mostly consistent with a theory of α2-receptor hypersensitivity, β-receptor hypofunction, and, perhaps most importantly, the inability to down-regulate β-receptors in the face of excessive stimulation (Piletz et al., 1990; Kay et al., 1993). This inability to respond adequately to stress might be a key factor to understanding the relationship of bipolar disorder and stress. Taken together, these findings are suggestive of a hyperresponsive noradrenergic system in bipolar disorder with an inept stress response, increased noradrenaline release - sometimes referred to as "synaptic leakiness" or "spill over" - and a shift towards extraneuronal metabolism during affective episodes.

Central changes of the Noradrenergic System

Measurements of noradrenaline and its metabolites in the cerebrospinal fluid cannot directly be interpreted to reflect the level of noradrenergic activation of the central nervous system, since peripheral epinephrine and noradrenaline metabolites readily cross the blood brain barrier and may even be one of their main sources (Kopin, 1985), reflecting a general sympathetic arousal. However, most findings from cerebrospinal fluid samples suggest that noradrenaline output is higher in mania than depression (Swann et al., 1987). The elevation appears to be positively correlated with total episode severity in general, and anxiety, dysphoria and hostility in particular. Studies of post mortem brains found an increased noradrenaline turnover (noradrenaline/MHPG ratio) in the frontal, temporal, and occipital cortices and the thalamus in bipolar patients (Young et al., 1994; Vawter et al., 2000). *In vivo* measurements of brain catecholamine release using catheters placed in an internal jugular vein showed clear signs of reduced noradrenaline turnover in therapy-resistant depressive patients (Lambert et al., 2000).

The Dopaminergic System

On a number of theoretical grounds, it seems surprising that the dopamine system has still not received greater study in bipolar disorder. Nearly opposite motoric changes in depression and mania (ranging from depressive immobility to manic hyperactivity) as well as loss of motivation versus "hyperhedonic states" are both iconic for the distinction between depression versus mania and dopamine deficiency versus dopamine excess. Even if dopamine metabolism might not be the primary cause of these symptoms, hyper- or hypofunction of this neurotransmitter system can explain many of the psychopathological symptoms observed during opposite episodes of bipolar disorder. A hallmark feature of bipolar depression, atypical depression, is characterized by a prominence of anhedonia, amotivation and psychomotor retardation and seems to have a close relation to dopaminergic hypofunction (Dunlop & Nemeroff, 2007).

The Dopamine Dysregulation Syndrome and Parkinson's Disease: A Proof of Concept for Bipolar Disorder?

Parkinson's disease is a common neurological disorder characterized by a degeneration of dopamine neurons in the substantia nigra and a loss of dopamine in the putamen. Depression is a frequent comorbidity and often precedes the onset of motor symptoms (Scappa et al., 1993). Dopamine dysregulation syndrome, also known as "hedonistic homeostatic dysregulation", can occur as a complication due to long-term exposure to dopamine replacement therapy. It is characterized by cyclical episodes of increased mood, activity, drive and sexual disinhibition followed by profound depression when the intake of dopamine precursors is reduced, mimicking the core symptoms of manic and depressive states in bipolar disorder, respectively (O'Sullivan et al., 2009). Moreover, episodic dyskinesia and Parkinsonism have been described in rapid cycling bipolar patients. In these cases, movement disorders began before the onset of depression, worsened during depressive episodes and resolved completely during manic states (Scappa et al., 1993). These examples showcase obvious connections of dopamine dysfunction and bipolar disorder. Dopamine dysregulation syndrome has been proposed as a mechanism underlying bipolar cyclicity. During mania, an increase of dopaminergic transmission may lead to a secondary downregulation of key system elements and receptors which eventually dampens the signal. The subsequent phase of decreased dopaminergic transmission induces a depressive state. Again, a secondary up-regulation may occur, terminate the episode and lead to the initiation of the next manic phase (Berk et al., 2007). One implication of this hypothesis is that agents increasing the amplitude of the dopaminergic cycle should also increase cyclicity in frequency or intensity (Figure 3). This phenomenon, also referred to as "phase acceleration", is indeed a well- known possible complication of antidepressants and drugs (e.g. amphetamine) that enhance catecholaminergic transmission and can worsen the course of bipolar disorder (Ghaemi et al., 2004).

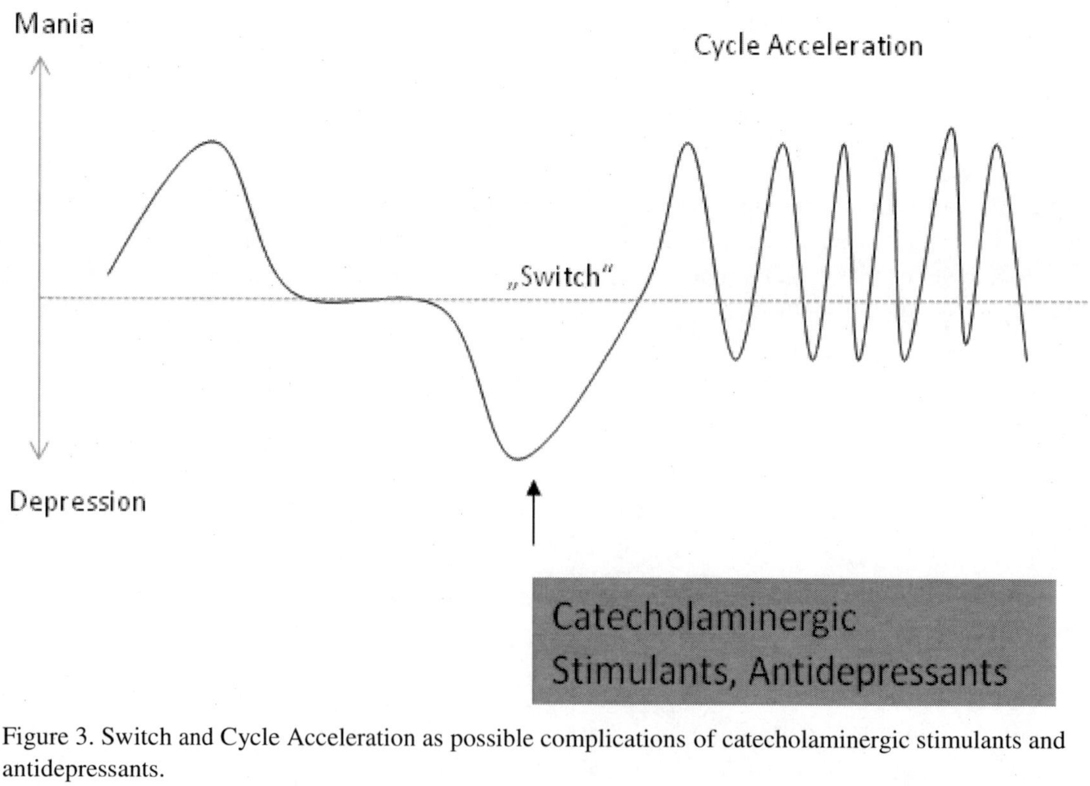

Figure 3. Switch and Cycle Acceleration as possible complications of catecholaminergic stimulants and antidepressants.

Changes of Dopamine Metabolites in Plasma and Cerebrospinal Fluid

One of the strongest findings implicating dopamine in depression is a reduction of the main metabolite homovanillic acid in cerebrospinal fluid, especially in depressive states characterized by psychomotor retardation and cognitive impairment (Willner, 1983; Wolfe et al., 1990; Manji et al., 1995). Low levels of homovanillic acid in cerebrospinal fluid are also associated with the lethality of suicide attempts in bipolar disorder (Sher et al., 2006). While many studies reported elevated levels of homovanillic acid in cerebrospinal fluid during manic episodes (Sjostrom & Roos, 1972; Gerner et al., 1984), these findings could not always be replicated (Swann et al., 1983). In plasma, homovanillic acid appears to be elevated during manic episodes, returning to lower levels after successful treatment (Chou et al., 2000).

Neuroimaging of the Dopamine System in Bipolar Disorder

Reduced D_1 receptor binding in the prefrontal cortex and increased D_2 receptor binding in the striatum was found in PET studies of drug-naïve bipolar patients, with the latter finding especially pronounced in psychotic versus non-psychotic bipolar patients (Suhara et al., 1992; Pearlson et al., 1995). In addition, vesicular monoamine transporter protein VMAT2 may be increased in bipolar patients, although this finding might be confounded by treatment effects (Zubieta et al., 2000). The habenula is an epithalamic structure that serves as a point of convergence for striatal and limbic input, and provides forebrain control over serotonergic and dopaminergic transmission from the midbrain. In comparison to healthy controls, unmedicated bipolar patients appear to have significantly reduced habenula volumes, which might be linked to disturbed reward processing and stress adaptation (Savitz et al., 2011). A recent fMRI study also found clear signs of abnormal reward system activation in manic patients during a delayed incentive paradigm. The expected pattern of activation of dopaminergic brain areas, like the ventral tegmentum and the nucleus accumbens, was significantly altered or missing altogether in manic patients compared to healthy controls and schizophrenic patients (Abler, Greenhouse, Ongur, Walter, & Heckers, 2008). These deficits may help to explain clinical symptoms of mania like disinhibition and abnormal goal pursuit regulation.

Mood Stabilizers and Catecholamines

Current treatment guidelines recommend the use of mood stabilizers, once a diagnosis of bipolar disorder is established. Mood stabilizers are a diverse group of drugs whose primary goal is the prevention of new manic or depressive phases in bipolar patients. The group comprises lithium, some antiepileptic drugs (valproic acid and carbamazepine) and a number of atypical antipsychotics. While the direct impact of atypical antipsychotics on catecholaminergic transmission is easily explained by their affinity to dopamine and serotonin receptors, other mood stabilizers appear to have a variety of indirect effects.

Lithium

Lithium targets various steps of intracellular signal transmission that are also part of signaling pathways in catecholaminergic neurons (Malhi et al., 2013). It inhibits several important enzymes in the normal recycling of membrane phosphoinositides, including conversion of IP_2 to IP_1 (inositol monophosphate) and the conversion of IP_1 to inositol. This block leads to a depletion of phosphatidylinositol-4, 5-bisphosphate (PIP_2), the membrane precursor of inositol-1,4,5-trisphosphate (IP_3) and diacylglycerol which are important second messengers in catecholaminergic transmission. Thus, lithium could cause a selective depression of the overactive catecholaminergic circuits seen in mania. Secondly, lithium is known to have indirect effects on stimulatory and inhibitory G-proteins, the formation of cyclic adenosine monophosphate and the activation of adenylate cyclase. The overall effect seems to be an elevation of basal adenylate cyclase activity but an attenuation of receptor-stimulated responses, to prevent "excessive excursions from the norm"(Jope, 1999). There is also evidence for an increase of tyrosine hydroxylase levels especially in limbic areas of the brain (Chen et al., 2000), a reduction of platelet mono amino oxydase activity and an increase in dopamine-beta-hydroxylase activity under chronic lithium treatment (Sofuoglu et al., 1995). Interestingly, lithium can prevent amphetamine-induced mania-like behavior and anti-hedonic effects of chronic stress in animal models without much effect on basal behavioral activity levels (Zheng et al., 2013; Marchese et al., 2013). These findings are consistent with the idea of lithium as a stabilizer of catecholaminergic function, although its effects are very diverse and by no means restricted to only one or two transmitter systems.

Valproic Acid

Valproic acid has a plethora of effects which are only partially understood. Apart from being a sodium channel inhibitor, it also enhances GABAergic function and various intracellular messenger systems. A distinctive feature is its action as a histone deacetylase inhibitor, thereby affecting gene expression. Valproic acid appears to increase basal tyrosine hydroxylase levels in the locus coeruleus while suppressing excessive stimulation under stress at the same time in animal models (Sands et al., 2000). Like lithium, valproic acid can attenuate the mania-like effects of stimulants in animals and prevent the development of sensitization to subsequent administration (Eckermann et al., 2001). After treatment with valproic acid, manic patients showed a decrease of presynaptic dopamine (Yatham et al., 2002).

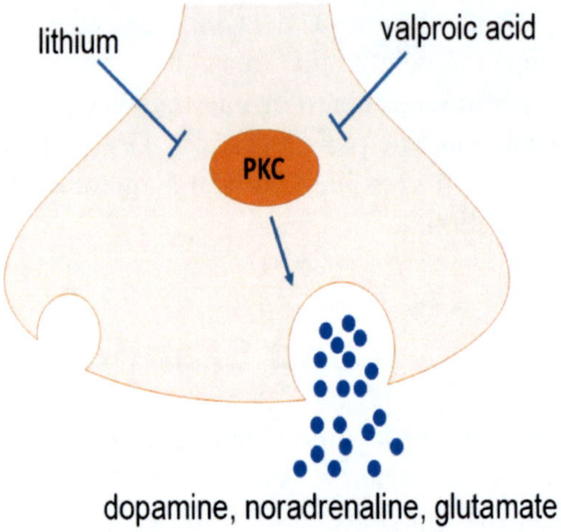

Figure 4. Lithium and valproic acid (VPA) inhibit protein kinase C (PKC), an important part in the signaling cascade which facilitates exocytosis of dopamine (DA), noradrenaline (NA) and glutamate.

Valproic acid also elicits a robust induction of prostate apoptosis response-4 (Par-4), an intracellular binding partner of dopamine D_2 receptors (DRD2) which significantly impacts DRD2-mediated signaling. Furthermore, the induction mechanism involves dynamic chromatin remodeling in the Par-4 promoter regions and indicates that part of the mood stabilizing efficacy of valproic acid is mediated by changes in DRD2-mediated signaling processes (Lee et al., 2012). Another possible mechanism, shared with lithium, is the inhibition of protein kinase C (Figure 4) and subsequent dampening of excessive release of noradrenaline and dopamine (Bachmann et al., 2005).

Carbamazepine

Carbamazepine's effects on catecholaminergic transmission are complex. It decreases catecholamine turnover (Waldmeier et al., 1984), acts as a weak reuptake inhibitor of noradrenaline (Purdy et al., 1977) and decreases β_2 adrenergic receptor-stimulated adenylate cyclase activity like lithium (Chen et al., 1996). Interestingly, carbamazepine also prevents cocaine-induced dopamine overflow in the nucleus accumbens (Baptista et al., 1993), which could explain its inhibitory effect on the reward system. In addition, carbamazepine appears to increase prefrontal dopamine release via the activation of serotoninergic $5HT_{1A}$ receptors, a mechanism shared with valproic acid and thought to contribute to its antidepressant effects (Ichikawa & Meltzer, 1999).

Summing up, mood stabilizers are used to prevent mania and depression. They appear to achieve this goal by partially different mechanisms. One point of convergence might be the ability to stabilize catecholaminergic function and prevent excessive stimulation.

Transcending Catecholamines

Catecholamines and Serotonin

Serotoninergic dysfunction is thought to play a key role in various psychiatric disorders, spanning the whole range from psychotic to affective disorders, from impulsivity and suicidality to eating and personality disorders. The spectrum of psychiatric symptoms thought to be associated with an imbalance of serotoninergic transmission is extremely broad and beyond the scope of this review. However, serotoninergic transmission is also interdependent on catecholamines. In many ways, there appear to be opponent interactions of serotonin and catecholamines with mostly antagonistic effects on a variety of psychiatric symptoms (Daw et al., 2002). Although the relationship between these transmitters is extremely complex and only partially understood, one important neuroanatomical substrate of the apparent partial antagonism can be found in serotoninergic fibers originating in the raphe nuclei and projecting to various dopaminergic and noradrenergic targets via inhibitory interneurons (Figure 5). These connections are thought to be part of an important feedback loop by which homeostasis between the different monoaminergic transmitters can be reinforced under normal conditions. In addition, a plethora of cross effects mediated by different types of pre- and postsynaptic dopamine, noradrenaline and serotonin receptors complement the interaction. As an example, inhibition of $5HT_{2C}$ receptors, a property commonly found in many atypical antipsychotics, disinhibits the release of dopamine and noradrenaline in the prefrontal cortex. Any interference with one part of the system is likely to affect the other parts. In this sense, catecholamines are closely intertwined with serotonin, and imbalances of any cause always have direct or indirect effects on both.

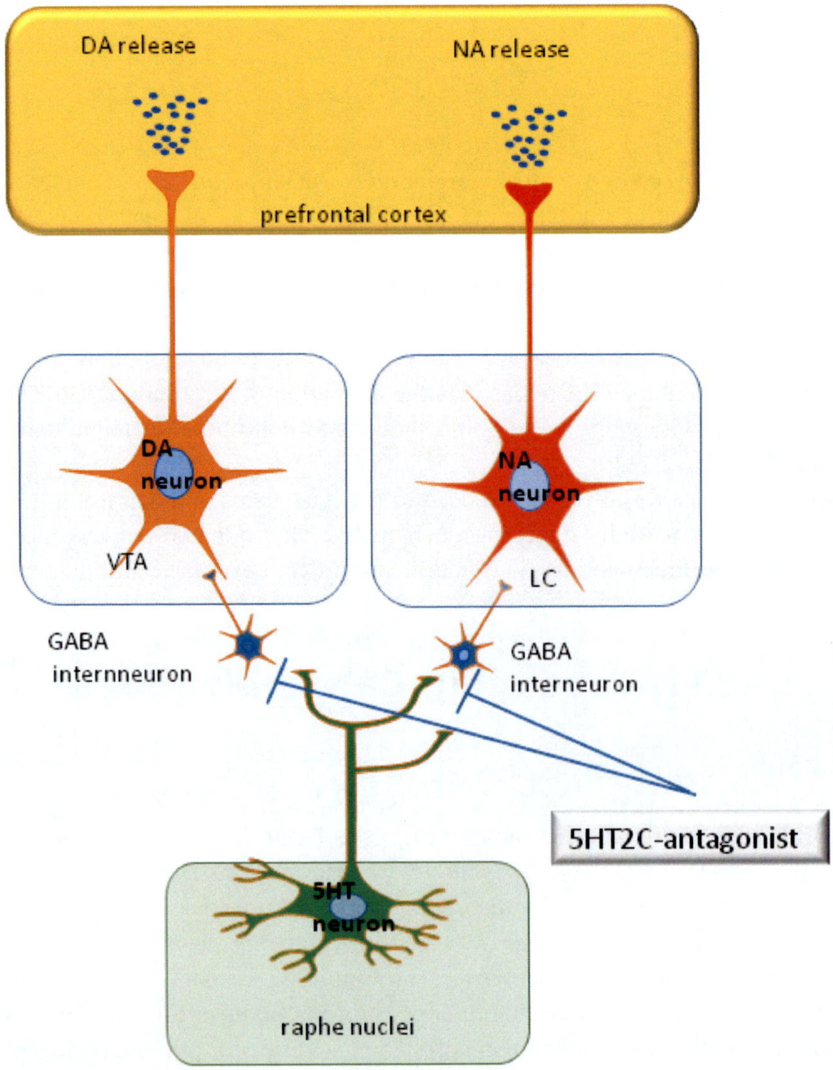

Figure 5. Interaction between serotonin (5HT) and catecholamines. Serotoninergic fibers originating in the raphe nuclei inhibit dopaminergic and noradrenergic neurons in the ventral tegmental area (VTA) and locus coerulaeus (LC) which project to the prefrontal cortex via gamma amino butyric acid (GABA) interneurons. Inhibitors of serontonin $5HT_2$-receptors can disinhibit this mechanism, resulting in an increase of dopamine (DA) and noradrenaline (NA) release in the prefrontal cortex.

Catecholamines and Glutamate

Glutamate is the main excitatory transmitter in the central nervous system and a precursor molecule for gamma amino butyric acid, the prime inhibitory neurotransmitter. Disequilibrium between these two neurotransmitters is prone to result in a plethora of possible consequences. Today, there is a large body of evidence supporting the role of glutamate in mood disorders (Javitt et al., 2011). The glutamatergic contribution is thought to lie further upstream in the causal chain than catecholaminergic transmission by playing the role of a superordinate regulator of dopamine (and serotonin) release. One important mechanism of this interaction is the dual glutamatergic brake/accelerator mechanism between the prefrontal cortex and dopaminergic centers in the brainstem (Figure 6). Direct glutamatergic projections increase dopamine release, whereas indirect connections via GABAergic interneurons dampen the response. Feedback loops probably exist, possibly via the striatum and thalamus.

Recent research suggests that a hypofunction of N-Methyl-D-Aspartate receptors, a subtype of glutamate receptors, and imbalance with other types of glutamate receptors may play a key role in psychosis. Hypofunction of N-Methyl-D-Aspartate receptors can not only lead to increased dopamine release in the limbic system but also can disturb dopamine function in the frontal cortex (Lisman et al., 2008). In contrast, glutamatergic hyperfunction in depression seems to be closely related to serotoninergic and catecholaminergic deficits and appears to correlate well with the clinical core symptoms (Muller & Schwarz, 2008; Hashimoto, 2009).

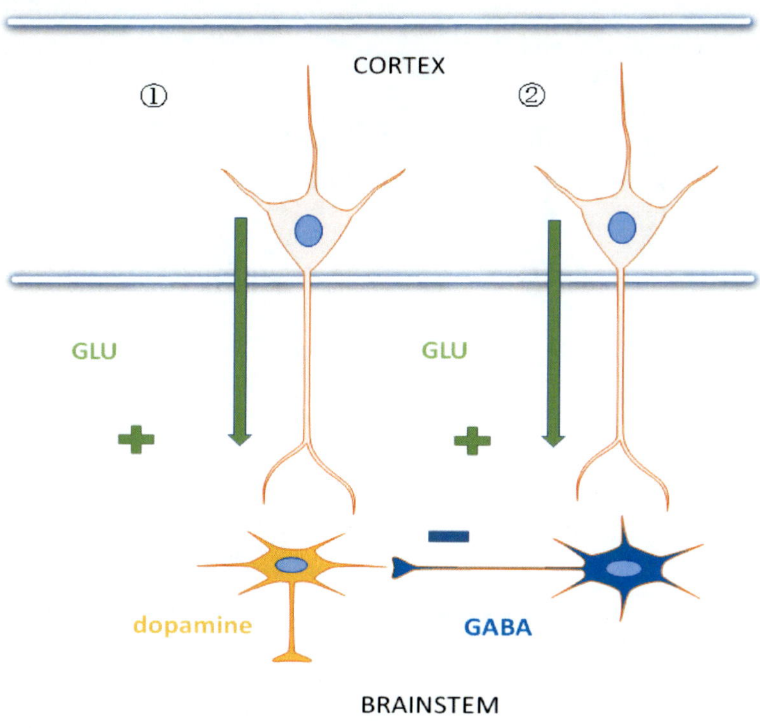

Figure 6. The glutamatergic accelerator/brake mechanism. (1) Glutamatergic fibers project from the cortex directly to dopaminergic neurons and enhance transmission. (2) Glutamatergic fibers can also inhibit dopaminergic neurons via inihibitory GABA-ergic interneurons.

Catecholamines and Stress

Throughout a wide range of psychiatric disorders, excessive stress and maladaptive stress management are well known risk factors that contribute unequivocally to their etiopathogenesis. The interaction of stress factors and catecholamines takes place on multiple levels (Leonard, 2001). Hypersecretion of corticotropin-releasing factor (CRF) occurs in both animal models of depression and depressed humans, with heightened CRF immunoreactivity in the cerebrospinal fluid (Nemeroff et al., 1984). In turn, tyrosine hydroxylase is activated and hastens noradrenaline turnover (Melia & Duman, 1991). The central noradrenergic system innervates vital parts of the immune system. Adrenoreceptors are found on a variety of immune cells like lymphocytes, macrophages and mast cells. When activated, these cells secrete pro-inflammatory cytokines. In affective disorders, a "pro-inflammatory" signature – an activation of inflammation-related genes - has been found in peripheral blood monocytes even before onset of the disorders, and pro-inflammatory cytokines are elevated during manic and depressive states (Drexhage et al., 2010; Goldstein et al., 2009). Increased inflammation and macrophage activity hasten noradrenaline turnover in the hypothalamus, increase CRF release and activate the hypothalamic-pituitary-adrenal axis to produce an excess of glucocorticoids (Figure 7). In addition, there is evidence that glucocorticoid receptors are desensitized in affective disorders, disabling the negative feedback loop. Thus, a vicious circle is established which involves stress, inflammation and catecholamines (Capuron & Miller, 2011).

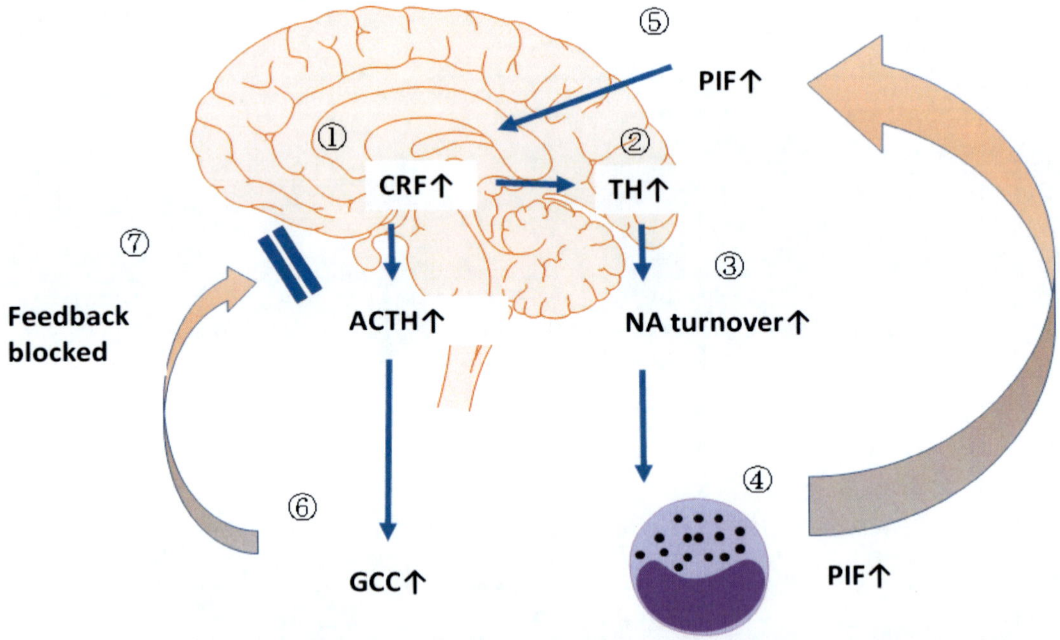

Figure 7. Catecholamines and stress. (1) Elevated levels of corticotropin releasing factor (CRF) increase tyrosine hydroxylase (TH) levels (2). As a consequence, noradrenaline (NA) levels rise (3) and acitvate different cells of the immune system to produce pro-inflammatory cytokines (PIF). (4) PIF create a positive feed back loop, further enhancing CRF production and noradrenaline turn over.(5). The hypothalamic pituitary adrenal axis is activated by CRF and levels of glucocorticoids (GCC) rise (6). Due to desensitized GCC-receptors, the negative feedback loop of the axis is interrupted, creating a vicious circle (7).

Catecholamines, Neuroprogression and Neurotoxicity

Increased lateral ventricular and cortical sulcal enlargement as well as a higher number of subcortical hyperintensities – mostly white matter lesions - have been found in bipolar patients (Figure 8) compared to healthy controls and confirmed in meta-analyses (Altshuler et al., 1995; Elkis et al., 1995; Raz & Raz, 1990).

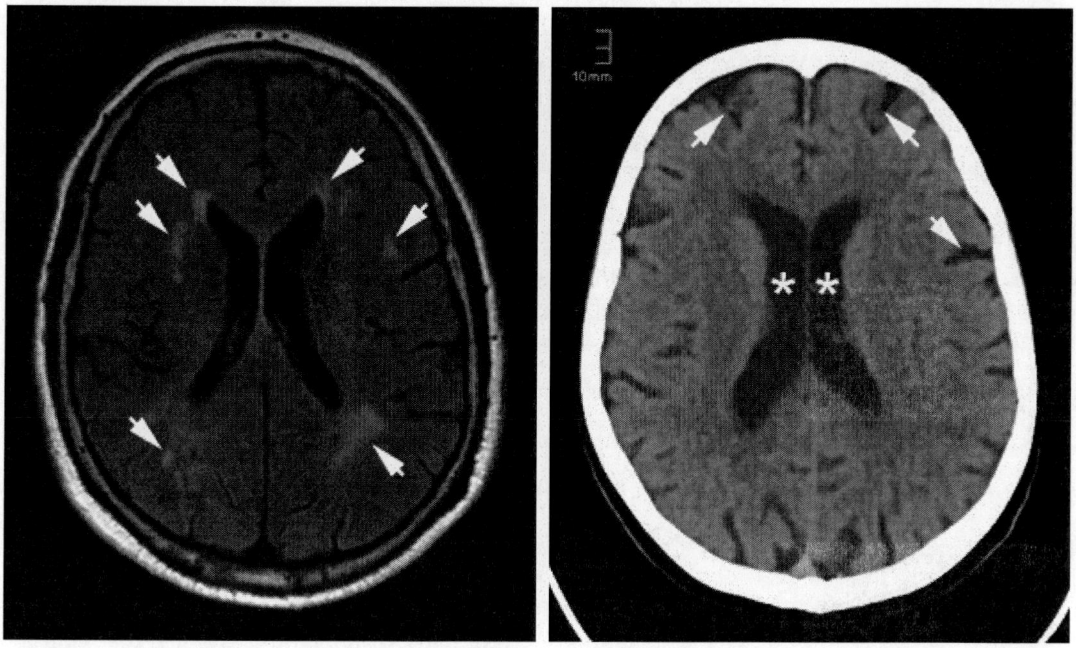

Figure 8. Subcortical hyperintensities (left insert, arrows), lateral ventricular enlargement (right insert, asterisks) and cortical sulcal enlargement (right insert, arrows) are common in bipolar patients. Cranial MRI scan (FLAIR). Reprinted with permission of Mark McCoy MD, Paracelsus Private Medical University, Salzburg, Austria.

In addition, there is evidence for a loss of grey matter in different regions of the brain, including the prefrontal cortex and different structures of the limbic system which are closely linked to catecholaminergic centers. Reduced regional brain volumes might partly be accounted for by hereditary and developmental factors linked to bipolar disorder. Accordingly, subcortical hyperintensities may partly be explained by comorbid conditions, especially cerebrovascular disease. However, progressive changes leading to a gradual escalation appear to play a key role as well (Schneider et al., 2012). These include a rising level of pro-inflammatory cytokines and a falling level of neurotrophins with detrimental effects on neuroplasticity as well as increasing oxidative stress. These factors have an impact on mitochondrial and endothelial function and result in protein and deoxyribonucleic acid damage or even cell death (Gama et al., 2013). Imbalances of catecholamine metabolism are entwined in these processes and might help to explain some of the observed effects. Both dopamine and noradrenaline have metabolites with neurotoxic properties. Increased overall catecholaminergic transmission or aberrant metabolic pathways may boost the formation of these products. As an example, 3, 4-dihydroxyphenylacetaldehyde is the aldehyde metabolite of dopamine, and 3, 4-dihydroxyphenylglycolaldehyde is the aldehyde metabolite of noradrenaline. Both of these aldehydes are highly reactive molecules, form reactive free radical intermediates under oxidative stress and enhance Ca^{2+}-mediated induction of the mitochondrial permeability transition (Burke et al., 1998). An additional source of oxidative stress that is unique to dopaminergic neurons is the (excess) presence of dopamine itself (Pedrosa & Soares-da-Silva, 2002). Metabolism of dopamine via monoamine oxidase or amine autoxidation can give rise to radical species, hydrogen peroxide (H_2O_2), semiquinones, and quinones (Graham, 1978). Interestingly, monoamine oxidase levels robustly increase with age, which might further exacerbate toxic effects (Glorioso et al., 2006). Quinones are thought to mediate toxicity by covalent binding to nucleophilic groups of biological macromolecules. The H_2O_2 resulting from the metabolism or autoxidation of L-dihydroxyphenylalanine (L-DOPA) and dopamine can be easily reduced in the presence of ferrous iron ($Fe2^{+}$) through the Fenton reaction originating the hydroxyl radical ($HO^{\cdot}$). This particle is considered the most damaging free radical for living cells. Dopamine *per se* is also known to induce apoptosis by a mechanism independent of oxidative stress and to regulate glial dystrophy-related pathways (Luo & Roth, 2000). In summary, there is a reasonably large body of evidence linking toxic catecholamine metabolites to neuroprogression in bipolar disorders.

Synopsis and Perspective

Bipolar disorder is a frequent and complex medical condition with a significant impact on the quality of life. It is often accompanied by a complexity of somatic and other psychiatric disorders. The catecholamine theory of affective disorders interprets depressive states as a relative lack of catecholamines and mania as a relative excess. These claims are corroborated by animal models and results from psychological studies in humans which clearly link core aspects of the opposite poles of mood to corresponding changes in the catecholaminergic system. Pharmacological challenge with compounds that boost or dampen dopamine or noradrenaline and correctly predict subsequent changes of mood provide additional evidence for the involvement of these transmitters in bipolar disorder. Furthermore, a relevant share of all currently licensed drugs used to treat bipolar disorder appears to have direct or indirect effects on catecholaminergic transmission. Intriguingly, many of the most frequent comorbidities seen in bipolar disorder seem to share the imbalance of catecholaminergic transmission as a common denominator from a partial overlap of the genetic background to altered levels of central and peripheral catecholamine metabolites. However, the metabolism of catecholamines is inextricably coupled with serotonin, glutamate, stress hormones, inflammatory signals, signal transmission and other regulatory systems. It seems possible or even likely that the changes found concerning catecholamines may ultimately only reflect detrimental alterations of superordinate factors located higher in the causal chain.

References

Abdolmaleky, H. M., Cheng, K. H., Faraone, S. V., Wilcox, M., Glatt, S. J., Gao, F. et al. (2006). Hypomethylation of MB-COMT promoter is a major risk factor for schizophrenia and bipolar disorder. *Hum.Mol.Genet., 15,* 3132-3145.

Abler, B., Greenhouse, I., Ongur, D., Walter, H., & Heckers, S. (2008). Abnormal reward system activation in mania. *Neuropsychopharmacology, 33,* 2217-2227.

Altshuler, L. L., Curran, J. G., Hauser, P., Mintz, J., Denicoff, K., & Post, R. (1995). T2 hyperintensities in bipolar disorder: magnetic resonance imaging comparison and literature meta-analysis. *Am.J.Psychiatry, 152,* 1139-1144.

Andrade, L., Caraveo-Anduaga, J. J., Berglund, P., Bijl, R. V., de, G. R., Vollebergh, W. et al. (2003). The epidemiology of major depressive episodes: results from the International Consortium of Psychiatric Epidemiology (ICPE) Surveys. *Int.J.Methods Psychiatr.Res., 12,* 3-21.

Angst, J., Sellaro, R., Stassen, H. H., & Gamma, A. (2005). Diagnostic conversion from depression to bipolar disorders: results of a long-term prospective study of hospital admissions. *J.Affect.Disord., 84,* 149-157.

Arnsten, A. F. (2007). Catecholamine and second messenger influences on prefrontal cortical networks of "representational knowledge": a rational bridge between genetics and the symptoms of mental illness. *Cereb.Cortex, 17 Suppl 1,* i6-15.

Avery, M. C., Dutt, N., & Krichmar, J. L. (2013). A large-scale neural network model of the influence of neuromodulatory levels on working memory and behavior. *Front Comput.Neurosci., 7,* 133.

Baarendse, P. J., Winstanley, C. A., & Vanderschuren, L. J. (2013). Simultaneous blockade of dopamine and noradrenaline reuptake promotes disadvantageous decision making in a rat gambling task. *Psychopharmacology (Berl), 225,* 719-731.

Bachmann, R. F., Schloesser, R. J., Gould, T. D., & Manji, H. K. (2005). Mood stabilizers target cellular plasticity and resilience cascades: implications for the development of novel therapeutics. *Mol.Neurobiol., 32,* 173-202.

Baptista, T., Weiss, S. R., & Post, R. M. (1993). Carbamazepine attenuates cocaine-induced increases in dopamine in the nucleus accumbens: an in vivo dialysis study. *Eur.J.Pharmacol., 236,* 39-42.

Basso, A. M., Gallagher, K. B., Bratcher, N. A., Brioni, J. D., Moreland, R. B., Hsieh, G. C. et al. (2005). Antidepressant-like effect of D(2/3) receptor-, but not D(4) receptor-activation in the rat forced swim test. *Neuropsychopharmacology, 30,* 1257-1268.

Beesdo, K., Hofler, M., Leibenluft, E., Lieb, R., Bauer, M., & Pfennig, A. (2009). Mood episodes and mood disorders: patterns of incidence and conversion in the first three decades of life. *Bipolar.Disord., 11,* 637-649.

Berk, M., Dodd, S., Kauer-Sant'anna, M., Malhi, G. S., Bourin, M., Kapczinski, F. et al. (2007). Dopamine dysregulation syndrome: implications for a dopamine hypothesis of bipolar disorder. *Acta Psychiatr.Scand.Suppl,* 41-49.

Berk, M., Kapczinski, F., Andreazza, A. C., Dean, O. M., Giorlando, F., Maes, M. et al. (2011). Pathways underlying neuroprogression in bipolar disorder: focus on inflammation, oxidative stress and neurotrophic factors. *Neurosci.Biobehav.Rev., 35,* 804-817.

Buckholtz, J. W. & Meyer-Lindenberg, A. (2008). MAOA and the neurogenetic architecture of human aggression. *Trends Neurosci., 31,* 120-129.

Buckholtz, J. W. & Meyer-Lindenberg, A. (2012). Psychopathology and the human connectome: toward a transdiagnostic model of risk for mental illness. *Neuron, 74,* 990-1004.

Burke, W. J., Kristal, B. S., Yu, B. P., Li, S. W., & Lin, T. S. (1998). Norepinephrine transmitter metabolite generates free radicals and activates mitochondrial permeability transition: a mechanism for DOPEGAL-induced apoptosis. *Brain Res., 787,* 328-332.

Capuron, L. & Miller, A. H. (2011). Immune system to brain signaling: neuropsychopharmacological implications. *Pharmacol.Ther., 130,* 226-238.

Chang, Y. H., Lee, S. Y., Chen, S. L., Tzeng, N. S., Wang, T. Y., Hui, L., I et al. (2013). Genetic variants of the BDNF and DRD3 genes in bipolar disorder comorbid with anxiety disorder. *J.Affect.Disord., 151,* 967-972.

Chen, G., Masana, M. I., & Manji, H. K. (2000). Lithium regulates PKC-mediated intracellular cross-talk and gene expression in the CNS in vivo. *Bipolar.Disord., 2,* 217-236.

Chen, G., Pan, B., Hawver, D. B., Wright, C. B., Potter, W. Z., & Manji, H. K. (1996). Attenuation of cyclic AMP production by carbamazepine. *J.Neurochem., 67,* 2079-2086.

Chou, J. C., Czobor, P., Tuma, I., Charles, O., Bebe, R., Cooper, T. B. et al. (2000). Pretreatment plasma HVA and haloperidol response in acute mania. *J.Affect.Disord., 59,* 55-59.

Coryell, W., Scheftner, W., Keller, M., Endicott, J., Maser, J., & Klerman, G. L. (1993). The enduring psychosocial consequences of mania and depression. *Am.J.Psychiatry, 150,* 720-727.

Daw, N. D., Kakade, S., & Dayan, P. (2002). Opponent interactions between serotonin and dopamine. *Neural Netw., 15,* 603-616.

Drexhage, R. C., Heul-Nieuwenhuijsen, L., Padmos, R. C., van, B. N., Cohen, D., Versnel, M. A. et al. (2010). Inflammatory gene expression in monocytes of patients with schizophrenia: overlap and difference with bipolar disorder. A study in naturalistically treated patients. *Int.J.Neuropsychopharmacol., 13,* 1369-1381.

Dunlop, B. W. & Nemeroff, C. B. (2007). The role of dopamine in the pathophysiology of depression. *Arch.Gen.Psychiatry, 64,* 327-337.

Eckermann, K., Beasley, A., Yang, P., Gaytan, O., Swann, A., & Dafny, N. (2001). Methylphenidate sensitization is modulated by valproate. *Life Sci., 69,* 47-57.

Elkis, H., Friedman, L., Wise, A., & Meltzer, H. Y. (1995). Meta-analyses of studies of ventricular enlargement and cortical sulcal prominence in mood disorders. Comparisons with controls or patients with schizophrenia. *Arch.Gen.Psychiatry, 52,* 735-746.

Ewald, H., Mors, O., Eiberg, H., Flint, T., & Kruse, T. A. (1995). No evidence of linkage between manic depressive illness and the dopa decarboxylase gene or nearby region on chromosome 7p. *Psychiatr.Genet., 5,* 161-169.

Ewald, H., Mors, O., Flint, T., Eiberg, H., & Kruse, T. A. (1994). Linkage analysis between manic depressive illness and the dopamine beta-hydroxylase gene. *Psychiatr.Genet., 4,* 177-183.

Fan, M., Liu, B., Jiang, T., Jiang, X., Zhao, H., & Zhang, J. (2010). Meta-analysis of the association between the monoamine oxidase-A gene and mood disorders. *Psychiatr.Genet., 20,* 1-7.

Ferrari, A. J., Baxter, A. J., & Whiteford, H. A. (2011). A systematic review of the global distribution and availability of prevalence data for bipolar disorder. *J.Affect.Disord., 134,* 1-13.

Fitzgerald, P. J. (2013a). Elevated Norepinephrine may be a Unifying Etiological Factor in the Abuse of a Broad Range of Substances: Alcohol, Nicotine, Marijuana, Heroin, Cocaine, and Caffeine. *Subst.Abuse, 7,* 171-183.

Fitzgerald, P. J. (2013b). Elevated norepinephrine may be an etiological factor in a wide range of diseases: age-related macular degeneration, systemic lupus erythematosus, atrial fibrillation, metabolic syndrome. *Med.Hypotheses, 80,* 558-563.

Gama, C. S., Kunz, M., Magalhaes, P. V., & Kapczinski, F. (2013). Staging and neuroprogression in bipolar disorder: a systematic review of the literature. *Rev.Bras.Psiquiatr., 35,* 70-74.

Gerner, R. H., Fairbanks, L., Anderson, G. M., Young, J. G., Scheinin, M., Linnoila, M. et al. (1984). CSF neurochemistry in depressed, manic, and schizophrenic patients compared with that of normal controls. *Am.J.Psychiatry, 141,* 1533-1540.

Ghaemi, S. N., Rosenquist, K. J., Ko, J. Y., Baldassano, C. F., Kontos, N. J., & Baldessarini, R. J. (2004). Antidepressant treatment in bipolar versus unipolar depression. *Am.J.Psychiatry, 161,* 163-165.

Glorioso, C., Sabatini, M., Unger, T., Hashimoto, T., Monteggia, L. M., Lewis, D. A. et al. (2006). Specificity and timing of neocortical transcriptome changes in response to BDNF gene ablation during embryogenesis or adulthood. *Mol.Psychiatry, 11,* 633-648.

Goldstein, B. I., Kemp, D. E., Soczynska, J. K., & McIntyre, R. S. (2009). Inflammation and the phenomenology, pathophysiology, comorbidity, and treatment of bipolar disorder: a systematic review of the literature. *J.Clin.Psychiatry, 70,* 1078-1090.

Graham, D. G. (1978). Oxidative pathways for catecholamines in the genesis of neuromelanin and cytotoxic quinones. *Mol.Pharmacol., 14,* 633-643.

Hashimoto, K. (2009). Emerging role of glutamate in the pathophysiology of major depressive disorder. *Brain Res.Rev., 61,* 105-123.

Huang, Y. Y., Cate, S. P., Battistuzzi, C., Oquendo, M. A., Brent, D., & Mann, J. J. (2004). An association between a functional polymorphism in the monoamine oxidase a gene promoter, impulsive traits and early abuse experiences. *Neuropsychopharmacology, 29,* 1498-1505.

Ichikawa, J. & Meltzer, H. Y. (1999). Valproate and carbamazepine increase prefrontal dopamine release by 5-HT1A receptor activation. *Eur.J.Pharmacol., 380,* R1-R3.

Javitt, D. C., Schoepp, D., Kalivas, P. W., Volkow, N. D., Zarate, C., Merchant, K. et al. (2011). Translating glutamate: from pathophysiology to treatment. *Sci.Transl.Med., 3,* 102mr2.

Jope, R. S. (1999). Anti-bipolar therapy: mechanism of action of lithium. *Mol.Psychiatry, 4,* 117-128.

Kay, G., Sargeant, M., McGuffin, P., Whatley, S., Marchbanks, R., Baldwin, D. et al. (1993). The lymphoblast beta-adrenergic receptor in bipolar depressed patients: characterization and down-regulation. *J.Affect.Disord., 27,* 163-172.

Kirov, G., Murphy, K. C., Arranz, M. J., Jones, I., McCandles, F., Kunugi, H. et al. (1998). Low activity allele of catechol-O-methyltransferase gene associated with rapid cycling bipolar disorder. *Mol.Psychiatry, 3,* 342-345.

Kopin, I. J. (1985). Catecholamine metabolism: basic aspects and clinical significance. *Pharmacol.Rev., 37,* 333-364.

Lachman, H. M., Morrow, B., Shprintzen, R., Veit, S., Parsia, S. S., Faedda, G. et al. (1996). Association of codon 108/158 catechol-O-methyltransferase gene polymorphism with the psychiatric manifestations of velo-cardio-facial syndrome. *Am.J.Med.Genet., 67,* 468-472.

Lambert, G., Johansson, M., Agren, H., & Friberg, P. (2000). Reduced brain norepinephrine and dopamine release in treatment-refractory depressive illness: evidence in support of the catecholamine hypothesis of mood disorders. *Arch.Gen.Psychiatry, 57,* 787-793.

Lee, H. Y. & Kim, Y. K. (2010). Catechol-O-methyltransferase Val158Met polymorphism affects therapeutic response to mood stabilizer in symptomatic manic patients. *Psychiatry Res., 175,* 63-66.

Lee, S., Jeong, J., Park, Y. U., Kwak, Y., Lee, S. A., Lee, H. et al. (2012). Valproate alters dopamine signaling in association with induction of Par-4 protein expression. *PLoS.One., 7,* e45618.

Lee, S. H., Ripke, S., Neale, B. M., Faraone, S. V., Purcell, S. M., Perlis, R. H. et al. (2013). Genetic relationship between five psychiatric disorders estimated from genome-wide SNPs. *Nat.Genet., 45,* 984-994.

Lee, S. Y., Chen, S. L., Chen, S. H., Huang, S. Y., Tzeng, N. S., Chang, Y. H. et al. (2011). The COMT and DRD3 genes interacted in bipolar I but not bipolar II disorder. *World J.Biol.Psychiatry, 12,* 385-391.

Lelli-Chiesa, G., Kempton, M. J., Jogia, J., Tatarelli, R., Girardi, P., Powell, J. et al. (2011). The impact of the Val158Met catechol-O-methyltransferase genotype on neural correlates of sad facial affect processing in patients with bipolar disorder and their relatives. *Psychol.Med., 41,* 779-788.

Leonard, B. E. (2001). Stress, norepinephrine and depression. *J.Psychiatry Neurosci., 26 Suppl,* S11-S16.

Lieberman, J. A., Kinon, B. J., & Loebel, A. D. (1990). Dopaminergic mechanisms in idiopathic and drug-induced psychoses. *Schizophr.Bull., 16,* 97-110.

Lisman, J. E., Coyle, J. T., Green, R. W., Javitt, D. C., Benes, F. M., Heckers, S. et al. (2008). Circuit-based framework for understanding neurotransmitter and risk gene interactions in schizophrenia. *Trends Neurosci., 31,* 234-242.

Luo, Y. & Roth, G. S. (2000). The roles of dopamine oxidative stress and dopamine receptor signaling in aging and age-related neurodegeneration. *Antioxid.Redox.Signal., 2,* 449-460.

Maas, J. W., Koslow, S. H., Davis, J., Katz, M., Frazer, A., Bowden, C. L. et al. (1987). Catecholamine metabolism and disposition in healthy and depressed subjects. *Arch.Gen.Psychiatry, 44,* 337-344.

Maj, M., Ariano, M. G., Arena, F., & Kemali, D. (1984). Plasma cortisol, catecholamine and cyclic AMP levels, response to dexamethasone suppression test and platelet MAO activity in manic-depressive patients. A longitudinal study. *Neuropsychobiology, 11,* 168-173.

Malhi, G. S., Tanious, M., Das, P., Coulston, C. M., & Berk, M. (2013). Potential mechanisms of action of lithium in bipolar disorder. Current understanding. *CNS.Drugs, 27,* 135-153.

Manji, H. K., Potter, W. Z., & Lenox, R. H. (1995). Signal transduction pathways. Molecular targets for lithium's actions. *Arch.Gen.Psychiatry, 52,* 531-543.

Marchese, G., Scheggi, S., Secci, M. E., De Montis, M. G., & Gambarana, C. (2013). Anti-anhedonic activity of long-term lithium treatment in rats exposed to repeated unavoidable stress. *Int.J.Neuropsychopharmacol., 16,* 1611-1621.

Massat, I., Kocabas, N. A., Crisafulli, C., Chiesa, A., Calati, R., Linotte, S. et al. (2011). COMT and age at onset in mood disorders: a replication and extension study. *Neurosci.Lett., 498,* 218-221.

Melia, K. R. & Duman, R. S. (1991). Involvement of corticotropin-releasing factor in chronic stress regulation of the brain noradrenergic system. *Proc.Natl.Acad.Sci.U.S.A, 88,* 8382-8386.

Mitchell, P. B., Wilhelm, K., Parker, G., Austin, M. P., Rutgers, P., & Malhi, G. S. (2001). The clinical features of bipolar depression: a comparison with matched major depressive disorder patients. *J.Clin.Psychiatry, 62,* 212-216.

Muller, N. & Schwarz, M. J. (2008). A psychoneuroimmunological perspective to Emil Kraepelins dichotomy: schizophrenia and major depression as inflammatory CNS disorders. *Eur.Arch.Psychiatry Clin.Neurosci., 258 Suppl 2,* 97-106.

Nemeroff, C. B., Widerlov, E., Bissette, G., Walleus, H., Karlsson, I., Eklund, K. et al. (1984). Elevated concentrations of CSF corticotropin-releasing factor-like immunoreactivity in depressed patients. *Science, 226,* 1342-1344.

O'Sullivan, S. S., Evans, A. H., & Lees, A. J. (2009). Dopamine dysregulation syndrome: an overview of its epidemiology, mechanisms and management. *CNS.Drugs, 23,* 157-170.

Pearlson, G. D., Wong, D. F., Tune, L. E., Ross, C. A., Chase, G. A., Links, J. M. et al. (1995). In vivo D2 dopamine receptor density in psychotic and nonpsychotic patients with bipolar disorder. *Arch.Gen.Psychiatry, 52,* 471-477.

Pedrosa, R. & Soares-da-Silva, P. (2002). Oxidative and non-oxidative mechanisms of neuronal cell death and apoptosis by L-3,4-dihydroxyphenylalanine (L-DOPA) and dopamine. *Br.J.Pharmacol., 137,* 1305-1313.

Peele, P. B., Xu, Y., & Kupfer, D. J. (2003). Insurance expenditures on bipolar disorder: clinical and parity implications. *Am.J.Psychiatry, 160,* 1286-1290.

Piletz, J. E., Halaris, A., Saran, A., & Marler, M. (1990). Elevated 3H-para-aminoclonidine binding to platelet purified plasma membranes from depressed patients. *Neuropsychopharmacology, 3,* 201-210.

Purdy, R. E., Julien, R. M., Fairhurst, A. S., & Terry, M. D. (1977). Effect of carbamazepine on the in vitro uptake and release of norepinephrine in adrenergic nerves of rabbit aorta and in whole brain synaptosomes. *Epilepsia, 18,* 251-257.

Ramos, B. P. & Arnsten, A. F. (2007). Adrenergic pharmacology and cognition: focus on the prefrontal cortex. *Pharmacol.Ther., 113,* 523-536.

Raz, S. & Raz, N. (1990). Structural brain abnormalities in the major psychoses: a quantitative review of the evidence from computerized imaging. *Psychol.Bull., 108,* 93-108.

Rotondo, A., Mazzanti, C., Dell'Osso, L., Rucci, P., Sullivan, P., Bouanani, S. et al. (2002). Catechol o-methyltransferase, serotonin transporter, and tryptophan hydroxylase gene polymorphisms in bipolar disorder patients with and without comorbid panic disorder. *Am.J.Psychiatry, 159,* 23-29.

Rudorfer, M. V., Ross, R. J., Linnoila, M., Sherer, M. A., & Potter, W. Z. (1985). Exaggerated orthostatic responsivity of plasma norepinephrine in depression. *Arch.Gen.Psychiatry, 42,* 1186-1192.

Sands, S. A., Guerra, V., & Morilak, D. A. (2000). Changes in tyrosine hydroxylase mRNA expression in the rat locus coeruleus following acute or chronic treatment with valproic acid. *Neuropsychopharmacology, 22,* 27-35.

Savitz, J. B., Nugent, A. C., Bogers, W., Roiser, J. P., Bain, E. E., Neumeister, A. et al. (2011). Habenula volume in bipolar disorder and major depressive disorder: a high-resolution magnetic resonance imaging study. *Biol.Psychiatry, 69,* 336-343.

Scappa, S., Teverbaugh, P., & Ananth, J. (1993). Episodic tardive dyskinesia and parkinsonism in bipolar disorder patients. *Can.J.Psychiatry, 38,* 633-634.

Schildkraut, J. J. (1965). The catecholamine hypothesis of affective disorders: a review of supporting evidence. *Am.J.Psychiatry, 122,* 509-522.

Schildkraut, J. J. (1995). The catecholamine hypothesis of affective disorders: a review of supporting evidence. 1965. *J.Neuropsychiatry Clin.Neurosci., 7,* 524-533.

Schneider, M. R., Delbello, M. P., McNamara, R. K., Strakowski, S. M., & Adler, C. M. (2012). Neuroprogression in bipolar disorder. *Bipolar.Disord., 14,* 356-374.

Schulze, T. G., Akula, N., Breuer, R., Steele, J., Nalls, M. A., Singleton, A. B. et al. (2012). Molecular genetic overlap in bipolar disorder, schizophrenia, and major depressive disorder. *World J.Biol.Psychiatry.*

Sher, L., Carballo, J. J., Grunebaum, M. F., Burke, A. K., Zalsman, G., Huang, Y. Y. et al. (2006). A prospective study of the association of cerebrospinal fluid monoamine metabolite levels with lethality of suicide attempts in patients with bipolar disorder. *Bipolar.Disord., 8,* 543-550.

Sjostrom, R. & Roos, B. E. (1972). 5-Hydroxyindolacetic acid and homovanillic acid in cerebrospinal fluid in manic-depressive psychosis. *Eur.J.Clin.Pharmacol., 4,* 170-176.

Soeiro-de-Souza, M. G., Bio, D. S., David, D. P., Rodrigues dos, S. D., Jr., Kerr, D. S., Gattaz, W. F. et al. (2012). COMT Met (158) modulates facial emotion recognition in bipolar I disorder mood episodes. *J.Affect.Disord., 136,* 370-376.

Sofuoglu, S., Dogan, P., Kose, K., Esel, E., Basturk, M., Oguz, H. et al. (1995). Changes in platelet monoamine oxidase and plasma dopamine-beta-hydroxylase activities in lithium-treated bipolar patients. *Psychiatry Res., 59,* 165-170.

Suhara, T., Nakayama, K., Inoue, O., Fukuda, H., Shimizu, M., Mori, A. et al. (1992). D1 dopamine receptor binding in mood disorders measured by positron emission tomography. *Psychopharmacology (Berl), 106,* 14-18.

Swann, A. C., Koslow, S. H., Katz, M. M., Maas, J. W., Javaid, J., Secunda, S. K. et al. (1987). Lithium carbonate treatment of mania. Cerebrospinal fluid and urinary monoamine metabolites and treatment outcome. *Arch.Gen.Psychiatry, 44,* 345-354.

Swann, A. C., Secunda, S., Davis, J. M., Robins, E., Hanin, I., Koslow, S. H. et al. (1983). CSF monoamine metabolites in mania. *Am.J.Psychiatry, 140,* 396-400.

Torack, R. M. & Morris, J. C. (1988). The association of ventral tegmental area histopathology with adult dementia. *Arch.Neurol., 45,* 497-501.

Turecki, G., Rouleau, G. A., Mari, J., Joober, R., & Morgan, K. (1997). Lack of association between bipolar disorder and tyrosine hydroxylase: a meta-analysis. *Am.J.Med.Genet., 74,* 348-352.

Valentini, V., Frau, R., & Di, C. G. (2004). Noradrenaline transporter blockers raise extracellular dopamine in medial prefrontal but not parietal and occipital cortex: differences with mianserin and clozapine. *J.Neurochem., 88,* 917-927.

Vawter, M. P., Freed, W. J., & Kleinman, J. E. (2000). Neuropathology of bipolar disorder. *Biol.Psychiatry, 48,* 486-504.

Waldmeier, P. C., Baumann, P. A., Fehr, B., De, H. P., & Maitre, L. (1984). Carbamazepine decreases catecholamine turnover in the rat brain. *J.Pharmacol.Exp.Ther., 231,* 166-172.

Wang, T. Y., Lee, S. Y., Chen, S. L., Chang, Y. H., Chen, S. H., Huang, S. Y. et al. (2013). Gender-specific association of the SLC6A4 and DRD2 gene variants in bipolar disorder. *Int.J.Neuropsychopharmacol.,* 1-12.

Willner, P. (1983). Dopamine and depression: a review of recent evidence. II. Theoretical approaches. *Brain Res., 287,* 225-236.

Wolfe, N., Katz, D. I., Albert, M. L., Almozlino, A., Durso, R., Smith, M. C. et al. (1990). Neuropsychological profile linked to low dopamine: in Alzheimer's disease, major depression, and Parkinson's disease. *J.Neurol.Neurosurg.Psychiatry, 53,* 915-917.

Yanowitch, R. & Coccaro, E. F. (2011). The neurochemistry of human aggression. *Adv.Genet., 75,* 151-169.

Yatham, L. N., Liddle, P. F., Shiah, I. S., Lam, R. W., Ngan, E., Scarrow, G. et al. (2002). PET study of [(18)F]6-fluoro-L-dopa uptake in neuroleptic- and mood-stabilizer-naive first-episode nonpsychotic mania: effects of treatment with divalproex sodium. *Am.J.Psychiatry, 159,* 768-774.

Young, A. H. & Grunze, H. (2013). Physical health of patients with bipolar disorder. *Acta Psychiatr.Scand.Suppl,* 3-10.

Young, L. T., Warsh, J. J., Kish, S. J., Shannak, K., & Hornykeiwicz, O. (1994). Reduced brain 5-HT and elevated NE turnover and metabolites in bipolar affective disorder. *Biol.Psychiatry, 35,* 121-127.

Zheng, W., Zeng, Z., Bhardwaj, S. K., Jamali, S., & Srivastava, L. K. (2013). Lithium normalizes amphetamine-induced changes in striatal FoxO1 phosphorylation and behaviors in rats. *Neuroreport, 24,* 560-565.

Zhou, Q. Y. & Palmiter, R. D. (1995). Dopamine-deficient mice are severely hypoactive, adipsic, and aphagic. *Cell, 83,* 1197-1209.

Zubieta, J. K., Huguelet, P., Ohl, L. E., Koeppe, R. A., Kilbourn, M. R., Carr, J. M. et al. (2000). High vesicular monoamine transporter binding in asymptomatic bipolar I disorder: sex differences and cognitive correlates. *Am.J.Psychiatry, 157,* 1619-1628.

In: The Central Catecholaminergic System
Editor: Bertalan Dudás
ISBN: 978-1-63117-937-2

Chapter 11

Catecholamines and Alzheimer's Disease

Michael S. Peroski and Bertalan Dudás

Introductory Comments

Alzheimer's disease (AD) is a progressive neurodegenerative condition for which there is currently no cure and is most well known for its deleterious effects on memory, behavior, and other cognitive functions. As the most common dementia, AD accounts for 60%-80% of all diagnoses of dementia (Thies & Bleiler, 2013). Understanding the pathogenesis of AD is of paramount importance given the projected future prevalence of cases. There are an estimated 5.2 million people over the age of 65 with AD in the United States presently (Thies & Bleiler, 2013); without any cure or new treatment, this will likely increase to 13.8 million people by 2050 (Hebert et al., 2013). Globally, it is anticipated that, without advancement in treatment, 115.4 million people will have dementia by 2050 (Prince et al., 2013). It has been projected that if a treatment was able to delay the onset of AD for five years in patients, it could decrease the expected prevalence of the disease by about 4.04 million cases in the United States after fifty years (Brookmeyer et al., 1998).

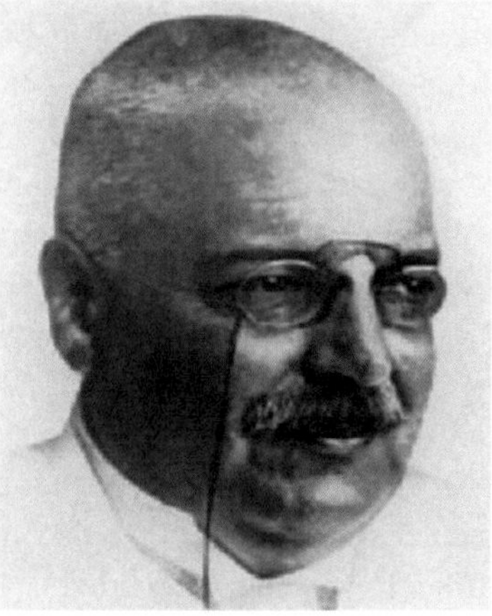

Figure 1. Aloysius Alzheimer (1864-1915), a German psychiatrist and neuropathologist

Alois Alzheimer (Figure 1) offered the first formal description of AD in 1906. He described a patient, Auguste D, who was a 51 year old female with cognitive impairment, language difficulty, psychiatric and other symptoms (Maurer et al., 1997). After Auguste's death in 1906, Alzheimer also described what would become some of the hallmark pathologic findings of AD: "miliary foci," later determined to be senile plaques, and "neurofibrillary degeneration," which was later defined as neurofibrillary tangles (Maurer et al., 1997; Zilka & Novak, 2006).

Diagnosis of Alzheimer's Disease

AD is a clinical diagnosis with *post-mortem* histopathologic confirmation. Commonly used guidelines for the clinical diagnosis of AD were established in 1984 by the National Institute of Neurological and Communicative Disorders and Stroke and the Alzheimer's Disease and Related Disorders Association (NINCDS-ADRDA) (McKhann et al., 1984). A series of National Institute of Ageing-Alzheimer's Association (NIA-AA) joint workgroups have proposed updates and changes to the diagnostic criteria for AD (McKhann et al., 2011) and have also suggested diagnostic criteria for preclinical AD (Sperling et al., 2011) and mild cognitive impairment (MCI) due to AD (Albert et al., 2011). There are several reasons that the organizations felt that an update was necessary, as detailed in an introductory article to the proposed updates (Jack, Jr. et al., 2011). Importantly, NIA-AA workgroups set forth criteria that recognize AD as a disease process that progresses from a preclinical phase in which pathology develops without clinical manifestations, to a stage of mild cognitive impairment (MCI) due to AD, in which baseline functioning is impaired but not to a degree that prevents independent functioning of a patient, and finally to AD, a final stage of dementia in which independent functioning is impaired. Although the NIA-AA diagnostic criteria are discussed herein, it is important to mention that other diagnostic criteria exist, notably the criteria of the International Working Group for New Research Criteria for the Diagnosis of AD (Dubois et al., 2007; Dubois et al., 2010; Visser et al., 2012). There are also criteria for major and minor neurocognitive disorder set forth in the "Diagnostic and Statistical Manual of Mental Disorders (DSM) V" (American Psychiatric Association, 2013). For a comparison between the international working group criteria and the NIA-AA criteria see Visser (Visser et al., 2012).

Preclinical Stage of AD

In the asymptomatic, preclinical stage of AD, pathology accumulates in the brain and neuronal damage may occur, without significant noticeable or detectable effect on the clinical presentation of the patient (Sperling et al., 2011). The NIA-AA workgroup's model relies on the detection of preclinical pathology reflective of AD pathology using biomarkers of the disease (Sperling et al., 2011). Sperling and his colleagues set forth a "draft operational research framework for staging preclinical AD" which uses biomarkers possibly suggestive of pathologic change in the brain to assess the progression of preclinical AD (Sperling et al., 2011). However, it is important to recognize that this was intended for research settings, as they explain: "...this framework is not intended to serve as diagnostic criteria for clinical purposes. Use of these biomarkers in the clinical setting is unwarranted because many individuals who satisfy the proposed research criteria may not develop the clinical features of AD in their lifetime"(Sperling et al., 2011). The proposed framework of preclinical AD includes three stages. In the first stage, the patient has asymptomatic amyloidosis detected through various biomarkers. In the second stage, the patient has biomarker evidence of amyloidosis and neurodegeneration. In the third stage, the patient has biomarker evidence of amyloidosis, neurodegeneration, and also a subtle cognitive decline that fails to meet criteria for MCI. The NIA-AA workgroup further emphasized the importance of additional research and study of biomarkers before they can be regularly applied in clinical context and also details the biomarkers that might prove useful in the aforementioned stages of preclinical AD (Sperling et al., 2011).

Mild Cognitive Impairment (MCI) due to AD

Although difficult to clinically establish the exact moment at which the transition from preclinical AD to MCI occurs in a patient, conceptually it happens when the accumulation of pathology is sufficient to cause detectible impairment in the patient's level of cognitive functioning [for review see (Petersen, 2011)]. Diagnostic criteria for MCI proposed by the NIA-AA workgroup include a departure from the patient's baseline level of cognitive functioning as reported by the patient or obtained from a collateral source with "impairment in one or more cognitive domains," that is clinically assessed and found to be a departure from the expected cognitive functioning of someone of the same age and educational level as the patient (Albert et al., 2011). Importantly, the criteria also emphasize the ability of the patient to function independently in daily living and also that the patient be free of dementia. The workgroup outlines a potential framework for using biomarkers in the assessment of MCI in research contexts as detailed in (Albert et al., 2011). Other potential causes for the cognitive impairment should also be excluded in the assessment of any patient suspected to have MCI due to AD. While being diagnosed with MCI certainly raises suspicion that a patient may have further cognitive decline, it does not necessarily mean that they will convert to dementia or full AD. A meta-analysis of forty-one cohort studies concluded that the annual rate of conversion from MCI to dementia is 5-10% with most patients not having converted to dementia after ten years of follow-up care (Mitchell & Shiri-Feshki, 2009). Patients with amnestic MCI, a subtype of MCI with memory loss being the main impairment, frequently show pathologic changes consistent with the early stages of AD (Jicha et al., 2006; Markesbery et al., 2006; Petersen et al., 2006) and also frequently progress to AD (Jicha et al., 2006; Markesbery et al., 2006; Petersen et al., 2006). However, patients with amnestic MCI do not always progress to AD, as one study demonstrated that, of patients diagnosed with amnestic MCI who progressed to dementia, up to 29% of the patients did not develop AD (Jicha et al., 2006).

AD

As mentioned, a NIA-AA workgroup recently proposed updates to the diagnostic criteria for AD (McKhann et al., 2011). This workgroup recommended criteria to diagnose dementia generally, specific criteria to further classify the dementia as AD, and criteria to establish whether the AD is probable or possible. They also set forth research criteria which incorporate biomarkers and specify AD as probable or possible with evidence of the AD pathophysiological process. It is important to recognize that, as outlined here, these diagnostic criteria are not intended to guide clinical decision making, but are rather intended to orient the reader. Please see (McKhann et al., 2011) for detailed description of the clinical and research diagnostic criteria for AD. According to the updated NIA-AA criteria, dementia is diagnosed when a patient has a departure from baseline cognitive functioning that interferes with daily activities and is detected through a combination of history from the patient or a collateral source and more objective testing such as a mental status examination or neuropsychological testing (McKhann et al., 2011). Notably, the patient must have cognitive impairment in at least two cognitive domains (McKhann et al., 2011). Other potential causes of cognitive impairment should also be excluded. This is distinguished from MCI most apparently in that the cognitive impairment is significant enough to interfere with independent functioning.

AD is diagnosed in a patient who meets the dementia criteria, and has a gradual onset of symptoms, a history of declining cognition, and who has amnestic or specific non-amnestic symptoms as the most obvious cognitive symptoms (McKhann et al., 2011). The non-amnestic cognitive symptoms include difficulties with language, visuospatial processing, or executive functioning. If a patient meets these criteria and also has documented cognitive decline or carries a genetic mutation known to be causative of AD they can be determined to have "probable AD" with increased certainty under the NIA-AA criteria (McKhann et al., 2011). "Possible AD" is present when either the course of the disease is unusual, such as sudden onset, or the etiology of the dementia is unclear. Evidence of the pathophysiological process is added to these diagnoses when biomarkers are utilized to yield findings suggestive of AD pathology; however, these biomarkers are intended to be used mainly in research settings.

Pathology

There are several hypotheses regarding the underlying cause of AD [for review see (Swerdlow, 2007)]. One of the most popular hypotheses is the "amyloid cascade hypothesis" that has an extensive literature (Hardy, 2006b; Hardy, 2006a; Hardy & Higgins, 1992; Karran et al., 2011; Pimplikar, 2009). This hypothesis suggests that the deposition of amyloid-β is the inciting event of AD that triggers the development of neurofibrillary tangles, cholinergic neuronal loss (Boller & Forette, 1989; Francis et al., 1999) and ultimately dementia (Hardy & Higgins, 1992). However, the exact cause of AD likely involves a complex set of events (Hardy & Selkoe, 2002; Hardy, 2006b; Hardy, 2006a; Hardy & Higgins, 1992; Karran et al., 2011; Lee et al., 2006; Pimplikar, 2009; Tanzi & Bertram, 2005)] that are beyond the scope of this chapter. The hallmark neuropathologic findings of AD are intracellular neurofibrillary tangles composed of hyperphosphorylated tau protein and extracellular senile plaques composed of amyloid-β (Figure 2). Due to the neural cell loss, reduction of the gray matter occurs (Figure 3). The guidelines commonly followed to establish a *post mortem* neuropathologic diagnosis of AD were established formally in 1985 and were updated in 1997 by the National Institute on Aging and Reagan Institute Working Group (Hyman & Trojanowski, 1997). A NIA-AA workgroup recently issued guidelines for neuropathologic assessment of AD (Hyman et al., 2012). These guidelines suggest ranking AD neuropathologic change by assigning an amyloid-β plaque score, a neurofibrillary tangle stage, and a neuritic plaque score based on neuropathologic findings in specified regions of the brain (Hyman et al., 2012). The neuropathologic findings are then compared with the patient's clinical history to determine the likelihood that AD pathology was the underlying cause of a patient's clinical symptoms.

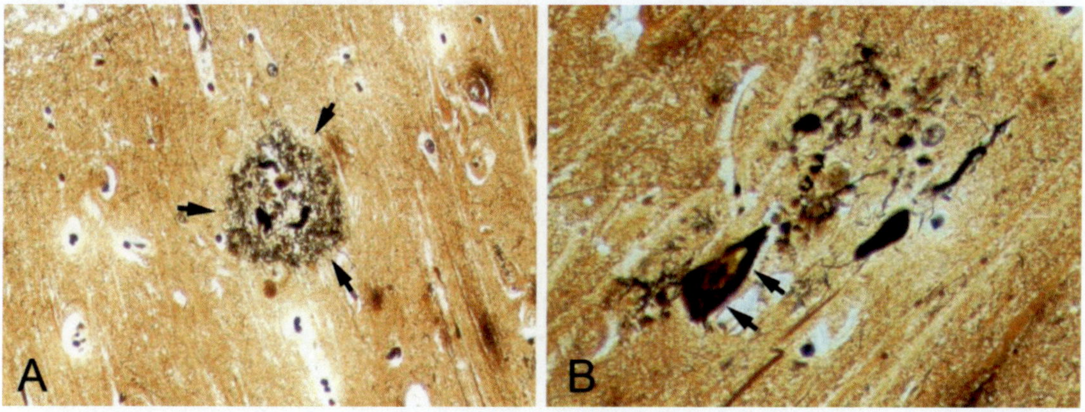

Figure 2. Characteristic neuropathological changes in Alzheimer's disease. (A) Amyloid plaques are abundant in the hippocampus (arrows). Magnification: 200x. (B) Flame-like tangles are located in the hippocampal pyramidal cells (arrows). Magnification: 400x.

Recently, there has been extensive interest in the potential application of biomarkers thought to be reflective of AD pathology to aid the *ante mortem* diagnosis of preclinical AD, MCI due to AD, and AD. At the present time, biomarkers are primarily used in research contexts. A detailed discussion of these technologies is beyond the scope of this chapter, however, there are several excellent reviews available (Blennow et al., 2010; Petrella et al., 2003; Risacher & Saykin, 2013; Shaw et al., 2007; Zhang, Jr. & Shi S Sr, 2013; Noel-Storr et al., 2013). The NIA-AA workgroup recommendations for the diagnosis of preclinical AD, MCI due to AD, and AD incorporate biomarkers into proposed diagnostic criteria for research settings (Albert et al., 2011; McKhann et al., 2011; Sperling et al., 2011). Notably, a joint task force of the Society of Nuclear Medicine and Molecular Imaging and the Alzheimer's Association, recently issued "appropriate use" criteria for amyloid PET imaging (Johnson et al., 2013).

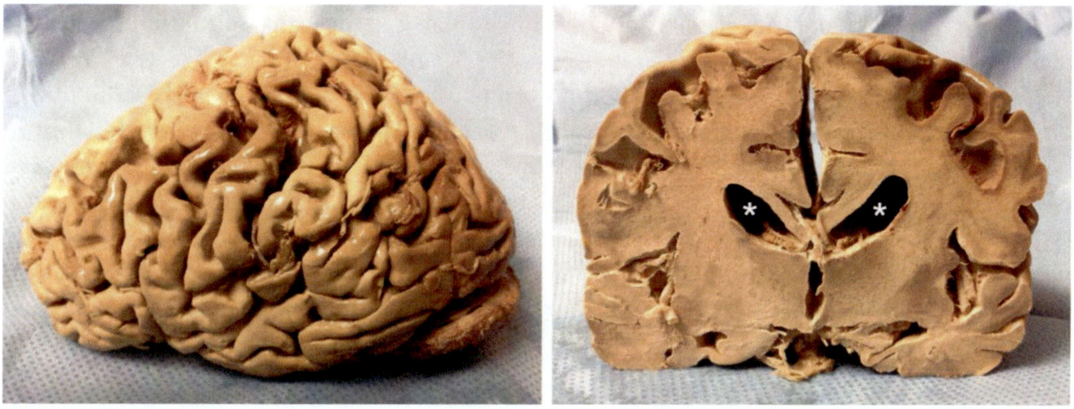

Figure 3. Characteristic features of the brain of a patient suffering in Alzheimer's disease. Significant declines in gray matter volume is represented by gyral atrophy (left insert) and the dilation of the lateral ventricles (asterisks, right insert).

Several studies using biomarkers of AD are available, including cerebrospinal fluid (CSF) analysis for amyloid-β and tau protein (Andreasen et al., 1999; Jack, Jr. et al., 2010; Morris et al., 2010; van Harten et al., 2013; Wallin et al., 2006; Mehta et al., 2000). Other techniques include amyloid PET scanning (Albert et al., 2011; Ikonomovic et al., 2008; Kemppainen et al., 2006; Kemppainen et al., 2007; Koivunen et al., 2008), MRI for cerebral atrophy (Dickerson et al., 2001; Fox et al., 1996; Jack, Jr. et al., 1997; Rabinovici et al., 2007; Scahill et al., 2002; Scheltens & van de Pol L., 2012), and fludeoxyglucose reuptake PET imaging (Chetelat et al., 2003; Edison et al., 2007; Herholz et al., 2002; Klunk et al., 2004; Mosconi et al., 2008). While this list of studies is by no means exhaustive, it is intended to offer the reader some exposure to the use of biomarkers in research settings.

Catecholamines and AD

There is emerging evidence that catecholamines may play a pivotal role in the pathogenesis of AD. Previous studies have shown that the noradrenergic system is substantially altered in AD (German et al., 1992; Iversen et al., 1983; Marcyniuk et al., 1986a; Marcyniuk et al., 1986b; Matthews et al., 2002; Storga et al., 1996; Tomlinson et al., 1981). Cell loss and morphological changes have been observed in the locus coeruleus, which is one of the largest noradrenergic cell groups in the brain. These morphological changes may be the result of retrograde pathological processes, originating from the terminal fields of neurons in the cortex and hippocampus (Fritschy & Grzanna, 1991; German et al., 1987; Marcyniuk et al., 1986a; Wang et al., 1994), changes within the locus coeruleus itself (Mann et al., 1982; Marien et al., 2004), or some combination of these factors. Indeed, the locus coeruleus projects to the temporal cortex and the hippocampus, where many of the histological hallmarks of AD can be observed. The morphological changes of the noradrenergic system are manifested as altered levels of noradrenaline in the brain, CSF and serum. Since noradrenaline has neuroprotective/anti-inflammatory properties, lower levels of noradrenaline at the initial stages of AD may further exacerbate inflammatory responses to amyloid deposition, setting up a *circulus vitiosus*; on the other hand, the compensatory increase of noradrenaline levels at later stages may play a significant role in the behavioral and psychological symptoms of AD.

Although the levels of adrenaline and dopamine often show changes in the brain tissue and body fluids of patients suffering from AD, the adrenergic and dopaminergic systems do not appear to be substantially altered in AD. However, the activity of the key and rate limiting enzymes of the catecholamine synthesis, tyrosine hydroxylase (TH), dopamine-β-hydroxylase (DBH), and phenylethanolamine-N-methyltransferase (PNMT) are frequently affected in AD patients along with alterations in the pattern of the adrenergic and dopaminergic receptors. In the next sections of the chapter we will discuss the role of noradrenaline, adrenaline and dopamine in AD.

Noradrenaline and AD

Noradrenergic Cell Loss

Advanced stages of AD are fundamentally associated with a reduction in the volume of noradrenergic neurons in the CNS. This neuronal loss may be triggered by retrograde pathological changes originating from the terminal fields of neurons from the temporal cortex and the hippocampus, where many of the pathological changes of AD can be observed (Fritschy & Grzanna, 1991; German et al., 1987; Marcyniuk et al., 1986a; Wang et al., 1994). Additionally, these changes may result from pathology within the LC itself (Mann et al., 1982; Marien et al., 2004), or may result from some combination of both pathological events. The toxicity of β-amyloid may play a significant role in these pathological events.

The most well-defined noradrenergic cell group, A6, is located in locus coeruleus in the pons. The locus coeruleus is composed of densely packed, pigmented perikarya representing about 50% of the central noradrenergic neurons (Nieuwenhuys, 1985). Due to its fundamental role in central noradrenergic innervation, the locus coeruleus has also been suggested as a central equivalent of a sympathetic ganglion (Amaral & Sinnamon, 1977). Loss of neurons in the locus coeruleus occurs with normal aging (Chan-Palay & Asan, 1989b; Manaye et al., 1995; Sturrock & Rao, 1985; Tomlinson et al., 1981). In fact, one study suggested that up to 50% of neurons in the locus coeruleus can be lost in ageing from the first through the tenth decades of life (Manaye et al., 1995). Cell loss in normal ageing has been observed to occur most predominately in the rostral end of the nucleus with neuronal loss occurring in a rostral-caudal gradient (Chan-Palay & Asan, 1989b; Manaye et al., 1995), however, at least one study observed diffuse loss of neurons throughout the entire locus (Marcyniuk et al., 1989).

While the rostral-caudal length of the locus coeruleus appears to be unchanged in normal ageing (Chan-Palay & Asan, 1989b), reduction of the length of thc nucleus has been reported in the brains of patients with AD (Chan-Palay & Asan, 1989a). Moreover, neuronal loss within the locus coeruleus in patients with AD deviates from age-related loss of neurons in the nucleus (German et al., 1992; Iversen et al., 1983; Marcyniuk et al., 1986a; Marcyniuk et al., 1986b; Matthews et al., 2002; Storga et al., 1996; Tomlinson et al., 1981). A significant decrease in the mean neuronal count of locus coeruleus has been reported in patients with AD (Tomlinson et al., 1981). Interestingly, the neuronal loss of many of the AD patients in two of these studies fell within the range values of the aged control patients, indicating that there may be variants of AD with greater loss of noradrenergic neurons than others (Tomlinson et al., 1981; Zarow et al., 2003). The mean total neuronal count in the locus coeruleus appears to correlate significantly with age, severity of dementia, and the length of the locus coeruleus in patients with AD (Bondareff & Mountjoy, 1986). The reduction of the volume of neurons in the nucleus appears to be greatest in AD patients less than 80 (Mann et al., 1984) or those younger at their age of diagnosis (Zarow et al., 2003).

The gradient of neuronal loss observed in normal ageing appears to be greatest at the rostral end of the locus coeruleus (Chan-Palay & Asan, 1989b; Manaye et al., 1995). While this gradual rostral cell loss may be maintained in AD during ageing, cell loss characteristic specifically to AD appears to be confined primarily to the dorsal and central areas of the nucleus, with the least loss of cells occurring in the ventral, rostral and caudal parts (Marcyniuk et al., 1986a; Marcyniuk et al., 1986b). It has been suggested that damage to the perikarya in the locus coeruleus in AD may represent a retrograde change from pathological events within the terminal fields of noradrenergic neurons (Fritschy & Grzanna, 1991; German et al., 1987; Marcyniuk et al., 1986a; Wang et al., 1994). Indeed, the central portion of the locus coeruleus is believed to project to the temporal cortex and hippocampus, where many of the characteristic AD pathology can be observed, while the rostral part targets the frontal cortex and the caudal part targets the occipital cortex (Marcyniuk et al., 1986a). However, it has also been suggested that the damage to the locus coeruleus might be mediated by events within the locus coeruleus itself rather than from retrograde changes secondary to damage outside of the locus coeruleus (Mann et al., 1982; Marien et al., 2004).

In addition to neuronal loss, the morphology of the locus coeruleus neurons also appears to be altered in AD. Previous studies reported reductions in the size of the perikarya of the neurons in the locus coeruleus associated with ageing (Chan-Palay & Asan, 1989a) with essentially unchanged dendritic arborization of these neurons in both young and old patients (Chan-Palay & Asan, 1989b; Mann et al., 1982). A significant divergence from these age-related changes has been reported in patients with AD including swollen and misshapen perikarya with shortened, thickened, and less branched dendrites (Chan-Palay & Asan, 1989a) and a reduction in the size of large pigmented neurons (Hoogendijk et al., 1995). In addition, significantly more neurofibrally tangles are observed in the locus coeruleus of patients with cognitive impairment (MCI or early AD) compared to normal controls (Grudzien et al., 2007). Moreover, a negative correlation has been noted between mini mental status examination scores and the markers for cytopathology of AD (Grudzien et al., 2007). There also appear to be changes in the projections of noradrenergic neurons to the hippocampus in AD with a reduction in the number of neurons as well as pathologic abnormalities noted in many of the remaining neurons (Powers et al., 1988).

Parallel to neuronal death and neurodegeneration, significant reductions in noradrenaline concentration can be observed in the cortices of patients with AD (German et al., 1992; Gottfries et al., 1983; Herrmann et al., 2004; Hoogendijk et al., 1999a; Hoogendijk et al., 1999b). These reductions have been found specifically in the caudate nucleus, substantia nigra, amygdala (Storga et al., 1996), cingulate gyrus (Arai et al., 1984; Storga et al., 1996), frontal cortex (Adolfsson et al., 1979; Cross et al., 1981; Kalaria et al., 1989a; Palmer et al., 1987b; Reinikainen et al., 1990), temporal cortex (Adolfsson et al., 1979; Cross et al., 1981; Kalaria & Andorn, 1991; Reinikainen et al., 1990), hippocampus (Cross et al., 1981; Powers et al., 1988), hypothalamus (Arai et al., 1984; Mann et al., 1980), substantia inominata, medial thalamic nucleus, raphe (Arai et al., 1984) and putamen (Adolfsson et al., 1979; Arai et al., 1984; Kalaria & Andorn, 1991; Reinikainen et al., 1990). Significant reductions in noradrenaline concentration in the brains of AD patients dying in their 60s and 70s have been described to be in the cingulate cortex, but they were also reported in the hippocampus and temporal cortex (Rossor et al., 1984). Interestingly, similar reductions in noradrenaline were not observed in AD patients dying in their 80s and 90s, suggesting that AD in younger patients might be a distinct form of early onset dementia (Mann et al., 1982; Rossor et al., 1984). In contrast, some studies were unable to demonstrate a correlation between the clinical or histopathologic severity of AD and the extent of noradrenergic neuronal loss (Palmer et al., 1987a; Haglund et al., 2006), indicating that there may be forms of AD where the degradation of noradrenergic system is less progressive.

Cell Loss and Inflammation in AD

Noradrenaline has been implicated as having a significant neuroprotective/anti-inflammatory role (Feinstein et al., 2002; Galea et al., 2003; Heneka & O'Banion, 2007; Marien et al., 2004). Noradrenaline has also been found to play a possible role in the deposition of amyloid-β (Heneka et al., 2002; Kalinin et al., 2007). Since noradrenaline has anti-inflammatory properties, noradrenergic neuronal loss may further exacerbate inflammatory responses to amyloid-β deposition, setting up a *circulus vitiosus* in neurodegenerative disorders, including AD (Heneka et al., 2002; Heneka & O'Banion, 2007; Jardanhazi-Kurutz et al., 2011; Marien et al., 2004). Indeed, a selective locus coeruleus lesion induced an elevation of glial inflammatory responses and augmented amyloid deposition (Heneka et al., 2006) and also increased levels of interleukin-1α, numbers of astrocytes in the cortex and hippocampus, and levels of β-amyloid 1-42 in a mouse model of AD (Jardanhazi-Kurutz et al., 2011). Reduced noradrenaline production due to noradrenergic cell loss in an AD mouse model impaired the migration of microglia and their phagocytic action which could decrease amyloid-β clearance (Heneka et al., 2010). Noradrenaline administration to mouse microglia suppressed cytokine and chemokine production promoted by amyloid-β and also increased the migration of these microglia (Heneka et al., 2010). Moreover, administering noradrenaline to rat microglia reduced microglial expression of nitric oxide synthase and decreased the production of interleukin-1β, which is a mediator of inflammation (Dello-Russo C. et al., 2004), and decreased the expression of cytokines in astrocytes, microglia and brain endothelial cells (Feinstein et al., 2002). Reductions in TH positive neurons in the locus coeruleus and reductions in brainstem levels of TH gene expression have been noted in rats in response to ageing and continuous exposure to inflammation, suggesting that these factors might negatively affect the functioning of the locus coeruleus (Bardou et al., 2013). In addition, it has been suggested that noradrenaline is involved in the regulation cerebral blood flow and that disruption of the noradrenergic system might therefore have further negative implications on the brain (Bekar et al., 2012). A detailed review of the inflammatory pathways that might play a significant role in the development of AD certainly exceeds the scope of the present chapter and is available elsewhere (Chalermpalanupap et al., 2013; Heneka & O'Banion, 2007; Marien et al., 2004). However, there is a general consensus that due to its anti-inflammatory effects, noradrenaline may act as an endogenous immunomodulator of the brain (Feinstein et al., 2002) and may also play a significant role in the pathogenesis of neurodegenerative conditions like AD.

Compensatory NE Elevation and Its Effects

The loss of noradrenergic neurons and the subsequent noradrenaline deficit with the progression of AD appears to be compensated for by increased noradrenaline levels in the CSF and plasma and/or hypersensitivity of the adrenoreceptors, all of which might contribute to the behavioral and psychological symptoms present in some cases of AD. Indeed, one study highlighted changes consistent with compensatory mechanisms in the locus coeruleus of AD patients (Szot et al., 2006). These changes included increased TH mRNA expression in the remaining locus coeruleus neurons, extension of the dendrites of the remaining neurons into the peri-nuclear dendritic zone, and the formation of axonal projections to the hippocampus (Szot et al., 2006). In AD patients who were ambulatory prior to death, TH mRNA expression per neuron has been found to be increased in the caudal half of the locus coeruleus as compared to non-demented patients (Szot et al., 2000).

CSF noradrenaline levels have been shown to increase in normal aging (Peskind et al., 1998). However, CSF noradrenaline has been also found to be significantly increased in patients with advanced AD compared to patients with mild to moderate AD and normal controls (Elrod et al., 1997; Raskind et al., 1984). However, this has not been the case in all studies to date with one study noting equivocal results (Tohgi et al., 1992) and another noting a significant decrease in CSF noradrenaline in patients with AD (Martignoni et al., 1992). Interestingly, in the study showing equivocal results, although increased CSF noradrenaline was not observed in AD patients relative to controls, it was noted that there was a significant increase in CSF noradrenaline as AD progressed (Tohgi et al., 1992). Interestingly, CSF noradrenaline has been found to correlate negatively with scores on mini-mental status examination (Elrod et al., 1997).

It is uncertain what significant changes, if any, plasma noradrenaline levels might have in AD. It was shown that plasma noradrenaline levels are significantly elevated in advanced AD and that patients with mild to moderate AD do not have significantly different levels of plasma noradrenaline than controls (Raskind et al., 1984). However, a later follow-up study with a larger sample size was unable to confirm these findings, reporting that while plasma noradrenaline appears to be significantly elevated in cases of AD relative to young controls, no significant difference between plasma noradrenaline levels in patients with advanced AD, mild to moderate AD, or normal controls with advanced age can be observed (Elrod et al., 1997). The finding that destruction of the peripheral sympathetic nervous system and adrenal medulla did not affect rat CSF noradrenaline (Peskind et al., 1986) suggests that peripheral sources of noradrenaline do not contribute significantly to the elevated CSF noradrenaline levels noted in AD. The results showing no significant difference in plasma noradrenaline between AD patients and aged controls, might be interpreted as being reflective of the lack of a contribution of locus coeruleus destruction to peripheral noradrenergic activity.

The idea that there is an increased noradrenergic neuronal activity in the remaining neurons in AD is supported by the finding that the level of 3-methoxy-4-hydroxyphenylglycol (MOPEG or MHPG), a noradrenaline metabolite, also appears to be altered in AD. Increases in MOPEG have been noted in the frontal and temporal cortices (Palmer et al., 1987b), and in the putamen, amygdala, caudate nucleus, substantia nigra, cingulate gyrus, and raphe of patients with AD (Storga et al., 1996), suggesting increased noradrenaline turnover. An inverse relationship between the remaining locus coeruleus neurons and the MOPEG/noradrenaline ratio in the locus coeruleus and frontal cortex has been observed (Hoogendijk et al., 1999a), supporting the idea that the remaining noradrenergic neurons are compensating for the cell loss in the locus coeruleus. Additionally, an increased MOPEG/noradrenaline ratio was found in the temporal cortex of patients with AD (Palmer et al., 1987a). CSF noradrenaline and MOPEG were shown to be significantly higher in patients with advanced AD when compared to patients with moderate AD or controls (Raskind et al., 1984). Notably, a direct correlation was found between CSF MOPEG in AD patients and the severity of a patient's cognitive impairment and an inverse correlation with the length of the patient's illness (Martignoni et al. 1992), however, other studies were unable to confirm these findings (Palmer et al., 1987a). There are studies that have noted decreased CSF MOPEG in AD patients relative to controls (Czech et al., 2012) and that have had equivocal results in patients with probable AD relative to controls (Molchan et al., 1991). Some caution must be used in interpreting findings of altered CSF metabolites of noradrenaline as being directly reflective of central changes to noradrenergic turnover. Catecholamines are generally unable to cross the blood brain barrier, however, some of their metabolites, including MOPEG can cross the blood brain barrier (Kopin, 1985). MOPEG specifically is able to flow between the CSF and plasma (Faull et al., 1990; Greene & Faull, 1989; Kopin, 1985). Therefore, if CSF MOPEG is to be interpreted as an index of central noradrenaline breakdown, the contribution of plasma MOPEG must be factored out (Kopin, 1985). It has been emphasized, however, that the effects of MOPEG crossing from the plasma into brain regions might not be considerably important in noradrenergic rich areas of the brain, but could confound interpretation of MOPEG levels in areas of the brain deficient in MOPEG (Kopin, 1985). Interestingly, levels of MOPEG in saliva have also been investigated in AD with some correlations to age and neurocognitive tests observed (Li et al., 2008).

Compensatory changes to the noradrenergic system reviewed previously are believed to play a role in the development of behavioral and psychological symptoms, particularly agitation/aggression, depression, or cognitive deficits in late AD (Haller et al., 1998; Herrmann et al., 2004). A significant correlation was shown between plasma MOPEG levels and the extent of cognitive impairment in patients with probable AD (Lawlor et al., 1995). Hallucinations, delusions, depression, and other psychiatric issues are known to be common in AD, especially in late stages of the condition (Lyketsos et al., 2001; Lyketsos et al., 2002; Lyketsos et al., 2003). It is a general consensus that noradrenaline plays a role in the development of these behavioral and psychiatric symptoms. Preservation of noradrenaline in the substantia nigra has been found to be associated with psychotic symptoms in patients with AD and psychosis (Zubenko et al., 1991). Although no significant difference was found between the locus coeruleus pigmented neuron counts in patients with AD who had depression, transient depression, or no depression, patients with depression at the onset of AD had more pigmented neurons in the locus coeruleus than those of other AD patients (Hoogendijk et al., 1999b). In addition, a positive correlation has been found between aggression in patients with dementia and the amount of cell loss in the rostral locus coeruleus (Matthews et al., 2002). Although beyond the scope of the present article, an extensive review of the role of noradrenaline in the behavioral and psychological symptoms of AD is readily available (Herrmann et al., 2004).

Dopamine β Hydroxylase and AD

Dopamine β Hydroxylase (DBH) is an important enzyme in the synthesis of noradrenaline from dopamine. Although plasma DBH activity varies based on the genetic makeup of an individual (Mustapic et al., 2013; Cubells & Zabetian, 2004; Weinshilboum et al., 1975), it has been previously established that the level of DBH may also change with ageing. However, the results of different studies are rather contradictory. While one study has noted that serum DBH has increased with age from the 20s to the 80s and then decreased in the 80s (Miyata et al., 1984), other studies indicated stable plasma DBH from age 21-60 (Paclt & Koudelova, 2004), equally high serum DBH activity in three different age groups (Ogihara et al., 1975), and no association between decreased plasma DBH and age in healthy controls from 60-90 years of age or between plasma DBH levels and age in AD patients 65 to 98 (Mustapic et al., 2013).

Despite the conflicting data regarding the correlation between DBH levels and age, patients with AD appear to have reduced DBH in serum and plasma relative to normal controls (Miyata et al., 1984; Nakamura et al., 1984) and the extent of the reduction in DBH has been shown to be related to the severity of brain atrophy or dementia (Miyata et al., 1984). Plasma DBH activity is most reduced in early stages as compared to later stages of AD (Mustapic et al., 2013). Interestingly, the reduction in plasma DBH that occurs in AD is independent of a patient's DBH genotype (Mustapic et al., 2013). As with many changes noted previously in patients with AD, this change in DBH is thought to be reflective of compensation for noradrenergic neuronal death in AD. As the disease progresses, plasma DBH activity appears to increase to compensate for the cellular loss and to increase the level of noradrenaline (Mustapic et al., 2013), and thus, treatment with noradrenaline reuptake inhibitors may offer some therapeutic advantage in early stages of AD (Mustapic et al., 2013).

Ageing does not appear to alter the DBH level in CSF, however, patients with AD appear to have lower CSF DBH levels than controls (Miyata et al., 1984; Nakamura et al., 1984), although some studies failed to confirm altered DBH activity in CSF in AD patients (Soininen et al. 1984) or show any relationship between DBH activity in the CSF and severity of dementia (Soininen et al., 1984). Significant reductions in DBH have been noted in AD patients in the temporal cortex, frontal cortex, and hippocampus when compared to *post mortem* brain tissue of patients with depression, multiinfarct dementia, terminal coma, and normal controls (Cross et al., 1981). It has been suggested that the reduction in DBH in these brain regions is related to the degeneration of the noradrenergic neurons in the locus coeruleus (Cross et al., 1981). There also might be a reduction in DBH activity in the temporal lobes of patients in later stages of AD (Perry et al., 1981a). In contrast, there does not appear to be a correlation between cortical DBH activity reduction and the number of locus coeruleus neurons lost in AD subjects or between markers of AD severity and DBH activity (Perry et al., 1981b). A complete review of the genetics of DBH is certainly beyond the scope of this chapter, but is readily available elsewhere (Cubells & Zabetian, 2004). It has been suggested that certain conditions, including congenital noradrenaline deficiency, might result from mutations in DBH genes, and that DBH genetic polymorphisms may be related to the pathogenesis of AD as well as behavioral and psychiatric symptoms in AD (Combarros et al., 2010; Cubells et al., 2000; Cubells & Zabetian, 2004; Kim et al., 2002). The DBH gene is located at chromosome 9q34 and has at least 71 known genetic polymorphisms, 68 of which are single nucleotide polymorphisms (Craig et al., 1988; Chen et al., 2011). One of these, the -1021 C→T polymorphism has been suggested to play a significant role in plasma DBH activity (Bhaduri & Mukhopadhyay, 2008; Kohnke et al., 2002; Tang et al., 2005; Tang et al., 2007; Zabetian et al., 2001) and might even play a role in AD (Combarros et al., 2010; Kohnke et al., 2002; Zabetian et al., 2001). Previous studies found an association between the -1021T (TT and CT genotypes) genetic polymorphism and AD in males under the age of 75 (Combarros et al., 2010). Associations between the -1021T allele and alleles associated with pro-inflammatory cytokines have also been found which might have implications for the role of noradrenaline in inflammatory processes that contributes to the pathogenesis of AD (Combarros et al., 2010; Mateo et al., 2006). In contrast, no association was found between TT homozygosity at the C-970T DBH allele and the risk of AD, indicating that a number of different factors, such as ethnic origin, gender, must be taken into consideration (Mustapic et al. 2013).

Adrenaline and AD

Similar to the noradrenergic system, the adrenergic system is also affected in the AD brain; however, it does not appear to be as substantially altered as the noradrenergic system. Nevertheless, adrenergic cell loss is characteristic of AD and may be responsible for a compensatory elevation of adrenaline in the CSF that, in turn, may contribute to the underlying mechanism of agitation characteristic of many AD patients. The largest of the adrenergic cell clusters in the brain, C1, is affected in AD, with reductions in both the average area occupied by C1 neurons and the size of these neurons in the brains of AD patients compared to normal, age-matched controls (Burke et al., 1994b). The C1 cluster of adrenergic neurons is located between the inferior olivary complex and the nucleus funiculi lateralis in the medulla (Nieuwenhuys, 1985). This cluster has been implicated in cardiac function, including cardiac reflexes (Granata et al., 1985; Reis et al., 1984; Reis et al., 1989). It has been suggested that the loss of these C1 neurons might contribute to alterations in systolic blood pressure and mean arterial pressure in AD patients (Burke et al., 1994a). Indeed, blood pressure and dementia appear to be linked in several cases (Qiu et al., 2005; Skoog, 1997).

Hypertension has been recognized to play a role in the pathophysiological process of dementia and AD (Forette et al., 1998; Forette et al., 2002). It has been suggested that low blood pressure might potentially be either a complication of AD or a factor that contributes to the AD pathophysiological process in some cases (Guo et al., 1996; Landin et al., 1993). However, while one study revealed that ageing affected blood pressure, it did not find an association between either AD and blood pressure or CSF adrenaline and blood pressure (Peskind et al. 1998). These results raise the possibility that while hypertension prior to the onset of AD might contribute to the pathophysiological process of AD, blood pressure is not necessarily affected by AD itself, and that alteration of CSF adrenaline levels specific to some cases of AD do not necessarily relate to blood pressure changes. However, the results might rather reflect that CSF adrenaline is not indicative of the state of the C1 neurons that project to the CNS areas and regulate the cardiovascular system (Peskind et al., 1998).

When measured with high pressure liquid chromatography, the concentrations of adrenaline are not significantly different in the globus pallidus, putamen, amygdala, caudate nucleus, substantia nigra, cingulate gyrus or raphe of patients with histopathologically confirmed AD as compared to controls (Storga et al., 1996). In contrast, CSF levels of adrenaline appear to be increased in patients with AD compared to old and young patients without AD and also seem to increase with the severity of the AD (Peskind et al., 1998). In addition, higher plasma adrenaline level was noted in patients with AD as compared to controls (Peskind et al. 1998). However, there have been reports of increased, decreased, and equivocal plasma adrenaline clearance with aging, which, in the event of decreased adrenaline clearance, could yield the resultant increased plasma adrenaline (Peskind et al., 1998).

The elevated adrenaline levels may represent a compensatory response to adrenergic cell loss characteristic in AD and may play a role in the development of agitation in some patients with AD (Peskind et al., 1998). CNS adrenergic activity appears to increase as AD progresses

(Peskind et al., 1998). It is possible that the adrenergic neurons in the CNS become more sensitive to α_2 antagonism with ageing, given that, regardless of AD diagnosis, older patients had an increased response to yohimbine relative to normal young controls as reflected through increased CSF adrenaline (Peskind et al., 1998). Interestingly, while yohimbine increases adrenaline in CSF, clonidine, an α_2 agonist did not alter CSF adrenaline levels in older subjects relative to controls (Peskind et al., 1998). These findings may be explained by endogenous tonic inhibition of adrenergic neurons that cannot be altered expressively by administering an alpha-2-agonist (Peskind et al., 1998). It was also noted that there was a significant correlation between CSF adrenaline and agitation with the administration of yohimbine in patients with advanced AD (Peskind et al., 1998). In support of a possible role of the adrenergic systems in agitation in AD, beta adrenergic blockade with propranolol has also been explored as a possible treatment for agitation in dementia (Hersch & Falzgraf, 2007; Shankle et al., 1995; Summers, 2006; Weiler et al., 1988; Yudofsky et al., 1981).

Phenylethanolamine N-methyltransferase (PNMT) is the rate limiting enzyme in the production of adrenaline that catalyzes the methylation of noradrenaline to produce adrenaline. It appears that PNMT activity is decreased in several areas of the brain affected by AD and that the decrease in PNMT activity is due to a loss in PNMT enzyme protein itself (Burke et al., 1987; Burke et al., 1988; Guan et al., 1999). The underlying cause for the reduction in PNMT protein has been suggested to be the retrograde degeneration of adrenergic neurons (Burke et al., 1988). The loss of PNMT activity also correlates with the amount of locus coeruleus neurons lost and there is also a correlation between the loss of neurons in adrenergic nuclei and the loss of neurons in the locus coeruleus (Burke et al., 1988). It appears that PNMT activity varies by the time course of AD with decreased PNMT in axon terminals and decreased total PNMT in adrenergic cell bodies of early AD patients (Burke et al., 1990). In advanced stages of AD, PNMT activity is significantly increased in adrenergic neuronal cell bodies as compared to controls, which is possibly due to increased PNMT enzyme protein (Burke et al., 1990). These findings support the hypothesis that early AD involves either reduced synthesis or increased breakdown of PNMT containing neurons and that late AD could involve a reduction in the transport of PNMT to nerve terminals making it seem as though PNMT is increased in the perikarya (Burke et al., 1990). Genetic variation in the promoter region of PNMT may also play a role in the development of "sporadic" early onset AD (Mann et al., 2001).

Adrenergic Receptors in AD

Adrenergic receptors appear to play a significant role in cognition and therefore, they are believed to be involved in the pathogenesis of AD. The beneficial actions of noradrenaline on cognitive functioning has been suggested to result from the stimulation of post-junctional α_2 receptors (Friedman et al., 1999). Indeed, a high density of α_2 receptors can be found in the prefrontal cortex and these receptors have been shown to overlap with other catecholaminergic receptors in primates (Goldman-Rakic et al., 1990). At the same time, α_1 receptor stimulation in the prefrontal cortex has been shown to impair prefrontal cortical cognitive function (Arnsten et al., 1999). Additionally, it has been suggested that the amygdala may modulate hippocampal activity in rats (Ikegaya et al., 1996a; Ikegaya et al.,

1996b) possibly via β receptors (Ikegaya et al., 1997). Indeed, β receptor antagonists impair hippocampal long-term potentiation (Ikegaya et al., 1997) and the consequent memory formation (Izquierdo et al., 1998). Noradrenaline has also been shown to enhance short term memory and long term memory when infused into the entorhinal cortex in rats (Izquierdo et al., 1998).

The significant loss of locus coeruleus neurons is considered one of the hallmarks of AD. It appears that the remaining neurons may compensate for this neuronal loss manifested frequently by sprouting axonal projections into the terminal fields of neurons in the hippocampus and prefrontal cortex, as determined by α_2 receptor binding site density (Szot et al., 2007). At the same time, neuronal loss in dementia may explain the loss of α_{1A}, α_{1D} and α_{2C} receptor subtype mRNA expression in the prefrontal cortex (Szot et al., 2007). There also appears to be a reduction in α_{2A} receptor density in the frontal cortex of patients with AD noted, which is absent in patients with dementia who do not meet neuropathologic criteria for AD (Meana et al., 1992). Additionally, there appears to be a negative correlation between α_2 receptor density and age of death in control subjects (Meana et al. 1992). This cortical neuronal loss may contribute to the loss of memory and behavioral changes. Moreover, AD patients appear to have a reduction in α_1 receptors in the hippocampus and cerebellum and decreased α_2 receptors in the nucleus basalis of Meynert, as determined through the binding of α_1 antagonist, [3H]prazosin, and the α_2 antagonist [3H]yohimbine (Shimohama et al., 1986). The binding of [3H]p-aminoclonidine, an α_2 agonist, to the prefrontal cortex is reduced with normal ageing; additionally, there is a 50% reduction in its binding in AD patients compared to controls (Kalaria & Andorn, 1991).

Receptor binding site changes may be reflective of the symptoms of AD, rather than being a diagnostic tool for the disease itself. Using receptor autoradiography, no significant difference in adrenergic receptor concentration can be observed between AD cases and control patients; however, AD patients with aggressive behavior have been found to have markedly increased concentrations of α_2 receptors in the cerebellar cortex compared with nonaggressive AD patients matched for levels of cognitive deficit (Russo-Neustadt & Cotman, 1997). In contrast, no differences were noted in α_2 receptor levels in the frontal cortex and hypothalamus of patients with AD, AD with aggression or agitation, and normal controls (Russo-Neustadt & Cotman, 1997). Similarly, no difference was found in α_2 adrenergic receptor density in cortical areas in AD patients compared to controls (Matthews et al., 2002), suggesting that other factors may play a role in the alteration of adrenergic receptor distribution; however, the functional consequence of these receptor pattern changes is still unclear. In a study investigating the presence of adrenergic receptors on cerebral microvasculature, no changes were found in the amount of α_1 receptors in AD patients relative to controls and an increase in α_2 receptors was noted in AD patients relative to controls (Kalaria & Harik, 1989).

There also appears to be an alteration of the β adrenergic receptors in AD. The β_1 and β_2 receptors are increased in the cerebellar cortex of aggressive AD patients as compared to non-aggressive AD patients (Russo-Neustadt & Cotman, 1997). The β_1 adrenoceptors are decreased and β_2 adrenoceptors are increased in number in AD subjects as compared to controls (Kalaria et al., 1989b). Studies have also found increased total, β_1 and β_2 receptors in the hippocampi of AD patients with decreases in the putamen noted (Kalaria et al., 1989b). Receptor binding studies investigating the alterations of β receptors in patients with AD did not note any changes in the total number of β receptors in the prefrontal cortices of controls nor did they observe any significant differences between age-matched controls and patients with AD (Kalaria et al., 1989b; Kalaria et al., 1989a). Reductions in total β receptor counts in the thalamus, reductions of β_1 receptor counts in the hippocampus, increases in β_1 receptor counts in the nucleus basalis of Meynert, reductions in β_2 receptors in the thalamus, NbM, cerebellar hemisphere and increases in β_2 receptors in the hippocampus and putamen of patients with AD relative to normal controls have all been noted (Shimohama et al., 1986). In the Han Chinese population, one study noted increased risk of late onset AD with two genetic polymorphisms of the β_2 adrenergic receptor (Yu et al., 2008). Significant increases in total β receptors and β_2 receptors have been observed in cerebral microvessels of patients with AD relative to controls (Kalaria & Harik, 1989). However, the ratio of β_1/ β_2 receptors appears to be decreased in AD (Kalaria et al., 1989b; Kalaria et al., 1989a). There have also been differences observed in total β receptor density in the cerebellum among all AD patients with small increases in β receptor density in aggressive AD patients, small increases in β_1 receptor density in the granule cell layer, Purkinje cell layer, and white matter, and increases in β_2 receptors in the subcortical white matter (Russo-Neustadt & Cotman, 1997). No differences have been noted among AD patients without agitation or aggression, AD patients with aggression or agitation, and normal controls in terms of β receptor density in the frontal cortex or the hypothalamus nor has there been a difference in total β receptor density in the cerebellum among all AD patients relative to controls (Russo-Neustadt & Cotman, 1997). As mentioned previously, β adrenergic blockade with propranolol has also been explored as a possible treatment for agitation in dementia (Hersch & Falzgraf, 2007; Shankle et al., 1995; Summers, 2006; Weiler et al., 1988; Yudofsky et al., 1981). For a review of the role of β receptors and β receptor antagonism in AD see (Luong & Nguyen, 2013; Yu et al., 2011).

Dopamine and AD

Levels of DA and Its Products

Several studies have investigated the levels of dopamine and its precursors, enzymes and metabolites in AD, including tyrosine, L-3,4- dihydroxyphenylalanine (L-DOPA), tyrosine hydroxylase (TH), 3,4- dihydroxyphenylacetic acid (DOPAC), 3-methoxytyramine (3-MT), and homovanillic acid (HVA). Tyrosine hydroxylase and aromatic acid decarboxylase enzyme activities decrease in normal aging; however there is an increase in monoamine oxidase activity with ageing and lowered dopamine and HVA levels in CSF of the elderly (Czech et al., 2012). These changes are expected to be even more marked as AD progresses (Czech et al., 2012). Indeed, slightly lowered dopamine levels have been reported in cortical tissues and the hippocampi of AD patients (Czech et al., 2012; Reinikainen et al., 1988; Reinikainen et al., 1990). The remaining neurons may be able to compensate for this cell loss, and consequently, dopamine or HVA levels in CSF may appear normal, or even increased in the initial stages of AD (Volicer et al., 1985; Beal & Growdon, 1986; Zubenko et al., 1986; Tohgi et al., 1992; Zimmer et al., 1984). Nevertheless, since slightly lowered levels of dopamine can usually observed in AD patients , dopamine appears to be one of the metabolic markers that can differentiate AD from controls (Tohgi et al., 1992; Czech et al., 2012). While there are alterations in the levels of dopamine, its metabolites as well as in the pattern of the dopaminergic receptors in cases of AD, the dopaminergic system does not appear to be substantially altered in AD (Arai et al., 1984). However, both dopamine and L-DOPA have been suggested to play a possible role in the pathogenesis of AD by possibly inhibiting the formation of and/or dissolving amyloid fibrils (Li et al., 2004).

Increased mean levels of tyrosine have been found in the globus pallidus, putamen, amygdala, caudate nucleus, substantia nigra, cingulate gyrus and raphe of patients with AD (Storga et al., 1996). The activity of TH, the rate limiting enzyme of catecholamine synthesis, has been found to be reduced in the substantia nigra (Sawada et al., 1987) and in the ventral tegmental area (Kastner et al., 1993) in patients with AD relative to controls. The concentration of L-DOPA , a precursor to dopamine, has also been found to be decreased in the amygdala and caudate nucleus of patients with AD (Storga et al., 1996).

Reductions of dopamine have been noted in the putamen (Allard et al., 1990; Arai et al., 1984; Storga et al., 1996), amygdala, caudate nucleus, cingulate gyrus and raphe (Storga et al., 1996). There are several areas of the brain where dopamine content is not altered including the cortex generally (Iversen et al., 1983), the temporal and frontal cortices (Palmer et al., 1987a; Palmer et al., 1987b) and substantia nigra in late-onset AD (Mann et al., 1980). Although there is no reduction in the number of neurons or the size of their perikarya, nuclei, and nucleoli in the substantia nigra pars compacta of patients with AD without Lewy body pathology, decreased neuromelanin content was found in the cell bodies of the substantia nigra pars compacta in these patients (Reyes et al., 2003).

CSF levels of dopamine are decreased in patients with "presenile" AD (Argentiero & Tavolato, 1980) and AD (Tohgi et al., 1992; Czech et al., 2012). However, no significant differences between AD patients and controls in plasma dopamine levels have been observed (Umegaki et al., 2000). One study noted severe atrophy, neurofibrillary degeneration, and loss of pigmented dopamine neurons in the ventral tegmental area in AD patients with changes also to the substantia nigra, but to a lesser extent (Mann et al., 1987). Indeed, 54% of AD patients had neurofibrillary tangles without Lewy Bodies in the substantia nigra with half of these patients showing significant neurodegeneration in one study (Gibb et al., 1989). The authors also observed that patients with tangles in the SN tended to be younger, had more plaques and tangles in the hippocampus and cortex, and had lower activities of cortical choline acetyltransferase (Gibb et al. 1989). In contrast, an additional study found no significant neuronal loss and only mild TH fiber loss in the ventral tegmental area of AD patients (Torack & Morris, 1992).

Dopamine can be metabolized through two pathways (see chapter 2 for more detail). In the first, dopamine is converted to 3,4-dihydroxyphenylacetaldehyde (DOPAL) and then on to 3,4-dishydroxyphenylacetic acid (DOPAC) in a coupled reaction catalyzed by monoamine oxidase and aldehyde dehydrogenase (ALDH). DOPAC is then converted to HVA by catechol-o-methyl transferase (COMT). In the second possible pathway of dopamine metabolism, dopamine is converted into 3-methoxytyramine (3-MT) by COMT. 3-MT is then converted to 3-methoxy-4-hydroxy-phenylacetaldehyde (MOPAL) then on to HVA by MAO and ALDH. DOPAC levels are not significantly altered in the temporal and frontal cortices of "presenile" AD patients compared to controls (Palmer et al., 1987a). However, reductions in DOPAC have been noted in several areas of the brain in AD including the globus pallidus (Storga et al., 1996), putamen (Allard et al., 1990; Storga et al., 1996), amygdala, caudate nucleus, substantia nigra, cingulate gyrus, and raphe (Storga et al., 1996). CSF DOPAC levels have been reported to be lower in AD patients than controls (Volicer et al., 1985). Patients who were noted to have symptoms of AD before age 65 tended to have lower CSF DOPAC levels and increased HVA/DOPAC ratio as compared to controls (Volicer et al., 1985). Reduced HVA concentrations have been found in the amygdala (Arai et al., 1984), caudate nucleus (Adolfsson et al., 1979; Nazarali & Reynolds, 1992), and putamen (Adolfsson et al., 1979) of patients with AD. However, no changes in HVA levels were detected in numerous areas of the cerebral cortex (Palmer et al., 1988) or in the temporal and frontal cortices of presenile AD patients compared to controls (Palmer et al., 1987a). Additionally, 3-MT concentration is reduced in the putamen of patients with AD (Allard et al., 1990).

Significant reductions of CSF HVA in AD patients relative to controls appear to be dependent on the severity of the dementia indicating a reduction in dopamine turnover in severe dementia (Soininen et al., 1981). Indeed, reductions in TH activity and increases in monoamine oxidase activity with ageing suggest that dopamine and HVA would be lower in the CSF of older patients and that these levels would be even lower in AD, especially late in the disease when compensatory mechanisms fail (Czech et al., 2012).

In patients with low CSF HVA and AD, neurocognitive deficits can be observed along with more extrapyramidal symptoms, and greater incidences of depression (Wolfe et al., 1990). Indeed, a significant correlation has been found between CSF HVA and geriatric depression scale of AD patients (Stuerenburg et al., 2004). The HVA/dopamine ratio is increased in the putamen and medial globus pallidus in patients with AD. In addition, decreased CSF DOPAC has been reported in AD (Zubenko et al., 1986).

In interpreting the various findings regarding dopamine and dopamine metabolites in the CSF and plasma of AD, it is important to excersise a degree of caution. CSF HVA has been reported to be a useful index of central dopamine metabolism; however, there appears to be a significant difference in the gradient of CSF HVA concentration of when it is sampled from brain CSF or lumbar CSF (Kopin, 1985).

Dopamine Receptors

Several studies have investigated the state of dopamine receptors in AD. Some of these studies have implicated dopamine receptors in the unique features of the "Lewy body Variant" of AD which is noted to have both characteristic AD pathology as well as Lewy bodies; others have suggested that receptor modification might play a role in cognitive functioning of patients. There is also an interest in the role that genetic polymorphisms of dopamine receptors might play in the development of the behavioral and psychiatric symptoms in AD.

While the density of D_1 receptors appears to be elevated in the putamen of patients with Parkinson's Disease (PD), normal levels of D_1 receptors have been noted in patients with AD and AD with extrapyramidal or parkinsonian features (AD/Park) (Joyce et al., 1998a). Similarly, no reduction in D_1 receptors in the putamen has been noted in some studies (Cross et al., 1984). Increased striatal D_1 receptor density has been shown in patients with AD with Lewy bodies compared to AD patients without Lewy body pathology (Sweet et al., 2001). Although D_1 receptor concentration does not seem to be altered in AD patients, a reduction in high affinity binding sites for dopamine agonists has been noted, suggesting a possible cell membrane alteration in AD which might explain some of the problems with developing dopaminergic therapies for AD (De Keyser J. et al., 1990). D_1 receptors have also been noted to be reduced in the hippocampus, molecular layer of the dentate gyrus and in the putamen in AD patients (Cortes et al., 1988). Decreased dopamine binding sites in the substantia nigra and nucleus accumbens have been reported in AD, with no changes to the striatal D_1 binding sites (Rinne et al., 1986a). However, a reduction in the D_1 receptor activity in the caudate nucleus and putamen was found in patients with AD, as denoted by reductions in the uptake of a D_1 receptor antagonist (Kemppainen et al., 2000).

D_2 receptors have been found to have decreased availability in the hippocampus of AD patients (Kemppainen et al., 2003; Ryoo & Joyce, 1994). Interestingly, there appears to be a greater reduction in the right hippocampal D_2 receptor availability (Kemppainen et al., 2003). The binding potential of the D_2 receptors in the right hippocampus had a positive correlation with performance on the Wechsler Memory Scale-Revised and picture naming in the Boston Naming Test (Kemppainen et al., 2003). In AD, reduction in D_2 receptors has been noted in the caudate nucleus (Rinne et al., 1986b), putamen (Cross et al., 1984; Rinne et al., 1986b), amygdala and dentate gyrus (Joyce et al., 1993), temporal cortex (Joyce et al., 1998b) and the striatum generally (Pizzolato et al., 1996). The finding that the areas of the brain with D_2 receptor loss did not usually contain plaques, tangles, nor did these areas show significant neuronal loss suggests that other pathophysiological process may be responsible for the loss of D_2 receptors in these regions (Ryoo & Joyce, 1994).

It appears that in dementia with Lewy bodies, the D_2 receptor pattern is more affected than in AD (Piggott et al. 1999). Indeed, decreased D_2 density has been observed in patients with AD with Lewy bodies compared to AD patients (Sweet et al. 2001). D_2 receptors were found to be significantly reduced in the caudate nucleus and putamen of AD/Park patients; these findings might explain the extrapyramidal symptoms in AD/Park and possibly also its lack of responsiveness to L-Dopa (Joyce et al., 1998a).

It has been suggested that alterations of the D_2 receptor system might play a role in the behavioral and psychological symptoms of dementia (Tanaka et al., 2003). Higher binding of D_2 antagonist ligand in the striatum was associated with increased motor speed and poorer performance on tests of attention in patients with mild to moderate AD, indicating that D_2 agonists might have a role in the treatment of AD (Reeves 2010).

The pattern of D_3 receptors also appears to be altered in AD. Increases in D_3 binding in the nucleus accumbens have been noted in AD (Piggott et al., 1999). Patients with AD with Lewy bodies have been noted to have decreased D_3 density in the striatum compared to AD patients (Sweet et al. 2001). D_3 receptors have also been suggested to play a possible role in cognition; therefore, D_3 receptor antagonism may enhance cognitive performance in patients (Nakajima et al., 2013). Moreover, D_3 receptor density is increased in the striatum of AD patients with a history of psychosis (Sweet et al., 2001). Association with D_1 and D_3 receptor genes and behavioral and psychological symptoms in AD has also been suggested (Sweet et al., 1998).

Conclusion

Catecholaminergic transmission appears to play a significant role in AD. Among the catecholaminergic systems, the noradrenergic system seems to be fundamentally affected in AD patients. Neuronal loss in the locus coeruleus, possibly due to the retrograde pathologic changes originating from the terminal fields of neurons or pathology within the locus coeruleus itself is a characteristic hallmark of AD. The initial lesion of the noradrenergic system due to cell loss is compensated by the remaining neurons in later stages of the disease and changes in the pattern of adrenergic receptors. These changes, in turn, may trigger or exacerbate the neurologic and psychiatric symptoms associated with AD. Although adrenergic and dopaminergic systems appear to exhibit functional and morphological changes, they do not seem to be fundamentally altered in AD. However, it is a general consensus that understanding the role of the catecholamines in AD may open up entirely new avenues in the treatment of this devastating disease.

References

Adolfsson, R., Gottfries, C. G., Roos, B. E., & Winblad, B. (1979). Changes in the brain catecholamines in patients with dementia of Alzheimer type. *Br.J Psychiatry, 135,* 216-223.

Albert, M. S., DeKosky, S. T., Dickson, D., Dubois, B., Feldman, H. H., Fox, N. C. et al. (2011). The diagnosis of mild cognitive impairment due to Alzheimer's disease: recommendations from the National Institute on Aging-Alzheimer's Association workgroups on diagnostic guidelines for Alzheimer's disease. *Alzheimers.Dement., 7,* 270-279.

Allard, P., Alafuzoff, I., Carlsson, A., Eriksson, K., Ericson, E., Gottfries, C. G. et al. (1990). Loss of dopamine uptake sites labeled with [3H]GBR-12935 in Alzheimer's disease. *Eur.Neurol., 30,* 181-185.

Amaral, D. G. & Sinnamon, H. M. (1977). The locus coeruleus: neurobiology of a central noradrenergic nucleus. *Prog.Neurobiol., 9,* 147-196.

American Psychiatric Association (2013). *Diagnostic and statistical manual of mental disorders*. (5th ed.) Arlington, VA: American Psychiatric Publishing.

Andreasen, N., Hesse, C., Davidsson, P., Minthon, L., Wallin, A., Winblad, B. et al. (1999). Cerebrospinal fluid beta-amyloid(1-42) in Alzheimer disease: differences between early- and late-onset Alzheimer disease and stability during the course of disease. *Arch.Neurol., 56,* 673-680.

Arai, H., Kosaka, K., & Iizuka, R. (1984). Changes of biogenic amines and their metabolites in postmortem brains from patients with Alzheimer-type dementia. *J Neurochem., 43,* 388-393.

Argentiero, V. & Tavolato, B. (1980). Dopamine (DA) and serotonin metabolic levels in the cerebrospinal fluid (CSF) in Alzheimer's presenile dementia under basic conditions and after stimulation with cerebral cortex phospholipids (BC-PL). *J Neurol., 224,* 53-58.

Arnsten, A. F., Mathew, R., Ubriani, R., Taylor, J. R., & Li, B. M. (1999). Alpha-1 noradrenergic receptor stimulation impairs prefrontal cortical cognitive function. *Biol.Psychiatry, 45,* 26-31.

Bardou, I., Kaercher, R. M., Brothers, H. M., Hopp, S. C., Royer, S., & Wenk, G. L. (2013). Age and duration of inflammatory environment differentially affect the neuroimmune response and catecholaminergic neurons in the midbrain and brainstem. *Neurobiol.Aging.*

Beal, M. F. & Growdon, J. H. (1986). CSF neurotransmitter markers in Alzheimer's disease. *Prog.Neuropsychopharmacol.Biol.Psychiatry, 10,* 259-270.

Bekar, L. K., Wei, H. S., & Nedergaard, M. (2012). The locus coeruleus-norepinephrine network optimizes coupling of cerebral blood volume with oxygen demand. *J Cereb.Blood Flow Metab, 32,* 2135-2145.

Bhaduri, N. & Mukhopadhyay, K. (2008). Correlation of plasma dopamine beta-hydroxylase activity with polymorphisms in DBH gene: a study on Eastern Indian population. *Cell Mol.Neurobiol., 28,* 343-350.

Blennow, K., Hampel, H., Weiner, M., & Zetterberg, H. (2010). Cerebrospinal fluid and plasma biomarkers in Alzheimer disease. *Nat.Rev.Neurol., 6,* 131-144.

Boller, F. & Forette, F. (1989). Alzheimer's disease and THA: a review of the cholinergic theory and of preliminary results. *Biomed.Pharmacother., 43,* 487-491.

Bondareff, W. & Mountjoy, C. Q. (1986). Number of neurons in nucleus locus ceruleus in demented and non-demented patients: rapid estimation and correlated parameters. *Neurobiol Aging, 7,* 297-300.

Brookmeyer, R., Gray, S., & Kawas, C. (1998). Projections of Alzheimer's disease in the United States and the public health impact of delaying disease onset. *Am.J Public Health, 88,* 1337-1342.

Burke, W. J., Chung, H. D., Huang, J. S., Huang, S. S., Haring, J. H., Strong, R. et al. (1988). Evidence for retrograde degeneration of epinephrine neurons in Alzheimer's disease. *Ann.Neurol., 24,* 532-536.

Burke, W. J., Chung, H. D., Marshall, G. L., Gillespie, K. N., & Joh, T. H. (1990). Evidence for decreased transport of PNMT protein in advanced Alzheimer's disease. *J Am.Geriatr.Soc., 38,* 1275-1282.

Burke, W. J., Chung, H. D., Nakra, B. R., Grossberg, G. T., & Joh, T. H. (1987). Phenylethanolamine N-methyltransferase activity is decreased in Alzheimer's disease brains. *Ann.Neurol., 22,* 278-280.

Burke, W. J., Coronado, P. G., Schmitt, C. A., Gillespie, K. M., & Chung, H. D. (1994a). Blood pressure regulation in Alzheimer's disease. *J Auton.Nerv.Syst., 48,* 65-71.

Burke, W. J., Galvin, N. J., Chung, H. D., Stoff, S. A., Gillespie, K. N., Cataldo, A. M. et al. (1994b). Degenerative changes in epinephrine tonic vasomotor neurons in Alzheimer's disease. *Brain Res, 661,* 35-42.

Chalermpalanupap, T., Kinkead, B., Hu, W. T., Kummer, M. P., Hammerschmidt, T., Heneka, M. T. et al. (2013). Targeting norepinephrine in mild cognitive impairment and Alzheimer's disease. *Alzheimers.Res.Ther., 5,* 21.

Chan-Palay, V. & Asan, E. (1989a). Alterations in catecholamine neurons of the locus coeruleus in senile dementia of the Alzheimer type and in Parkinson's disease with and without dementia and depression. *J Comp Neurol., 287,* 373-392.

Chan-Palay, V. & Asan, E. (1989b). Quantitation of catecholamine neurons in the locus coeruleus in human brains of normal young and older adults and in depression. *J Comp Neurol., 287,* 357-372.

Chen, Y., Zhang, K., Wen, G., Rao, F., Sanchez, A. P., Wang, L. et al. (2011). Human dopamine beta-hydroxylase promoter variant alters transcription in chromaffin cells, enzyme secretion, and blood pressure. *Am.J.Hypertens., 24,* 24-32.

Chetelat, G., Desgranges, B., de, l. S., V, Viader, F., Eustache, F., & Baron, J. C. (2003). Mild cognitive impairment: Can FDG-PET predict who is to rapidly convert to Alzheimer's disease? *Neurology, 60,* 1374-1377.

Combarros, O., Warden, D. R., Hammond, N., Cortina-Borja, M., Belbin, O., Lehmann, M. G. et al. (2010). The dopamine beta-hydroxylase -1021C/T polymorphism is associated with the risk of Alzheimer's disease in the Epistasis Project. *BMC.Med.Genet., 11,* 162.

Cortes, R., Probst, A., & Palacios, J. M. (1988). Decreased densities of dopamine D1 receptors in the putamen and hippocampus in senile dementia of the Alzheimer type. *Brain Res, 475,* 164-167.

Craig, S. P., Buckle, V. J., Lamouroux, A., Mallet, J., & Craig, I. W. (1988). Localization of the human dopamine beta hydroxylase (DBH) gene to chromosome 9q34. *Cytogenet.Cell Genet., 48,* 48-50.

Cross, A. J., Crow, T. J., Ferrier, I. N., Johnson, J. A., & Markakis, D. (1984). Striatal dopamine receptors in Alzheimer-type dementia. *Neurosci.Lett., 52,* 1-6.

Cross, A. J., Crow, T. J., Perry, E. K., Perry, R. H., Blessed, G., & Tomlinson, B. E. (1981). Reduced dopamine-beta-hydroxylase activity in Alzheimer's disease. *Br.Med.J (Clin Res Ed), 282,* 93-94.

Cubells, J. F., Kranzler, H. R., Cance-Katz, E., Anderson, G. M., Malison, R. T., Price, L. H. et al. (2000). A haplotype at the DBH locus, associated with low plasma dopamine beta-hydroxylase activity, also associates with cocaine-induced paranoia. *Mol.Psychiatry, 5,* 56-63.

Cubells, J. F. & Zabetian, C. P. (2004). Human genetics of plasma dopamine beta-hydroxylase activity: applications to research in psychiatry and neurology. *Psychopharmacology (Berl), 174,* 463-476.

Czech, C., Berndt, P., Busch, K., Schmitz, O., Wiemer, J., Most, V. et al. (2012). Metabolite profiling of Alzheimer's disease cerebrospinal fluid. *PLoS.One., 7,* e31501.

De Keyser J., Ebinger, G., & Vauquelin, G. (1990). D1-dopamine receptor abnormality in frontal cortex points to a functional alteration of cortical cell membranes in Alzheimer's disease. *Arch.Neurol., 47,* 761-763.

Dello-Russo C., Boullerne, A. I., Gavrilyuk, V., & Feinstein, D. L. (2004). Inhibition of microglial inflammatory responses by norepinephrine: effects on nitric oxide and interleukin-1beta production. *J Neuroinflammation., 1,* 9.

Dickerson, B. C., Goncharova, I., Sullivan, M. P., Forchetti, C., Wilson, R. S., Bennett, D. A. et al. (2001). MRI-derived entorhinal and hippocampal atrophy in incipient and very mild Alzheimer's disease. *Neurobiol Aging, 22,* 747-754.

Dubois, B., Feldman, H. H., Jacova, C., Cummings, J. L., DeKosky, S. T., Barberger-Gateau, P. et al. (2010). Revising the definition of Alzheimer's disease: a new lexicon. *Lancet Neurol., 9,* 1118-1127.

Dubois, B., Feldman, H. H., Jacova, C., DeKosky, S. T., Barberger-Gateau, P., Cummings, J. et al. (2007). Research criteria for the diagnosis of Alzheimer's disease: revising the NINCDS-ADRDA criteria. *Lancet Neurol., 6,* 734-746.

Edison, P., Archer, H. A., Hinz, R., Hammers, A., Pavese, N., Tai, Y. F. et al. (2007). Amyloid, hypometabolism, and cognition in Alzheimer disease: an [11C]PIB and [18F]FDG PET study. *Neurology, 68,* 501-508.

Elrod, R., Peskind, E. R., DiGiacomo, L., Brodkin, K. I., Veith, R. C., & Raskind, M. A. (1997). Effects of Alzheimer's disease severity on cerebrospinal fluid norepinephrine concentration. *Am.J Psychiatry, 154,* 25-30.

Faull, K. F., Pascoe, N., Maddaluno, J., Greene, K. A., & Wiener, S. G. (1990). Passage of MHPG from plasma to CSF in a non-human primate. *J.Neurosci.Res., 27,* 533-540.

Feinstein, D. L., Heneka, M. T., Gavrilyuk, V., Dello, R. C., Weinberg, G., & Galea, E. (2002). Noradrenergic regulation of inflammatory gene expression in brain. *Neurochem.Int., 41,* 357-365.

Forette, F., Seux, M. L., Staessen, J. A., Thijs, L., Babarskiene, M. R., Babeanu, S. et al. (2002). The prevention of dementia with antihypertensive treatment: new evidence from the Systolic Hypertension in Europe (Syst-Eur) study. *Arch.Intern.Med., 162,* 2046-2052.

Forette, F., Seux, M. L., Staessen, J. A., Thijs, L., Birkenhager, W. H., Babarskiene, M. R. et al. (1998). Prevention of dementia in randomised double-blind placebo-controlled Systolic Hypertension in Europe (Syst-Eur) trial. *Lancet, 352,* 1347-1351.

Fox, N. C., Warrington, E. K., Freeborough, P. A., Hartikainen, P., Kennedy, A. M., Stevens, J. M. et al. (1996). Presymptomatic hippocampal atrophy in Alzheimer's disease. A longitudinal MRI study. *Brain, 119 (Pt 6),* 2001-2007.

Francis, P. T., Palmer, A. M., Snape, M., & Wilcock, G. K. (1999). The cholinergic hypothesis of Alzheimer's disease: a review of progress. *J Neurol.Neurosurg.Psychiatry, 66,* 137-147.

Friedman, J. I., Adler, D. N., & Davis, K. L. (1999). The role of norepinephrine in the pathophysiology of cognitive disorders: potential applications to the treatment of cognitive dysfunction in schizophrenia and Alzheimer's disease. *Biol.Psychiatry, 46,* 1243-1252.

Fritschy, J. M. & Grzanna, R. (1991). Experimentally-induced neuron loss in the locus coeruleus of adult rats. *Exp.Neurol., 111,* 123-127.

Galea, E., Heneka, M. T., Dello, R. C., & Feinstein, D. L. (2003). Intrinsic regulation of brain inflammatory responses. *Cell Mol.Neurobiol., 23,* 625-635.

German, D. C., Manaye, K. F., White, C. L., III, Woodward, D. J., McIntire, D. D., Smith, W. K. et al. (1992). Disease-specific patterns of locus coeruleus cell loss. *Ann.Neurol., 32,* 667-676.

German, D. C., White, C. L., III, & Sparkman, D. R. (1987). Alzheimer's disease: neurofibrillary tangles in nuclei that project to the cerebral cortex. *Neuroscience, 21,* 305-312.

Gibb, W. R., Mountjoy, C. Q., Mann, D. M., & Lees, A. J. (1989). The substantia nigra and ventral tegmental area in Alzheimer's disease and Down's syndrome. *J.Neurol.Neurosurg.Psychiatry, 52,* 193-200.

Goldman-Rakic, P. S., Lidow, M. S., & Gallager, D. W. (1990). Overlap of dopaminergic, adrenergic, and serotoninergic receptors and complementarity of their subtypes in primate prefrontal cortex. *J.Neurosci., 10,* 2125-2138.

Gottfries, C. G., Adolfsson, R., Aquilonius, S. M., Carlsson, A., Eckernas, S. A., Nordberg, A. et al. (1983). Biochemical changes in dementia disorders of Alzheimer type (AD/SDAT). *Neurobiol Aging, 4,* 261-271.

Granata, A. R., Ruggiero, D. A., Park, D. H., Joh, T. H., & Reis, D. J. (1985). Brain stem area with C1 epinephrine neurons mediates baroreflex vasodepressor responses. *Am.J Physiol, 248,* H547-H567.

Greene, K. A. & Faull, K. F. (1989). Relationship between plasma and cerebrospinal fluid norepinephrine and dopamine metabolites in a nonhuman primate. *J.Neurochem., 53,* 1007-1013.

Grudzien, A., Shaw, P., Weintraub, S., Bigio, E., Mash, D. C., & Mesulam, M. M. (2007). Locus coeruleus neurofibrillary degeneration in aging, mild cognitive impairment and early Alzheimer's disease. *Neurobiol Aging, 28,* 327-335.

Guan, Z. Z., Wang, Y. N., Xiao, K. Q., Hu, P. S., & Liu, J. L. (1999). Activity of phosphatidylethanolamine-N-methyltransferase in brain affected by Alzheimer's disease. *Neurochem.Int., 34,* 41-47.

Guo, Z., Viitanen, M., Fratiglioni, L., & Winblad, B. (1996). Low blood pressure and dementia in elderly people: the Kungsholmen project. *BMJ, 312,* 805-808.

Haglund, M., Sjobeck, M., & Englund, E. (2006). Locus ceruleus degeneration is ubiquitous in Alzheimer's disease: possible implications for diagnosis and treatment. *Neuropathology., 26,* 528-532.

Haller, J., Makara, G. B., & Kruk, M. R. (1998). Catecholaminergic involvement in the control of aggression: hormones, the peripheral sympathetic, and central noradrenergic systems. *Neurosci.Biobehav.Rev., 22,* 85-97.

Hardy, J. (2006a). Alzheimer's disease: the amyloid cascade hypothesis: an update and reappraisal. *J Alzheimers.Dis., 9,* 151-153.

Hardy, J. (2006b). Has the amyloid cascade hypothesis for Alzheimer's disease been proved? *Curr.Alzheimer Res, 3,* 71-73.

Hardy, J. & Selkoe, D. J. (2002). The amyloid hypothesis of Alzheimer's disease: progress and problems on the road to therapeutics. *Science, 297,* 353-356.

Hardy, J. A. & Higgins, G. A. (1992). Alzheimer's disease: the amyloid cascade hypothesis. *Science, 256,* 184-185.

Hebert, L. E., Weuve, J., Scherr, P. A., & Evans, D. A. (2013). Alzheimer disease in the United States (2010-2050) estimated using the 2010 census. *Neurology, 80,* 1778-1783.

Heneka, M. T., Galea, E., Gavriluyk, V., Dumitrescu-Ozimek, L., Daeschner, J., O'Banion, M. K. et al. (2002). Noradrenergic depletion potentiates beta -amyloid-induced cortical inflammation: implications for Alzheimer's disease. *J Neurosci., 22,* 2434-2442.

Heneka, M. T., Nadrigny, F., Regen, T., Martinez-Hernandez, A., Dumitrescu-Ozimek, L., Terwel, D. et al. (2010). Locus ceruleus controls Alzheimer's disease pathology by modulating microglial functions through norepinephrine. *Proc.Natl.Acad.Sci.U.S.A, 107,* 6058-6063.

Heneka, M. T. & O'Banion, M. K. (2007). Inflammatory processes in Alzheimer's disease. *J Neuroimmunol., 184,* 69-91.

Heneka, M. T., Ramanathan, M., Jacobs, A. H., Dumitrescu-Ozimek, L., Bilkei-Gorzo, A., Debeir, T. et al. (2006). Locus ceruleus degeneration promotes Alzheimer pathogenesis in amyloid precursor protein 23 transgenic mice. *J Neurosci., 26,* 1343-1354.

Herholz, K., Salmon, E., Perani, D., Baron, J. C., Holthoff, V., Frolich, L. et al. (2002). Discrimination between Alzheimer dementia and controls by automated analysis of multicenter FDG PET. *Neuroimage., 17,* 302-316.

Herrmann, N., Lanctot, K. L., & Khan, L. R. (2004). The role of norepinephrine in the behavioral and psychological symptoms of dementia. *J Neuropsychiatry Clin Neurosci., 16,* 261-276.

Hersch, E. C. & Falzgraf, S. (2007). Management of the behavioral and psychological symptoms of dementia. *Clin.Interv.Aging, 2,* 611-621.

Hoogendijk, W. J., Feenstra, M. G., Botterblom, M. H., Gilhuis, J., Sommer, I. E., Kamphorst, W. et al. (1999a). Increased activity of surviving locus ceruleus neurons in Alzheimer's disease. *Ann.Neurol., 45,* 82-91.

Hoogendijk, W. J., Pool, C. W., Troost, D., van, Z. E., & Swaab, D. F. (1995). Image analyser-assisted morphometry of the locus coeruleus in Alzheimer's disease, Parkinson's disease and amyotrophic lateral sclerosis. *Brain, 118 (Pt 1),* 131-143.

Hoogendijk, W. J., Sommer, I. E., Pool, C. W., Kamphorst, W., Hofman, M. A., Eikelenboom, P. et al. (1999b). Lack of association between depression and loss of neurons in the locus coeruleus in Alzheimer disease. *Arch.Gen.Psychiatry, 56,* 45-51.

Hyman, B. T., Phelps, C. H., Beach, T. G., Bigio, E. H., Cairns, N. J., Carrillo, M. C. et al. (2012). National Institute on Aging-Alzheimer's Association guidelines for the neuropathologic assessment of Alzheimer's disease. *Alzheimers.Dement., 8,* 1-13.

Hyman, B. T. & Trojanowski, J. Q. (1997). Consensus recommendations for the postmortem diagnosis of Alzheimer disease from the National Institute on Aging and the Reagan Institute Working Group on diagnostic criteria for the neuropathological assessment of Alzheimer disease. *J.Neuropathol.Exp.Neurol., 56,* 1095-1097.

Ikegaya, Y., Nakanishi, K., Saito, H., & Abe, K. (1997). Amygdala beta-noradrenergic influence on hippocampal long-term potentiation in vivo. *Neuroreport, 8,* 3143-3146.

Ikegaya, Y., Saito, H., & Abe, K. (1996a). Dentate gyrus field potentials evoked by stimulation of the basolateral amygdaloid nucleus in anesthetized rats. *Brain Res., 718,* 53-60.

Ikegaya, Y., Saito, H., & Abe, K. (1996b). The basomedial and basolateral amygdaloid nuclei contribute to the induction of long-term potentiation in the dentate gyrus in vivo. *Eur.J.Neurosci., 8,* 1833-1839.

Ikonomovic, M. D., Klunk, W. E., Abrahamson, E. E., Mathis, C. A., Price, J. C., Tsopelas, N. D. et al. (2008). Post-mortem correlates of in vivo PiB-PET amyloid imaging in a typical case of Alzheimer's disease. *Brain, 131,* 1630-1645.

Iversen, L. L., Rossor, M. N., Reynolds, G. P., Hills, R., Roth, M., Mountjoy, C. Q. et al. (1983). Loss of pigmented dopamine-beta-hydroxylase positive cells from locus coeruleus in senile dementia of Alzheimer's type. *Neurosci.Lett., 39,* 95-100.

Izquierdo, I., Medina, J. H., Izquierdo, L. A., Barros, D. M., de Souza, M. M., & Mello e Souza (1998). Short- and long-term memory are differentially regulated by monoaminergic systems in the rat brain. *Neurobiol.Learn.Mem., 69,* 219-224.

Jack, C. R., Jr., Albert, M. S., Knopman, D. S., McKhann, G. M., Sperling, R. A., Carrillo, M. C. et al. (2011). Introduction to the recommendations from the National Institute on Aging-Alzheimer's Association workgroups on diagnostic guidelines for Alzheimer's disease. *Alzheimers.Dement., 7,* 257-262.

Jack, C. R., Jr., Knopman, D. S., Jagust, W. J., Shaw, L. M., Aisen, P. S., Weiner, M. W. et al. (2010). Hypothetical model of dynamic biomarkers of the Alzheimer's pathological cascade. *Lancet Neurol., 9,* 119-128.

Jack, C. R., Jr., Petersen, R. C., Xu, Y. C., Waring, S. C., O'Brien, P. C., Tangalos, E. G. et al. (1997). Medial temporal atrophy on MRI in normal aging and very mild Alzheimer's disease. *Neurology, 49,* 786-794.

Jardanhazi-Kurutz, D., Kummer, M. P., Terwel, D., Vogel, K., Thiele, A., & Heneka, M. T. (2011). Distinct adrenergic system changes and neuroinflammation in response to induced locus ceruleus degeneration in APP/PS1 transgenic mice. *Neuroscience, 176,* 396-407.

Jicha, G. A., Parisi, J. E., Dickson, D. W., Johnson, K., Cha, R., Ivnik, R. J. et al. (2006). Neuropathologic outcome of mild cognitive impairment following progression to clinical dementia. *Arch.Neurol., 63,* 674-681.

Johnson, K. A., Minoshima, S., Bohnen, N. I., Donohoe, K. J., Foster, N. L., Herscovitch, P. et al. (2013). Appropriate use criteria for amyloid PET: a report of the Amyloid Imaging Task Force, the Society of Nuclear Medicine and Molecular Imaging, and the Alzheimer's Association. *Alzheimers.Dement., 9,* e-16.

Joyce, J. N., Kaeger, C., Ryoo, H., & Goldsmith, S. (1993). Dopamine D2 receptors in the hippocampus and amygdala in Alzheimer's disease. *Neurosci.Lett., 154,* 171-174.

Joyce, J. N., Murray, A. M., Hurtig, H. I., Gottlieb, G. L., & Trojanowski, J. Q. (1998a). Loss of dopamine D2 receptors in Alzheimer's disease with parkinsonism but not Parkinson's or Alzheimer's disease. *Neuropsychopharmacology, 19,* 472-480.

Joyce, J. N., Myers, A. J., & Gurevich, E. (1998b). Dopamine D2 receptor bands in normal human temporal cortex are absent in Alzheimer's disease. *Brain Res, 784,* 7-17.

Kalaria, R. N. & Andorn, A. C. (1991). Adrenergic receptors in aging and Alzheimer's disease: decreased alpha 2-receptors demonstrated by [3H]p-aminoclonidine binding in prefrontal cortex. *Neurobiol Aging, 12,* 131-136.

Kalaria, R. N., Andorn, A. C., & Harik, S. I. (1989a). Alterations in adrenergic receptors of frontal cortex and cerebral microvessels in Alzheimer's disease and aging. *Prog.Clin.Biol.Res., 317,* 367-374.

Kalaria, R. N., Andorn, A. C., Tabaton, M., Whitehouse, P. J., Harik, S. I., & Unnerstall, J. R. (1989b). Adrenergic receptors in aging and Alzheimer's disease: increased beta 2-receptors in prefrontal cortex and hippocampus. *J.Neurochem., 53,* 1772-1781.

Kalaria, R. N. & Harik, S. I. (1989). Increased alpha 2- and beta 2-adrenergic receptors in cerebral microvessels in Alzheimer disease. *Neurosci.Lett., 106,* 233-238.

Kalinin, S., Gavrilyuk, V., Polak, P. E., Vasser, R., Zhao, J., Heneka, M. T. et al. (2007). Noradrenaline deficiency in brain increases beta-amyloid plaque burden in an animal model of Alzheimer's disease. *Neurobiol.Aging, 28,* 1206-1214.

Karran, E., Mercken, M., & De, S. B. (2011). The amyloid cascade hypothesis for Alzheimer's disease: an appraisal for the development of therapeutics. *Nat.Rev.Drug Discov., 10,* 698-712.

Kastner, A., Hirsch, E. C., Herrero, M. T., Javoy-Agid, F., & Agid, Y. (1993). Immunocytochemical quantification of tyrosine hydroxylase at a cellular level in the mesencephalon of control subjects and patients with Parkinson's and Alzheimer's disease. *J.Neurochem., 61,* 1024-1034.

Kemppainen, N., Laine, M., Laakso, M. P., Kaasinen, V., Nagren, K., Vahlberg, T. et al. (2003). Hippocampal dopamine D2 receptors correlate with memory functions in Alzheimer's disease. *Eur.J Neurosci., 18,* 149-154.

Kemppainen, N., Ruottinen, H., Nagren, K., & Rinne, J. O. (2000). PET shows that striatal dopamine D1 and D2 receptors are differentially affected in AD. *Neurology, 55,* 205-209.

Kemppainen, N. M., Aalto, S., Wilson, I. A., Nagren, K., Helin, S., Bruck, A. et al. (2006). Voxel-based analysis of PET amyloid ligand [11C]PIB uptake in Alzheimer disease. *Neurology, 67,* 1575-1580.

Kemppainen, N. M., Aalto, S., Wilson, I. A., Nagren, K., Helin, S., Bruck, A. et al. (2007). PET amyloid ligand [11C]PIB uptake is increased in mild cognitive impairment. *Neurology, 68,* 1603-1606.

Kim, C. H., Zabetian, C. P., Cubells, J. F., Cho, S., Biaggioni, I., Cohen, B. M. et al. (2002). Mutations in the dopamine beta-hydroxylase gene are associated with human norepinephrine deficiency. *Am.J Med.Genet., 108,* 140-147.

Klunk, W. E., Engler, H., Nordberg, A., Wang, Y., Blomqvist, G., Holt, D. P. et al. (2004). Imaging brain amyloid in Alzheimer's disease with Pittsburgh Compound-B. *Ann.Neurol., 55,* 306-319.

Kohnke, M. D., Zabetian, C. P., Anderson, G. M., Kolb, W., Gaertner, I., Buchkremer, G. et al. (2002). A genotype-controlled analysis of plasma dopamine beta-hydroxylase in healthy and alcoholic subjects: evidence for alcohol-related differences in noradrenergic function. *Biol.Psychiatry, 52,* 1151-1158.

Koivunen, J., Verkkoniemi, A., Aalto, S., Paetau, A., Ahonen, J. P., Viitanen, M. et al. (2008). PET amyloid ligand [11C]PIB uptake shows predominantly striatal increase in variant Alzheimer's disease. *Brain, 131,* 1845-1853.

Kopin, I. J. (1985). Catecholamine metabolism: basic aspects and clinical significance. *Pharmacol.Rev., 37,* 333-364.

Landin, K., Blennow, K., Wallin, A., & Gottfries, C. G. (1993). Low blood pressure and blood glucose levels in Alzheimer's disease. Evidence for a hypometabolic disorder? *J Intern.Med., 233,* 357-363.

Lawlor, B. A., Bierer, L. M., Ryan, T. M., Schmeidler, J., Knott, P. J., Williams, L. L. et al. (1995). Plasma 3-methoxy-4-hydroxyphenylglycol (MHPG) and clinical symptoms in Alzheimer's disease. *Biol.Psychiatry, 38,* 185-188.

Lee, H. G., Zhu, X., Nunomura, A., Perry, G., & Smith, M. A. (2006). Amyloid beta: the alternate hypothesis. *Curr.Alzheimer Res, 3,* 75-80.

Li, G. Y., Watanabe, I., Kunitake, Y., Sugataka, K., Muraoka, T., Kojima, N. et al. (2008). Relationship between saliva level of 3-methoxy-4-hydroxyphenylglycol and mental health in the elderly general population. *Psychiatry Clin.Neurosci., 62,* 562-567.

Li, J., Zhu, M., Manning-Bog, A. B., Di Monte, D. A., & Fink, A. L. (2004). Dopamine and L-dopa disaggregate amyloid fibrils: implications for Parkinson's and Alzheimer's disease. *FASEB J, 18,* 962-964.

Luong, K. & Nguyen, L. T. (2013). The role of Beta-adrenergic receptor blockers in Alzheimer's disease: potential genetic and cellular signaling mechanisms. *Am.J.Alzheimers.Dis.Other Demen., 28,* 427-439.

Lyketsos, C. G., DelCampo, L., Steinberg, M., Miles, Q., Steele, C. D., Munro, C. et al. (2003). Treating depression in Alzheimer disease: efficacy and safety of sertraline therapy, and the benefits of depression reduction: the DIADS. *Arch.Gen.Psychiatry, 60,* 737-746.

Lyketsos, C. G., Lopez, O., Jones, B., Fitzpatrick, A. L., Breitner, J., & DeKosky, S. (2002). Prevalence of neuropsychiatric symptoms in dementia and mild cognitive impairment: results from the cardiovascular health study. *JAMA, 288,* 1475-1483.

Lyketsos, C. G., Sheppard, J. M., Steinberg, M., Tschanz, J. A., Norton, M. C., Steffens, D. C. et al. (2001). Neuropsychiatric disturbance in Alzheimer's disease clusters into three groups: the Cache County study. *Int.J Geriatr.Psychiatry, 16,* 1043-1053.

Manaye, K. F., McIntire, D. D., Mann, D. M., & German, D. C. (1995). Locus coeruleus cell loss in the aging human brain: a non-random process. *J Comp Neurol., 358,* 79-87.

Mann, D. M., Lincoln, J., Yates, P. O., Stamp, J. E., & Toper, S. (1980). Changes in the monoamine containing neurones of the human CNS in senile dementia. *Br.J Psychiatry, 136,* 533-541.

Mann, D. M., Yates, P. O., & Hawkes, J. (1982). The noradrenergic system in Alzheimer and multi-infarct dementias. *J Neurol.Neurosurg.Psychiatry, 45,* 113-119.

Mann, D. M., Yates, P. O., & Marcyniuk, B. (1984). A comparison of changes in the nucleus basalis and locus caeruleus in Alzheimer's disease. *J Neurol.Neurosurg.Psychiatry, 47,* 201-203.

Mann, D. M., Yates, P. O., & Marcyniuk, B. (1987). Dopaminergic neurotransmitter systems in Alzheimer's disease and in Down's syndrome at middle age. *J.Neurol.Neurosurg.Psychiatry, 50,* 341-344.

Mann, M. B., Wu, S., Rostamkhani, M., Tourtellotte, W., MacMurray, J., & Comings, D. E. (2001). Phenylethanolamine N-methyltransferase (PNMT) gene and early-onset Alzheimer disease. *Am.J Med.Genet., 105,* 312-316.

Marcyniuk, B., Mann, D. M., & Yates, P. O. (1986a). Loss of nerve cells from locus coeruleus in Alzheimer's disease is topographically arranged. *Neurosci.Lett., 64,* 247-252.

Marcyniuk, B., Mann, D. M., & Yates, P. O. (1986b). The topography of cell loss from locus caeruleus in Alzheimer's disease. *J Neurol.Sci., 76,* 335-345.

Marcyniuk, B., Mann, D. M., & Yates, P. O. (1989). The topography of nerve cell loss from the locus caeruleus in elderly persons. *Neurobiol Aging, 10,* 5-9.

Marien, M. R., Colpaert, F. C., & Rosenquist, A. C. (2004). Noradrenergic mechanisms in neurodegenerative diseases: a theory. *Brain Res Brain Res Rev., 45,* 38-78.

Markesbery, W. R., Schmitt, F. A., Kryscio, R. J., Davis, D. G., Smith, C. D., & Wekstein, D. R. (2006). Neuropathologic substrate of mild cognitive impairment. *Arch.Neurol., 63,* 38-46.

Martignoni, E., Blandini, F., Petraglia, F., Pacchetti, C., Bono, G., & Nappi, G. (1992). Cerebrospinal fluid norepinephrine, 3-methoxy-4-hydroxyphenylglycol and neuropeptide Y levels in Parkinson's disease, multiple system atrophy and dementia of the Alzheimer type. *J.Neural Transm.Park Dis.Dement.Sect., 4,* 191-205.

Mateo, I., Infante, J., Rodriguez, E., Berciano, J., Combarros, O., & Llorca, J. (2006). Interaction between dopamine beta-hydroxylase and interleukin genes increases Alzheimer's disease risk. *J.Neurol.Neurosurg.Psychiatry, 77,* 278-279.

Matthews, K. L., Chen, C. P., Esiri, M. M., Keene, J., Minger, S. L., & Francis, P. T. (2002). Noradrenergic changes, aggressive behavior, and cognition in patients with dementia. *Biol.Psychiatry, 51,* 407-416.

Maurer, K., Volk, S., & Gerbaldo, H. (1997). Auguste D and Alzheimer's disease. *Lancet, 349,* 1546-1549.

McKhann, G., Drachman, D., Folstein, M., Katzman, R., Price, D., & Stadlan, E. M. (1984). Clinical diagnosis of Alzheimer's disease: report of the NINCDS-ADRDA Work Group under the auspices of Department of Health and Human Services Task Force on Alzheimer's Disease. *Neurology, 34,* 939-944.

McKhann, G. M., Knopman, D. S., Chertkow, H., Hyman, B. T., Jack, C. R., Jr., Kawas, C. H. et al. (2011). The diagnosis of dementia due to Alzheimer's disease: recommendations from the National Institute on Aging-Alzheimer's Association workgroups on diagnostic guidelines for Alzheimer's disease. *Alzheimers.Dement., 7,* 263-269.

Meana, J. J., Barturen, F., Garro, M. A., Garcia-Sevilla, J. A., Fontan, A., & Zarranz, J. J. (1992). Decreased density of presynaptic alpha 2-adrenoceptors in postmortem brains of patients with Alzheimer's disease. *J.Neurochem., 58,* 1896-1904.

Mehta, P. D., Pirttila, T., Mehta, S. P., Sersen, E. A., Aisen, P. S., & Wisniewski, H. M. (2000). Plasma and cerebrospinal fluid levels of amyloid beta proteins 1-40 and 1-42 in Alzheimer disease. *Arch.Neurol., 57,* 100-105.

Mitchell, A. J. & Shiri-Feshki, M. (2009). Rate of progression of mild cognitive impairment to dementia--meta-analysis of 41 robust inception cohort studies. *Acta Psychiatr.Scand., 119,* 252-265.

Miyata, S., Nagata, H., Yamao, S., Nakamura, S., & Kameyama, M. (1984). Dopamine-beta-hydroxylase activities in serum and cerebrospinal fluid of aged and demented patients. *J Neurol.Sci., 63,* 403-409.

Molchan, S. E., Lawlor, B. A., Hill, J. L., Martinez, R. A., Davis, C. L., Mellow, A. M. et al. (1991). CSF monoamine metabolites and somatostatin in Alzheimer's disease and major depression. *Biol.Psychiatry, 29,* 1110-1118.

Morris, J. C., Roe, C. M., Xiong, C., Fagan, A. M., Goate, A. M., Holtzman, D. M. et al. (2010). APOE predicts amyloid-beta but not tau Alzheimer pathology in cognitively normal aging. *Ann.Neurol., 67,* 122-131.

Mosconi, L., Tsui, W. H., Herholz, K., Pupi, A., Drzezga, A., Lucignani, G. et al. (2008). Multicenter standardized 18F-FDG PET diagnosis of mild cognitive impairment, Alzheimer's disease, and other dementias. *J Nucl.Med., 49,* 390-398.

Mustapic, M., Presecki, P., Pivac, N., Mimica, N., Hof, P. R., Simic, G. et al. (2013). Genotype-independent decrease in plasma dopamine beta-hydroxylase activity in Alzheimer's disease. *Prog.Neuropsychopharmacol.Biol.Psychiatry, 44,* 94-99.

Nakajima, S., Gerretsen, P., Takeuchi, H., Caravaggio, F., Chow, T., Le, F. B. et al. (2013). The potential role of dopamine D(3) receptor neurotransmission in cognition. *Eur.Neuropsychopharmacol., 23,* 799-813.

Nakamura, S., Koshimura, K., Kato, T., Yamao, S., Iijima, S., Nagata, H. et al. (1984). Neurotransmitters in dementia. *Clin Ther., 7 Spec No,* 18-34.

Nazarali, A. J. & Reynolds, G. P. (1992). Monoamine neurotransmitters and their metabolites in brain regions in Alzheimer's disease: a postmortem study. *Cell Mol.Neurobiol, 12,* 581-587.

Nieuwenhuys, R. (1985). *Chemoarchitecture of the brain*. Berlin Heidelberg: Springer-Verlag.

Noel-Storr, A. H., Flicker, L., Ritchie, C. W., Nguyen, G. H., Gupta, T., Wood, P. et al. (2013). Systematic review of the body of evidence for the use of biomarkers in the diagnosis of dementia. *Alzheimers.Dement., 9,* e96-e105.

Ogihara, T., Nugent, C. A., Shen, S. W., & Goldfein, S. (1975). Serum dopamine-beta-hydroxylase activity in parents and children. *J.Lab Clin.Med., 85,* 566-573.

Paclt, I. & Koudelova, J. (2004). Changes of dopamine-beta-hydroxylase activity during ontogenesis in healthy subjects and in an experimental model (rats). *Physiol Res., 53,* 661-667.

Palmer, A. M., Francis, P. T., Bowen, D. M., Benton, J. S., Neary, D., Mann, D. M. et al. (1987a). Catecholaminergic neurones assessed ante-mortem in Alzheimer's disease. *Brain Res, 414,* 365-375.

Palmer, A. M., Stratmann, G. C., Procter, A. W., & Bowen, D. M. (1988). Possible neurotransmitter basis of behavioral changes in Alzheimer's disease. *Ann.Neurol., 23,* 616-620.

Palmer, A. M., Wilcock, G. K., Esiri, M. M., Francis, P. T., & Bowen, D. M. (1987b). Monoaminergic innervation of the frontal and temporal lobes in Alzheimer's disease. *Brain Res, 401,* 231-238.

Perry, E. K., Blessed, G., Tomlinson, B. E., Perry, R. H., Crow, T. J., Cross, A. J. et al. (1981a). Neurochemical activities in human temporal lobe related to aging and Alzheimer-type changes. *Neurobiol Aging, 2,* 251-256.

Perry, E. K., Tomlinson, B. E., Blessed, G., Perry, R. H., Cross, A. J., & Crow, T. J. (1981b). Neuropathological and biochemical observations on the noradrenergic system in Alzheimer's disease. *J Neurol.Sci., 51,* 279-287.

Peskind, E. R., Elrod, R., Dobie, D. J., Pascualy, M., Petrie, E., Jensen, C. et al. (1998). Cerebrospinal fluid epinephrine in Alzheimer's disease and normal aging. *Neuropsychopharmacology, 19,* 465-471.

Peskind, E. R., Raskind, M. A., Wilkinson, C. W., Flatness, D. E., & Halter, J. B. (1986). Peripheral sympathectomy and adrenal medullectomy do not alter cerebrospinal fluid norepinephrine. *Brain Res, 367,* 258-264.

Petersen, R. C. (2011). Clinical practice. Mild cognitive impairment. *N.Engl.J.Med., 364,* 2227-2234.

Petersen, R. C., Parisi, J. E., Dickson, D. W., Johnson, K. A., Knopman, D. S., Boeve, B. F. et al. (2006). Neuropathologic features of amnestic mild cognitive impairment. *Arch.Neurol., 63,* 665-672.

Petrella, J. R., Coleman, R. E., & Doraiswamy, P. M. (2003). Neuroimaging and early diagnosis of Alzheimer disease: a look to the future. *Radiology, 226,* 315-336.

Piggott, M. A., Marshall, E. F., Thomas, N., Lloyd, S., Court JA, Jaros, E. et al. (1999). Striatal dopaminergic markers in dementia with Lewy bodies, Alzheimer's and Parkinson's diseases: rostrocaudal distribution. *Brain, 122 (Pt 8),* 1449-1468.

Pimplikar, S. W. (2009). Reassessing the amyloid cascade hypothesis of Alzheimer's disease. *Int.J Biochem.Cell Biol., 41,* 1261-1268.

Pizzolato, G., Chierichetti, F., Fabbri, M., Cagnin, A., Dam, M., Ferlin, G. et al. (1996). Reduced striatal dopamine receptors in Alzheimer's disease: single photon emission tomography study with the D2 tracer [123I]-IBZM. *Neurology, 47,* 1065-1068.

Powers, R. E., Struble, R. G., Casanova, M. F., O'Connor, D. T., Kitt, C. A., & Price, D. L. (1988). Innervation of human hippocampus by noradrenergic systems: normal anatomy and structural abnormalities in aging and in Alzheimer's disease. *Neuroscience, 25,* 401-417.

Prince, M., Bryce, R., Albanese, E., Wimo, A., Ribeiro, W., & Ferri, C. P. (2013). The global prevalence of dementia: a systematic review and metaanalysis. *Alzheimers.Dement., 9,* 63-75.

Qiu, C., Winblad, B., & Fratiglioni, L. (2005). The age-dependent relation of blood pressure to cognitive function and dementia. *Lancet Neurol., 4,* 487-499.

Rabinovici, G. D., Seeley, W. W., Kim, E. J., Gorno-Tempini, M. L., Rascovsky, K., Pagliaro, T. A. et al. (2007). Distinct MRI atrophy patterns in autopsy-proven Alzheimer's disease and frontotemporal lobar degeneration. *Am.J Alzheimers.Dis.Other Demen., 22,* 474-488.

Raskind, M. A., Peskind, E. R., Halter, J. B., & Jimerson, D. C. (1984). Norepinephrine and MHPG levels in CSF and plasma in Alzheimer's disease. *Arch.Gen.Psychiatry, 41,* 343-346.

Reinikainen, K. J., Paljarvi, L., Halonen, T., Malminen, O., Kosma, V. M., Laakso, M. et al. (1988). Dopaminergic system and monoamine oxidase-B activity in Alzheimer's disease. *Neurobiol.Aging, 9,* 245-252.

Reinikainen, K. J., Soininen, H., & Riekkinen, P. J. (1990). Neurotransmitter changes in Alzheimer's disease: implications to diagnostics and therapy. *J Neurosci.Res, 27,* 576-586.

Reis, D. J., Granata, A. R., Joh, T. H., Ross, C. A., Ruggiero, D. A., & Park, D. H. (1984). Brain stem catecholamine mechanisms in tonic and reflex control of blood pressure. *Hypertension, 6,* II7-15.

Reis, D. J., Ruggiero, D. A., & Morrison, S. F. (1989). The C1 area of the rostral ventrolateral medulla oblongata. A critical brainstem region for control of resting and reflex integration of arterial pressure. *Am.J Hypertens., 2,* 363S-374S.

Reyes, M. G., Faraldi, F., Rydman, R., & Wang, C. C. (2003). Decreased nigral neuromelanin in Alzheimer's disease. *Neurol.Res., 25,* 179-182.

Rinne, J. O., Sako, E., Paljarvi, L., Molsa, P. K., & Rinne, U. K. (1986a). Brain dopamine D-1 receptors in senile dementia. *J.Neurol.Sci., 73,* 219-230.

Rinne, J. O., Sako, E., Paljarvi, L., Molsa, P. K., & Rinne, U. K. (1986b). Brain dopamine D-2 receptors in senile dementia. *J.Neural Transm., 65,* 51-62.

Risacher, S. L. & Saykin, A. J. (2013). Neuroimaging and other biomarkers for Alzheimer's disease: the changing landscape of early detection. *Annu.Rev.Clin Psychol., 9,* 621-648.

Rossor, M. N., Iversen, L. L., Reynolds, G. P., Mountjoy, C. Q., & Roth, M. (1984). Neurochemical characteristics of early and late onset types of Alzheimer's disease. *Br.Med.J (Clin Res Ed), 288,* 961-964.

Russo-Neustadt, A. & Cotman, C. W. (1997). Adrenergic receptors in Alzheimer's disease brain: selective increases in the cerebella of aggressive patients. *J Neurosci., 17,* 5573-5580.

Ryoo, H. L. & Joyce, J. N. (1994). Loss of dopamine D2 receptors varies along the rostrocaudal axis of the hippocampal complex in Alzheimer's disease. *J.Comp Neurol., 348,* 94-110.

Sawada, M., Hirata, Y., Arai, H., Iizuka, R., & Nagatsu, T. (1987). Tyrosine hydroxylase, tryptophan hydroxylase, biopterin, and neopterin in the brains of normal controls and patients with senile dementia of Alzheimer type. *J Neurochem., 48,* 760-764.

Scahill, R. I., Schott, J. M., Stevens, J. M., Rossor, M. N., & Fox, N. C. (2002). Mapping the evolution of regional atrophy in Alzheimer's disease: unbiased analysis of fluid-registered serial MRI. *Proc.Natl.Acad.Sci.U.S.A, 99,* 4703-4707.

Scheltens, P. & van de Pol L. (2012). Impact commentaries. Atrophy of medial temporal lobes on MRI in "probable" Alzheimer's disease and normal ageing: diagnostic value and neuropsychological correlates. *J Neurol.Neurosurg.Psychiatry, 83,* 1038-1040.

Shankle, W. R., Nielson, K. A., & Cotman, C. W. (1995). Low-dose propranolol reduces aggression and agitation resembling that associated with orbitofrontal dysfunction in elderly demented patients. *Alzheimer Dis.Assoc.Disord., 9,* 233-237.

Shaw, L. M., Korecka, M., Clark, C. M., Lee, V. M., & Trojanowski, J. Q. (2007). Biomarkers of neurodegeneration for diagnosis and monitoring therapeutics. *Nat.Rev.Drug Discov., 6,* 295-303.

Shimohama, S., Taniguchi, T., Fujiwara, M., & Kameyama, M. (1986). Biochemical characterization of alpha-adrenergic receptors in human brain and changes in Alzheimer-type dementia. *J Neurochem., 47,* 1295-1301.

Skoog, I. (1997). The relationship between blood pressure and dementia: a review. *Biomed.Pharmacother., 51,* 367-375.

Soininen, H., MacDonald, E., Rekonen, M., & Riekkinen, P. J. (1981). Homovanillic acid and 5-hydroxyindoleacetic acid levels in cerebrospinal fluid of patients with senile dementia of Alzheimer type. *Acta Neurol.Scand., 64,* 101-107.

Soininen, H., Pitkanen, A., Halonen, T., & Riekkinen, P. J. (1984). Dopamine-beta-hydroxylase and acetylcholinesterase activities of cerebrospinal fluid in Alzheimer's disease. *Acta Neurol.Scand., 70,* 29-34.

Sperling, R. A., Aisen, P. S., Beckett, L. A., Bennett, D. A., Craft, S., Fagan, A. M. et al. (2011). Toward defining the preclinical stages of Alzheimer's disease: recommendations from the National Institute on Aging-Alzheimer's Association workgroups on diagnostic guidelines for Alzheimer's disease. *Alzheimers.Dement., 7,* 280-292.

Storga, D., Vrecko, K., Birkmayer, J. G., & Reibnegger, G. (1996). Monoaminergic neurotransmitters, their precursors and metabolites in brains of Alzheimer patients. *Neurosci.Lett., 203,* 29-32.

Stuerenburg, H. J., Ganzer, S., & Muller-Thomsen, T. (2004). 5-Hydroxyindoleacetic acid and homovanillic acid concentrations in cerebrospinal fluid in patients with Alzheimer's disease, depression and mild cognitive impairment. *Neuro.Endocrinol.Lett., 25,* 435-437.

Sturrock, R. R. & Rao, K. A. (1985). A quantitative histological study of neuronal loss from the locus coeruleus of ageing mice. *Neuropathol.Appl.Neurobiol, 11,* 55-60.

Summers, W. K. (2006). The management of agitation in demented patients with propranolol. *J.Alzheimers.Dis., 9,* 69-75.

Sweet, R. A., Hamilton, R. L., Healy, M. T., Wisniewski, S. R., Henteleff, R., Pollock, B. G. et al. (2001). Alterations of striatal dopamine receptor binding in Alzheimer disease are associated with Lewy body pathology and antemortem psychosis. *Arch.Neurol., 58,* 466-472.

Sweet, R. A., Nimgaonkar, V. L., Kamboh, M. I., Lopez, O. L., Zhang, F., & DeKosky, S. T. (1998). Dopamine receptor genetic variation, psychosis, and aggression in Alzheimer disease. *Arch.Neurol., 55,* 1335-1340.

Swerdlow, R. H. (2007). Pathogenesis of Alzheimer's disease. *Clin Interv.Aging, 2,* 347-359.

Szot, P., Leverenz, J. B., Peskind, E. R., Kiyasu, E., Rohde, K., Miller, M. A. et al. (2000). Tyrosine hydroxylase and norepinephrine transporter mRNA expression in the locus coeruleus in Alzheimer's disease. *Brain Res.Mol.Brain Res., 84,* 135-140.

Szot, P., White, S. S., Greenup, J. L., Leverenz, J. B., Peskind, E. R., & Raskind, M. A. (2006). Compensatory changes in the noradrenergic nervous system in the locus ceruleus and hippocampus of postmortem subjects with Alzheimer's disease and dementia with Lewy bodies. *J Neurosci., 26,* 467-478.

Szot, P., White, S. S., Greenup, J. L., Leverenz, J. B., Peskind, E. R., & Raskind, M. A. (2007). Changes in adrenoreceptors in the prefrontal cortex of subjects with dementia: evidence of compensatory changes. *Neuroscience, 146,* 471-480.

Tanaka, Y., Meguro, K., Yamaguchi, S., Ishii, H., Watanuki, S., Funaki, Y. et al. (2003). Decreased striatal D2 receptor density associated with severe behavioral abnormality in Alzheimer's disease. *Ann.Nucl.Med., 17,* 567-573.

Tang, Y., Anderson, G. M., Zabetian, C. P., Kohnke, M. D., & Cubells, J. F. (2005). Haplotype-controlled analysis of the association of a non-synonymous single nucleotide polymorphism at DBH (+ 1603C --> T) with plasma dopamine beta-hydroxylase activity. *Am.J.Med.Genet.B Neuropsychiatr.Genet., 139B,* 88-90.

Tang, Y. L., Epstein, M. P., Anderson, G. M., Zabetian, C. P., & Cubells, J. F. (2007). Genotypic and haplotypic associations of the DBH gene with plasma dopamine beta-hydroxylase activity in African Americans. *Eur.J Hum.Genet., 15,* 878-883.

Tanzi, R. E. & Bertram, L. (2005). Twenty years of the Alzheimer's disease amyloid hypothesis: a genetic perspective. *Cell, 120,* 545-555.

Thies, W. & Bleiler, L. (2013). 2013 Alzheimer's disease facts and figures. *Alzheimers.Dement., 9,* 208-245.

Tohgi, H., Ueno, M., Abe, T., Takahashi, S., & Nozaki, Y. (1992). Concentrations of monoamines and their metabolites in the cerebrospinal fluid from patients with senile dementia of the Alzheimer type and vascular dementia of the Binswanger type. *J.Neural Transm.Park Dis.Dement.Sect., 4,* 69-77.

Tomlinson, B. E., Irving, D., & Blessed, G. (1981). Cell loss in the locus coeruleus in senile dementia of Alzheimer type. *J Neurol.Sci., 49,* 419-428.

Torack, R. M. & Morris, J. C. (1992). Tyrosine hydroxylase-like (TH) immunoreactivity in Parkinson's disease and Alzheimer's disease. *J.Neural Transm.Park Dis.Dement.Sect., 4,* 165-171.

Umegaki, H., Ikari, H., Nakahata, H., Yoshimura, J., Endo, H., Yamamoto, T. et al. (2000). Low plasma epinephrine in elderly female subjects of dementia of Alzheimer type. *Brain Res, 858,* 67-70.

van Harten, A. C., Visser, P. J., Pijnenburg, Y. A., Teunissen, C. E., Blankenstein, M. A., Scheltens, P. et al. (2013). Cerebrospinal fluid Abeta42 is the best predictor of clinical progression in patients with subjective complaints. *Alzheimers.Dement., 9,* 481-487.

Visser, P. J., Vos, S., van, R., I, & Scheltens, P. (2012). Comparison of International Working Group criteria and National Institute on Aging-Alzheimer's Association criteria for Alzheimer's disease. *Alzheimers.Dement., 8,* 560-563.

Volicer, L., Direnfeld, L. K., Langlais, P. J., Freedman, M., Bird, E. D., & Albert, M. L. (1985). Catecholamine metabolites and cyclic nucleotides in cerebrospinal fluid in dementia of Alzheimer type. *J.Gerontol., 40,* 708-713.

Wallin, A. K., Blennow, K., Andreasen, N., & Minthon, L. (2006). CSF biomarkers for Alzheimer's Disease: levels of beta-amyloid, tau, phosphorylated tau relate to clinical symptoms and survival. *Dement.Geriatr.Cogn Disord., 21,* 131-138.

Wang, Z., Liu, R. H., Reddy, V. K., & Barnes, C. D. (1994). Hippocampal beta-amyloid reduces locus coeruleus glutamate and tyrosine hydroxylase. *Brain Res.Bull., 35,* 485-491.

Weiler, P. G., Mungas, D., & Bernick, C. (1988). Propranolol for the control of disruptive behavior in senile dementia. *J.Geriatr.Psychiatry Neurol., 1,* 226-230.

Weinshilboum, R. M., Schorott, H. G., Raymond, F. A., Weidman, W. H., & Elveback, L. R. (1975). Inheritance of very low serum dopamine-beta-hydroxylase activity. *Am.J Hum.Genet., 27,* 573-585.

Wolfe, N., Katz, D. I., Albert, M. L., Almozlino, A., Durso, R., Smith, M. C. et al. (1990). Neuropsychological profile linked to low dopamine: in Alzheimer's disease, major depression, and Parkinson's disease. *J Neurol.Neurosurg.Psychiatry, 53,* 915-917.

Yu, J. T., Tan, L., Ou, J. R., Zhu, J. X., Liu, K., Song, J. H. et al. (2008). Polymorphisms at the beta2-adrenergic receptor gene influence Alzheimer's disease susceptibility. *Brain Res., 1210,* 216-222.

Yu, J. T., Wang, N. D., Ma, T., Jiang, H., Guan, J., & Tan, L. (2011). Roles of beta-adrenergic receptors in Alzheimer's disease: implications for novel therapeutics. *Brain Res.Bull., 84,* 111-117.

Yudofsky, S., Williams, D., & Gorman, J. (1981). Propranolol in the treatment of rage and violent behavior in patients with chronic brain syndromes. *Am.J.Psychiatry, 138,* 218-220.

Zabetian, C. P., Anderson, G. M., Buxbaum, S. G., Elston, R. C., Ichinose, H., Nagatsu, T. et al. (2001). A quantitative-trait analysis of human plasma-dopamine beta-hydroxylase activity: evidence for a major functional polymorphism at the DBH locus. *Am.J Hum.Genet., 68,* 515-522.

Zarow, C., Lyness, S. A., Mortimer, J. A., & Chui, H. C. (2003). Neuronal loss is greater in the locus coeruleus than nucleus basalis and substantia nigra in Alzheimer and Parkinson diseases. *Arch.Neurol., 60,* 337-341.

Zhang, J., Jr. & Shi S Sr (2013). A literature review of AD7c-ntp as a biomarker for Alzheimer's disease. *Ann.Indian Acad.Neurol., 16,* 307-309.

Zilka, N. & Novak, M. (2006). The tangled story of Alois Alzheimer. *Bratisl.Lek.Listy, 107,* 343-345.

Zimmer, R., Teelken, A. W., Trieling, W. B., Weber, W., Weihmayr, T., & Lauter, H. (1984). Gamma-aminobutyric acid and homovanillic acid concentration in the CSF of patients with senile dementia of Alzheimer's type. *Arch.Neurol., 41,* 602-604.

Zubenko, G. S., Marquis, J. K., Volicer, L., Direnfeld, L. K., Langlais, P. J., & Nixon, R. A. (1986). Cerebrospinal fluid levels of angiotensin-converting enzyme, acetylcholinesterase, and dopamine metabolites in dementia associated with Alzheimer's disease and Parkinson's disease: a correlative study. *Biol.Psychiatry, 21,* 1365-1381.

Zubenko, G. S., Moossy, J., Martinez, A. J., Rao, G., Claassen, D., Rosen, J. et al. (1991). Neuropathologic and neurochemical correlates of psychosis in primary dementia. *Arch.Neurol., 48,* 619-624.

In: The Central Catecholaminergic System
Editor: Bertalan Dudás

ISBN: 978-1-63117-937-2

Chapter 12

Catecholamines and Tourette Syndrome: Frontal-Subcortical Circuits and Their Neurochemical Modulation

David G. Lichter

Introduction

Tourette syndrome (TS) is an inherited neuropsychiatric disorder characterized by a fluctuating pattern of multiple motor tics and at least one phonic tic (Leckman, 2002). Tics are involuntary abrupt stereotyped movements and sounds, which may be simple or complex in nature, including echo- and coprophenomena. Tics may also have a sensory prodrome. Sometimes called a "sensory tic", this consists either of an uncomfortable intrusive sensation which arises in the bodily region subsequently involved in the tic, or a more generalized premonitory psychic symptom, including increased tension or an urge to release the tic (Cohen & Leckman, 1992). Unlike other hyperkinetic disorders, tics can typically be suppressed for variable periods of time. TS usually has a childhood onset with greatest severity typically in the first two decades of life. Boys are more commonly affected than girls. Although tics are its hallmark, TS is a multifaceted disorder, additional problems in many patients including attention deficit hyperactivity disorder, obsessive-compulsive symptoms, anxiety, depression, mood lability and, in adults, substance abuse (Lichter, 2011).

Although the precise pathophysiological mechanism for TS remains unknown, neuroanatomical, neuroimaging and neurophysiological studies together with the sensorimotor, compulsive and impulsive features of the disorder have suggested dysfunction involving the integration of parallel segregated cortico-striato-thalamo-cortical (CSTC) circuits (Berardelli et al., 2003; Hoekstra et al., 2004; Singer & Minzer, 2003, Bloch et al., 2005, Harris & Singer, 2006). These frontal-subcortical circuits serve as principal organizational networks of the brain and play an essential role in voluntary movement and brain-behavior relationships.

Structure and Neurochemical Organization of Frontal-Subcortical Circuits Relevant to TS

At least five CSTC circuits have been identified (Alexander et al., 1986), which are named according to their cortical area of origin and function. In addition to the motor and oculomotor circuits, there are three major parallel segregated CSTC circuits which mediate cognitive, emotional, and motivational processes. These are the dorsolateral prefrontal and lateral orbitofrontal ("associative") circuits and the anterior cingulate ("limbic") circuit. Each of the five circuits has the same organizational structure, including the frontal lobe, striatum, globus pallidus, substantia nigra pars reticulata (SNr), and thalamus, and connecting links between these regions. The FSCs have two separate striatal pathways, referred to as "direct" and "indirect". The direct pathway, which starts with medium spiny striatal projection neurons (MSNs) that express the D_1 dopamine receptor, transmits striatal information via a monosynaptic link to the internal segment of the globus pallidus (GPi) and SNr. In comparison, the indirect system, which involves MSNs that express the D_2 dopamine receptor, projects to these same regions via a disynaptic relay from the globus pallidus externa to the subthalamic nucleus. Activation of the direct pathway facilitates motor activity via disinhibition of thalamocortical neurons, while indirect pathway activation reduces motor activity by increasing inhibition of thalamocortical neurons (Figure 1).

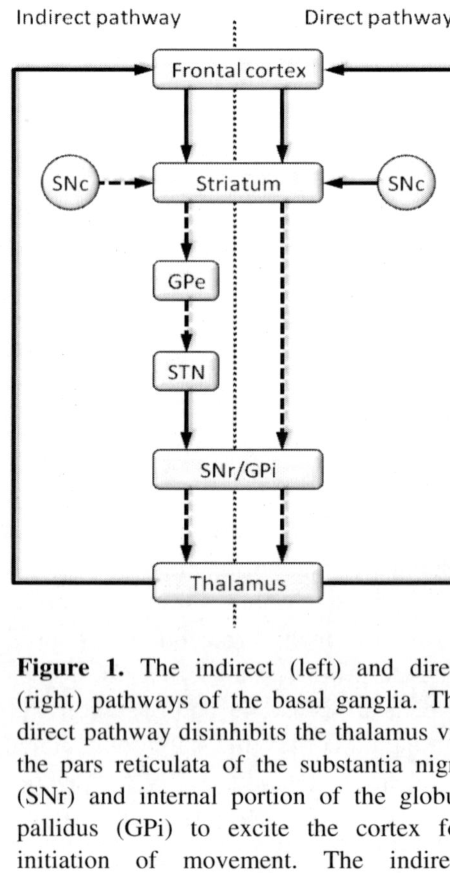

Figure 1. The indirect (left) and direct (right) pathways of the basal ganglia. The direct pathway disinhibits the thalamus via the pars reticulata of the substantia nigra (SNr) and internal portion of the globus pallidus (GPi) to excite the cortex for initiation of movement. The indirect pathway eventually inhibits the thalamus via the external portion of the globus pallidus (GPe) and the subthalamic nucleus (STN). Dopaminergic nigrostriatal projections from the pars compacta of the substantia nigra (SNc) excite the direct pathway via D_1 receptors and simultaneously inhibit the indirect pathway via D_2 receptors. Both of these processes result in excitation of the cortex.

Striatal nuclei, comprising the caudate, putamen, and ventral "limbic" striatum, play a critical role in the organization and function of frontal-subcortical circuits. The striatum has a mosaic structure characterized by specialized striosomes (striatal bodies) and an intervening matrix. Striosomes, which are clustered predominantly in the head of the caudate and rostral putamen, have a high density of opiate receptors, substance P, neurotensin, dynorphin, D_1 dopamine receptors, and tyrosine hydroxylase. Striosomes receive dense orbitofrontal and insular input, with dopaminergic projections from the ventral tier of the substantia nigra, pars compacta.

In contrast, the matrix compartment stains selectively for adenylate cyclase and is rich in D_2 dopamine receptors, cholinergic markers, and enkaphalin. Matrix cells receive afferents predominantly from the sensorimotor cortex and express primarily D_2 receptors, with dopaminergic input from the dorsal tier of the substantia nigra compacta (Lichter & Cummings, 2001).

Frontal-Subcortical Circuit Dysfunction in TS

It has been suggested that striosomes exert and maintain limbic control over behaviors driven by surrounding sensorimotor and associative parts of the striatal matrix. Consistent with this concept, imbalances between striatal stromosomal and matrix functions have been hypothesized to be central to the development of certain hyperkinetic movement disorders (Crittenden & Graybiel, 2011). A more specific model for the involuntary movements of TS has been proposed based upon the concept that there is aberrant activity in a subset of striatal neurons (Mink, 2001). This would then lead to increased inhibition of neurons in the internal segment of the GPi and SNr, releasing the thalamus from inhibition and ultimately leading to excitation of a set of cortical neurons which generate unwanted movements. Aberrant activity in several different sets of striatal neurons will result in the expression of multiple different tics.

The above model of TS is supported by postmortem data as well as micro-stimulation and micro-injection data. Examination of post-mortem TS brains has shown a loss of GABAergic and cholinergic parvalbumin-positive (PV+) interneurons in the caudate and putamen (Kalinithi et al., 2005; Kataoka et al., 2010). These PV+ cells inhibit the medium spiny output striatal neurons, to reduce the base-line firing rate of the striatum. Fewer PV+ interneurons would therefore result in an increased firing rate of the striatal output neurons which could represent the aberrant activity in the striatum proposed by Mink. Supporting the model, microstimulation of discrete regions of the putamen in rhesus monkeys results in movements of specific body parts (Alexander & DeLong, 1985), while microstimulation of the SNr, GPi and STN evokes no similar movement (Basso & Liu, 2007; Horak & Anderson, 1984; Wichmann et al., 1994). The finding by Alexander and DeLong of somatotopic organization in the putamen supports the notion that altered activity in discrete sets of striatal neurons may generate tics involving different body parts. Similarly, microinjection of the GABA-A antagonist bicuculline into the putamen of cynomolgus monkeys has elicited stereotyped tic-like movements (Bronfeld et al., 2011; McCairn et al., 2009), further supporting the Mink model.

A variety of neuroimaging studies have shown abnormalities in the structure and function of both subcortical and cortical components of the CSTC circuits. Reduced volume of the caudate nucleus has been the most consistent finding, with a reported correlation between caudate volume in children and symptom severity in later life (Bloch et al., 2005). With functional imaging, BOLD signal in the caudate is increased during active tic suppression, an increase which is attenuated in individuals with greater tic severity, suggesting impaired regulation of striatal activity in TS. Decreased activity and blood flow in the striatum has been shown with both SPECT and PET studies (Braun et al., 1993; Eidelberg et al., 1997; Moriarty et al., 1995), consistent with reduced striatal regulation.

Cortical areas that receive input from and project to the basal ganglia have also appeared abnormal in neuroimaging studies in TS patients. Cortical thinning has been noted in sensorimotor cortices in both children and adults with TS, increased thinning being associated with increased tic severity (Fahim et al., 2010) with specificity of regional cortical thinning determining TS phenotype (Worbe et al., 2010). A reduction in prefrontal volume has been observed in TS adults, which has been interpreted as reflecting a failure to develop frontal control over the striatum and therefore to regulate tics. Overall, while showing some inconsistencies, multiple lines of evidence, including functional neuroimaging data, suggest that disturbances in the development of the sensorimotor portions of CSTC circuits likely predispose to the development of TS, and that neuroplastic changes in the limbic and associative circuits may help to modulate the severity of symptom expression over the lifespan (Wang et al., 2011; Graybiel, 2008; Plessen et al., 2009; Leckman et al., 2010).

Neurochemical Modulation of Frontal-Subcortical Circuit Functioning

Neurochemical interactions occur at multiple levels within the CSTC circuits. The complex integration of multiple neurotransmitters, receptor subtypes and second messengers within the circuits provide a mechanism for balancing and fine-tuning the circuitry, mediating the complex control of movements and behavior (Bronstein & Cummings, 2001). While multiple neurotransmitters have been implicated in the pathophysiology of TS (Singer & Minzer, 2003), the strongest evidence suggests a major role for dopamine (Leckman et al., 2010).

Evidence Supporting a Role for Dopamine in the Pathogenesis of TS

The reconceptualization of TS from a psychological to a neuropsychiatric disorder with a primary organic basis (Kushner, 1999) started in 1968 with the publication by Arthur and Elaine Shapiro of the successful treatment of a young TS woman with haloperidol (Shapiro & Shapiro, 1968). Subsequent clinical experience with a wide variety of medications, including both typical and atypical neuroleptic (dopamine antagonist) drugs, which suppress tics in the majority of affected individuals (Singer, 2010; Bloch et al., 2011), has continued to support an important role for dopamine in TS. Symptomatic improvement may also be seen following the administration of drugs that block dopamine synthesis (e.g. alpha-methyl-para-tyrosine) or deplete dopamine from presynaptic storage vesicles, such as tetrabenazine (Porta et al., 2008; Sweet et al., 2008). Conversely, tic exacerbation may follow withdrawal of neuroleptic drugs or treatment with agents that increase central dopaminergic activity, such as L-dopa and central stimulants (Karagianis & Nagpurkar, 1990; Klawans et al., 1978).

Such clinical data notwithstanding, no consistent linkage or association has been demonstrated between TS patients and candidate genes such as the dopamine D_2-D_5 alleles, mutations in the D_1 receptor, or dopamine beta hydroxylase gene (O'Rourke et al., 2009). Similarly, no linkage has been demonstrated between TS and a functional polymorphism in the catechol-O-methyltransferase (COMT) gene (Barr et al., 1999). However, a significant association has been reported between TS and a dopamine transporter polymorphism (DAT1 *Ddel*) (Yoon et al., 2007b).

Postulated Dopamine Abnormalities in TS

The dopamine hypothesis of TS is predicated on increased signal transduction due to either increased sensitivity to dopamine (mediated, for example, by an increased number or affinity of dopamine receptors), or an increased amount of synaptic dopamine (via tonic or phasic release).

The Hypothesis of Dopamine Receptor Sensitivity in TS

A limited study of single-point binding assays in postmortem striatum showed no significant difference between TS and control membrane preparations for both D_1 ([^{3}H] SCH 23390) and D_2 ([^{3}H] spiperone) receptors (Singer et al., 1991). PET and SPECT studies comparing D_2 dopamine receptors in TS patients and controls have produced inconsistent results (Singer, 2013). In one study which utilized the ligand [^{123}I] IBZM, dopamine receptors were significantly different in medicated but not neuroleptic-naïve patients (Muller-Vahl et al., 2000). There is also inconsistency when comparing neuroimaging and postmortem analysis of extra-striatal dopamine receptor binding in TS, perhaps related to the limitation of PET binding to externalized surface receptors. Thus, two small studies have suggested reduced extrastriatal D_2/D_3 receptor dopamine binding potentials as measured by the high-affinity D_2/D_3 receptor antagonists [^{11}C] FLB 457 and [F18] fallypride (Gilbert et al., 2006; Steeves et al., 2010), while a study of postmortem tissue has revealed increased cortical dopamine receptors (Minzer et al., 2004; Yoon et al., 2007a). Heterogenous samples and methods hamper efforts to draw firm conclusion regarding possible changes in D_2 or D_3 receptor density or affinity in TS and the rather small sample sizes limit the validity of the findings.

The Hypothesis of Dopamine Hyperinnervation versus Abnormal Dopamine Reuptake in TS

In a small number of postmortem samples from subjects with TS, a significant increase in the number of striatal presynaptic dopamine carrier sites was shown with 3H-mazindole binding (Singer, 1991). Subsequent attempts to provide support for a postulated dopaminergic hyperinnervation of the striatum have utilized binding to the DA transporter (DAT). Although some studies using SPECT or PET in adult TS patients showed no difference in DAT binding compared to controls (Heinz et al., 1998; Stamenkovic et al., 2001, Hwang et al., 2008), most studies support increased levels of DAT binding (e.g. Mena et al., 2004; Liu et al., 2010). In one study, the mean striatal activity ratio was significantly higher in TS patients, with 5 of the 12 subjects showing striatum/occipital cortex ratios more than 2 standard deviations above the normal mean (Muller-Vahl et al., 2000). In a study of five TS adults with [^{123}I]beta-CIT

SPECT, striatal DAT binding was higher than in controls, but the correlations noted in the midbrain and thalamus could have been influenced by serotonin binding (Malison et al., 1995). In a second study, DAT binding using high-resolution scanning with [^{123}I]FP-CIT showed increased striatal binding but no association with TS-related behaviors (Serra-Mestres et al., 2004). Another smaller study showed similar results (Choen et al., 2004).

Binding to the vesicular monoamine transporter type 2 (VMAT2) has also been used to assess striatal dopaminergic innervation. In-vivo studies of VMAT2 using the ligand (+)-alpha-[^{11}C] dihydrotetrabenazine have shown no consistent differences between TS subjects and controls (Bohnen et al., 1999), an apparent increase in ventral striatal binding in one study (Albin et al., 2003) failing to be confirmed in a follow-up investigation (Albin et al., 2009). These studies suggest that, as opposed to increased striatal innervation, there may be an abnormality in the regulation of dopamine reuptake in TS.

Other Potential Presynaptic Dopamine Abnormalities in TS

Based on decreased dopamine uptake into platelet storage granules in 18 TS patients, a presynaptic abnormality, possibly involving the neuronal membrane, has been postulated (Rabey et al., 1995). A presynaptic dopamine abnormality has also been suggested involving dopa decarboxylase activity. This was suggested by a PET study involving 11 TS adolescents, whose [^{18}F]-fluorodopa accumulation was 25% higher in the left caudate nucleus and 53% higher in the right midbrain compared with control subjects (Ernst et al., 1999). The authors proposed that these differences could be explained by an up-regulation of dopa decarboxylase activity, leading to alterations in the dopamine system. However, in another study using the same methodology, no differences were found between 10 adult TS patients (three of whom were drug-naïve and seven of whom were receiving neuroleptic treatment) and healthy controls (Turjanski et al., 1994).

The Hypothesis of Disordered Tonic or Phasic Release of Dopamine in TS

Electrophysiologic and neurochemical data have indicated both a homeostatic (tonic) and spike-dependent (phasic) aspect to normal dopamine release in the brain (Grace, 1991; Grace, 1995). Recent interest has focused on a possible abnormality of either phasic or tonic dopamine release in TS, which could exist in either the striatum or cortex.

Tonic Dopamine Release

Tonic dopamine exists in low concentration extracellularly and determines long-term dopamine homeostasis. Dopamine D_2 and D_3 autoreceptors, located on pre-synaptic dopaminergic neurons, are considered to be regulators of tonic dopamine. A reduction in levels of tonic dopamine would be expected to produce an upregulation of postysynaptic dopamine receptors. A lower tonic dopamine level could result from a reduction in cortical glutamatergic afferent input, a disordered autoreceptor, or an overactive dopamine transporter system.

Initial studies in TS showed that basal and turnover levels of cerebrospinal fluid HVA, the major metabolite of dopamine, were reduced, not elevated, in TS subjects, and levels were normalized following administration of haloperidol (Singer, 1982). Subsequent findings of normal concentrations of dopamine, HVA and 3,4-dihydroxyphenylacetic acid (DOPAC) in postmortem striatal samples confirmed absence of excessive production or tonic release of dopamine. However, suggestions of a possible abnormality of regulation of tonic dopamine in TS have been provided by studies demonstrating a significant increase in the number of presynaptic dopamine transporter sites in post-mortem striatum (Singer et al., 1991), and frontal cortex (Minzer et al., 2004) as well as findings of increased dopamine transporter binding in pediatric and adult SPECT/PET imaging studies (Choen et al., 2004; Liu et al., 2010; Malison et al., 1995; Mena et al., 2004; Muller-Vahl et al., 2000, Serra-Mestres et al., 2004). An overactive dopamine transporter would result not only in diminished levels of extracellular dopamine but also in higher concentrations of dopamine in the axon terminal, which in turn might lead to an increase of stimulus-dependent (phasic) dopamine release (Buse et al., 2013).

Phasic Dopamine Release

Phasic dopamine refers to spike-dependent dopamine released into the synaptic cleft. With sufficient stimulation, or in response to high concentrations of an uptake blocker, phasic dopamine can diffuse more widely. A hyper-responsive spike-dependent (phasic) dopaminergic system could result from an alteration in afferent cortical inputs with or without an abnormality of dopamine transporters.

The hypothesis of altered phasic release of dopamine in TS is supported by several clinical findings. First, tics are not infrequently exacerbated by stimulant medications (Erenberg et al., 1985; Price et al., 1986), most likely secondary to enhanced dopamine release from the axon terminal. Second, tics are typically exacerbated by environmental stimuli such as stress, anxiety, and specific medications, stimuli which have been shown to increase phasic bursts of dopamine (Harris & Singer, 2006). Finally, tics may be suppressed by dopamine agonists administered in very low dose, likely secondary to preferential stimulation at such doses of the presynaptic dopamine autoreceptors, with resulting reduction of phasic dopamine release.

The intrasynaptic release of dopamine that can be induced by stimulant challenges, for example with amphetamine, has been used as a surrogate measure of phasic dopamine. Several studies have shown increased release of dopamine in the striatum following amphetamine stimulation (Singer et al., 2002; Wong et al., 2008). In one study of seven adult TS patients and five age-matched controls, using [^{11}C] raclopride PET, the mean value of intrasynaptic dopamine in the putamen increased by 21% in the TS subjects following amphetamine challenge, with no change in the controls (Singer et al., 2002). In a second study, dopamine release was significantly increased in the ventral striatum of TS subjects compared with controls (Wong et al., 2008). In addition, an [^{11}C]–FLB457 PET study incorporating amphetamine challenge showed increased dopamine release in the medial frontal gyri and anterior cingulate cortex in TS subjects (Steeves et al., 2010). A smaller reduction of the 99mT TRODAT-1 dopamine transporter binding ratio in the caudate nucleus of TS patients following methylphenidate challenge was also interpreted as evidence for a phasic dopamine abnormality (Yeh et al., 2007). Finally, in two preliminary reports of a small number of TS patients improved by deep brain stimulation (DBS) of the centromedian-parafascicular nucleus of the thalamus, the suggested mechanism of improvement was dopamine receptor upregulation associated with a decrease in dopamine release (Kuhn et al., 2012; Vernaleken et al., 2009). Thus, using [^{18}F] fallypride PET scans about 6 months after surgery, there was a dramatic decrease in D_2/D_3 receptor binding potential from the "stimulator-on" to the "stimulator-off" state, suggesting an increased release of endogenous dopamine in the "off" condition. In addition, a dramatic elevation of D_2/D_3 receptor availability in the thalamus caudate, putamen and temporal cortex was noted in the "on" condition in TS patients compared with healthy subjects.

Sensorimotor Integration and Dopamine in TS

Experimental data suggests that a core problem in TS is not merely an abnormality in pathways mediating voluntary movement, but abnormal sensorimotor processing. The relevance of disturbances in sensorimotor integration in TS is highlighted by the presence of premonitory sensory urges immediately prior to tics in 92% of patients (Kwak et al., 2003). This phenomenon has suggested a failure in the automatic "gating" of sensory stimuli in TS (Sutherland Owens et al., 2010).

The best studied example of a measure of sensorimotor gating is prepulse inhibition (PPI). PPI refers to the reduction of the startle reflex, measure with electromyography, when the startling stimulus is preceded by a weaker (prepulse) stimulus. Poor sensorimotor gating, as demonstrated by disrupted PPI, has been observed in several psychiatric disorders involving CSTC circuits, including TS (Braff et al., 2001). In TS patients with co-morbid ADHD, reductions of the electrically induced PPI have suggested deficient pallidal inhibition (Castellanos et al., 1996). Inhibitory deficits in TS have also been observed in PPI paradigms using acoustic or tactile conditioning stimuli (Swerdlow et al., 2001; Swerdlow, 2013). Using a tactile startle response, fMRI has shown nine regions where brain activity during PPI differs significantly in TS compared with controls, activation of the left caudate being significantly correlated with current tic severity (YGTSS) (Zebardast et al., 2013).

There is strong evidence that dopamine plays a major role in the regulation of PPI. Animal models have demonstrated the impact of dopamine modulating drugs on the expression of PPI (Swerdlow et al., 2006a). Thus, the dopamine agonist apomorphine disrupted PPI in rats (Davis et al., 1990), and this effect was block by dopamine antagonists (Hoffman & Donovan, 1994; Swerdlow et al., 1994). The antipsychotic potency of several psychopharmacological compounds has been shown to correlate with their ability to restore PPI in apomorphine-treated rats (Swerdlow et al., 1994). Furthermore, genes responsible for differences in forebrain D_2 receptor function may contribute to differences in PPI in rats (Swerdlow et al., 2006b); and COMT polymorphisms, which influence tonic dopamine signaling, determine PPI responsivity to COMT inhibition with tolcapone in healthy human subjects (Roussos et al., 2009). These and other studies suggest that D_2 receptors are positioned at a critical "node" within CSTC circuitry regulating sensorimotor gating (Swerdlow & Sutherland, 2005).

However, dopamine is not the only neurotransmitter involved in such regulation. In particular, sensorimotor gating abnormalities have been shown to be associated with altered noradrenergic regulation within distinct thalamocortical and ventral forebrain networks (Alsene et al., 2011).

Studies of sensorimotor integration using transcranial magnetic stimulation (TMS) have consistently found TS to be associated with impaired cortical inhibition. Both short intracortical inhibition (Orth et al., 2005: Heise et al., 2010) and short latency afferent inhibition (SAI) (Orth et al., 2005) are reduced in TS patients compared to healthy controls. The SAI findings, wherein a transient sensory input produces short-lasting inhibition of the motor cortex, indicates that impaired cortical inhibition in TS is probably not limited to the motor cortex but also involves circuits linking sensory input and motor output (Tokimura et al., 2000; Orth & Rothwell, 2009). The effect of dopaminergic medication on cortical inhibition measured with TMS has been demonstrated in a variety of neurological and psychiatric disorders as well as in healthy controls (Buse et al., 2013).

Such data suggests that dysfunction in catecholamine systems, primarily involving dopamine but also involving noradrenergic mechanisms, might play an important role not only in the motor dysfunction in TS but also in the impairment of sensorimotor processes in this condition.

TS and Stress

A characteristic feature of TS is its waxing and waning course, with episodes of tic exacerbation interspersed with periods of relative tic remission. Tics typically worsen during periods of increased psychosocial stress or anxiety (Silva et al., 1995; Conelea and Woods, 2008), a phenomenon that was reported by 96.8% of 763 TS patients surveyed by Bornstein et al. (1990). TS patients experience stress more often than controls (Findley et al., 2003; Lin et al., 2007). Normally, stress-related activation of several brain regions, including the prefrontal cortex and amygdala, results in release of corticotropin-releasing hormone (CRH) from the hypothalamus, which stimulates the pituitary to release ACTH, causing release of cortisol from the adrenal glands. Stress also results in a rapid and robust activation of the locus coeruleus/noradrenergic system. Relative to control subjects, TS patients show a stronger biochemical response to stress-producing stimuli. Thus, elevated corticotropin-releasing factor has been found in the CSF of TS patients (Chappell et al., 1996) and, compared with controls, TS adults have increased levels of CSF norepinephrine (Leckman et al., 1995) and excrete elevated levels of urinary norepinephrine in response to the stress of a lumbar puncture (Chappell et al., 1994).

Along with the hypothalamic-pituitary-adrenal (HPA) axis, the dopamine system is involved in the response to stress. Thus, stressors effect an increase in extracellular dopamine concentration in the prefrontal cortex, amygdala, hippocampus, and nucleus accumbens (Mora et al., 2012), regions involved in the organization and control of central stress responses and which receive projections from the mesocortical and mesolimbic dopamine systems. The relationship between stress and mesolimbic dopamine release has also been demonstrated in human subjects. Thus, in a PET study of ten healthy students, psychosocial stressors stimulated dopamine release in the ventral striatum (Pruessner et al., 2004).

The dopamine system interacts with the HPA axis, via projections from diencephalic dopamine neurons to the paraventricular nucleus of the hypothalamus (Lookingland & Moore, 2005). There is also evidence that stress-related CRH effects changes in the dopamine system, CRH administered to rats stimulating dopaminergic neuron terminals in the nucleus accumbens, paraventricular nucleus and the intermediate pituitary lobe, as measured by the dopamine metabolite DOPAC (Pan et al., 1995).

The precise mechanisms by which neurophysiologic and neurochemical responses to stress may induce changes in tic expression are incompletely understood. However, the close relationship between the neurobiological responses to stress and activity in the mesolimbic dopamine system and the evidence that tic expression may be modulated by changes in the dopamine system suggests at least one likely mechanism for the observed exacerbation of tics by psychosocial stress in TS.

Summary and Conclusion

- The pathobiology of TS involves dysfunction in integrated cortico-striato-thalamo-cortical (CSTC) circuits.
- Although dysfunction in TS may involve several neurotransmitter systems, consistent evidence suggests a major role for dopamine.
- Of the various dopaminergic hypotheses proposed, an alteration of the tonic-phasic neurotransmitter release system appears most likely.
- The activity of dopaminergic neurons modulating CSTC circuits, the impact on this circuitry of externally determined states (e.g. stress) and the resulting internal responses to such states (including activation of the HPA axis and changes in the mesolimbic dopaminergic system) play a major role in tic expression.

References

Albin, R.L., Koeppe, R.A., Bohnen, N.I., Nichols, T.E., Meyer, P., Wernette, K., Frey, K.A. (2003). Increased ventral striatal monoaminergic innervation in Tourette syndrome. *Neurology 61,* 310-315.

Albin, R.L., Koeppe, R.A., Wernette, K., Zhuang, W., Nichols, T., Kilbourn, M.R., & Frey, K.A. (2009). Striatal [^{11}C] dihydrotetrabenazine and [^{11}C] methylphenidate binding in Tourette syndrome. *Neurology 72,* 1390-1396.

Alexander, G.E., & DeLong, M.R. (1985). Microstimulation of the primate neostriatum. II. Somatotopic organization of striatal microexcitable zones and their relation to neuronal response properties. *J Neurophysiol, 53,* 1417-1430.

Alexander, G.E., DeLong, M.R., & Strick, P.L. (1986). Parallel organization of functionally segregated circuits linking basal ganglia and cortex. *Annu Rev Neurosci, 9*, 357-381.

Alsene, K.M., Rajbhandari, A.K., Ramaker, M.J., & Bakshi, V.P. (2011). Discrete forebrain neuronal networks supporting noradrenergic regulation of sensorimotor gating. *Neuropsychopharmacology, 36,* 1003-1014.

Barr, C.L., Wigg, K.G., & Sandor, P. (1999). Catechol-O-methyltransferase and Gilles de la Tourette syndrome. *Mol Psychiatry, 4,* 492-495.

Basso, M.A., & Liu, P. (2007). Context-dependent effects of substantia nigra stimulation on eye movements. *J Neurophysiol, 97,* 4129-4142.

Berardelli, A., Curra, A., Fabbrini G, Gilio, F., & Manfredi, M. (2003). Pathophysiology of tics and Tourette syndrome. *J Neurol, 250*, 781-787.

Block, M.H., Leckman, J.F., Zhu, H.,& Peterson, B.S. (2005). Caudate volumes in childhood predict symptom severity in adults with Tourette syndrome. *Neurology, 65*, 1253-1258.

Bloch, M., State, M., & Pittenger, C. (2011). Recent advances in Tourette syndrome. *Curr Opin Neurol , 24,* 119-125.

Bohnen, N.I., Minoshima, S., & Kilbourn, M.R. (1999). Presynaptic monoaminergic vesicular transporter imaging in Tourette syndrome using (+)-[alpha]-[^{11}C]DTBZ PET. *Neurology 52,* A176.

Bornstein, R.A., Stefl, M.E., & Hammond, L. (1990). A survey of Tourette syndrome patients and their families: the 1987 Ohio Tourette Survey. *J Neuropsychiatry Clin Neurosci, 2,* 275-281.

Braff, D.L., Geyer, M.A., & Swerdlow, N.R. (2001). Human studies of prepulse inhibition of startle: normal subjects , patient groups, and pharmacological studies. *Psychopharmacology (Berl), 156,* 234-258.

Braun, A.R., Stoetter, B., Randolph, C., Hsiao, J.K., Vladar, K., Gernet, J., …Chase, T.N. (1993). The functional neuroanatomy of Tourette's syndrome: an FDG-PET study. I. Regional changes in cerebral glucose metabolism differentiating patients and controls. *Neuropsychopharmacology, 9,* 277-291.

Bronfield, M., Belelovsky, K., & Bar-Gad., I. (2011). Spatial and temporal properties of tic-related neuronal activity in the cortico-basal ganglia loop. *J Neurosci, 31,* 8713-8721.

Bronstein, Y.L., & Cummings, J.L (2001). Neurochemistry of frontal-subcortical circuits. In D.G. Lichter & J.L. Cummings (Eds), *Frontal-subcortical circuits in psychiatric and neurological disorders* (pp. 59-91). New York, NY: The Guilford Press.

Buse, J., Schoenefeld, J., Munchau, A., & Roessner, V. (2013). Neuromodulation in Tourette syndrome: dopamine and beyond. *Neurosci Biobehav Rev, 37,* 1069-1084.

Castellanos, F.X., Fine, E.J., Kaysen, D., Marsh, W.L., Rapoport, J.L., & Hallett, M. (1996). Sensorimotor gating in boys with Tourette's syndrome and ADHD: preliminary results. *Biol Psychiatry, 39,* 33-41.

Chappell, P., Leckman, J., Goodman, W., Bisette, G., Pauls, D, Anderson, G.,….Cohen, D. (1996). Elevated cerebrospinal fluid corticotropin-releasing factor in Tourette's syndrome: comparison to obsessive compulsive disorder and normal controls. *Biol Psychiatry, 39,* 776-783.

Chappell, P., Riddle, M., Anderson, G., Scahill, L., Hardin, M., Walker, D.,…Leckman, J. (1994). Enhanced stress responsivity of Tourette patients undergoing lumbar puncture. *Biol Psychiatry, 36,* 35-43.

Choen, K.A., Ryu, Y.H., Namgoong, K., Kim, C.H., Kim, J.J., & Lee, J.D. (2004). Dopamine transporter density of the basal ganglia assessed with [^{123}I]IPT SPECT in drug-naïve children with Tourette's disorder. *Psychiatry Res 130,* 85-95.

Cohen, A.J., & Leckman, J.F. (1992). Sensory phenomena associated with Gilles de la Tourette's syndrome. *J Clin Psychiatry, 53,* 319-323.

Conelea, C.A., & Woods, D.W. (2008). The influence of contextual factors on tic expression in Tourette's syndrome: a review. *J Psychosom Res, 65,* 487-496.

Crittenden, J.R., & Graybiel, A.M. (2011). Basal ganglia disorders associated with imbalances in the striatal striosome and matrix compartments. *Front Neuroanat, 5,* 59.

Davis, M., Mansbach, R.S., Swerdlow, N.R., Campeau, S., Braff, D.L., & Geyer, M.A. (1990). Apomorphine disrupts the inhibition of acoustic startle induced by weak prepulses in rats. *Psychopharmacology (Berl), 102,* 1-4.

Eidelberg, D., Moeller J.R., Antonini, A., Kazumata, K., Dhawan, V., Budman, C., & Feigin, A. (1997). The metabolic anatomy of Tourette's syndrome. *Neurology, 48,* 927-934.

Erenberg, G., Cruse, R.P., & Rothner, A.D. (1985). Gilles de la Tourette syndrome: effects of stimulant drugs. Neurology 35, 1346-1348.

Ernst, M., Zametkin, A.J., Jons, P.H., et al. High presynaptic dopaminergic activity in children with Tourette's disorder. *J Am Acad Child Adolesc Psychiatry 38,* 86-94.

Fahim, C., Yoon, U., Das, S., Lyttelton, O., Chen, J., Arnaoutelis, R., Evans, A.C. (2010). Somatosensory-motor bodily representation cortical thinning in Tourette: effects of tic severity, age and gender. *Cortex, 46,* 750-760.

Findley, D.B., Leckman, J.F., Katsovich, L., Lin, H., Zhang, H., Grantz, H.,...King, R.A. (2003). Development of the Yale Children's Global Stress Index (YCGSI) and its application in children and adolescents with Tourette's syndrome and obsessive-compulsive disorder. *J Am Acad Child Adolesc Psychiatry, 42,* 450-457.

Gilbert, D.L, Christian, B.T., Gelfand, M.J., Shi, B., Mantil, J., & Sallee, F.R. (2006). Altered mesolimbocortical and thalamic dopamine in Tourette syndrome. *Neurology, 67,* 1695-1697.

Grace, A.A. (1991). Phasic versus tonic dopamine release and the modulation of dopamine system responsivity: a hypothesis for the etiology of schizophrenia. *Neuroscience, 41,* 1-24.

Grace, A.A., (1995). The tonic/phasic model of dopamine system regulation: its relevance for understanding how stimulant abuse can alter basal ganglia function. *Drug Alcohol Depend, 37,* 111-129.

Graybiel., A.M. (2008). Habits, rituals, and the evaluative brain. *Annu Rev Neurosci, 31,* 359-387.

Harris, K., & Singer, H.S. (2006). Tic disorders: neural circuits, neurochemistry, and neuroimmunology. *J Child Neurol, 21,* 678-689.

Heinz., A., Knable., M.B., Wolfe, S.S., Jones, D.W., Gorey, J.G., Hyde, T.M., & Weinberger, D.R. (1998). Tourette's syndrome: [I-123] beta-CIT SPECT correlates of vocal tic severity. *Neurology 51,* 1069-1074.

Heise, K-F., Steven, B., Liuzzi, G., Thomalla, G., Jonas, M., Muller-Vahl, K., ...Hummel, F.C. (2010). Altered modulation of intracortical excitability during movement preparation in Gilles de la Tourette syndrome. *Brain, 133,* 580-590.

Hoekstra, P.J., Anderson, G.M., Limburg, P.C., Korf, J., Kallenberg, C.G.M., & Minderaa, R.B. (2004). Neurobiology and neuroimmunology of Tourette's syndrome: an update. *Cell Mol Life Sci, 61,* 886-898.

Hoffman, D.C. & Donovan, H. (1994). D1 and D2 dopamine receptor antagonists reverse prepulse inhibition deficits in an animal model of schizophrenia. *Psychopharmacology (Berl), 115,* 447-453.

Horak, F.B., & Anderson, M.E. (1984). Influence of globus pallidus on arm movements in monkeys. II. Effects of stimulation. *J Neurophysiol, 52,* 305-322.

Hwang, W.J., Yao, W.J., Fu, Y.K., & Yang, A.S. (2008). [99mTc} TRODAT-1/[^{123}I]IBZM SPECT studies of the dopaminergic system in Tourette syndrome. *Psychiatry Res 162,* 159-166.

Kataoka, Y., Kalanithi, P.S. A., Grantz, H., Schwartz, M.L., Saper, C., Leckman, J.F., & Vaccarino, F.M. (2010). Decreased number of parvalbumin and cholinergic interneurons in the striatum of individuals with Tourette syndrome. *J Comp Neurol, 518,* 277-291.

Kalinthi, P.S., Zheng W., Kataoka, Y., DiFiglia, M., Grantz, H., Saper, C.B., …Vaccarino, F.M. (2005). Altered parvalbumin-positive neuron distribution in basal ganglia of individuals with Tourette syndrome. *Proc Natl Acad Sci USA, 102,* 13307-13312.

Karagianis, J.L., & Nagpurkar, R. (1990). A case of Tourette syndrome developing during haloperidol treatment. *Can J Psychiatry, 35,* 228-232.

Klawans, H.L., Falk, D.K., Nausieda, P.A., & Weiner, W.J. (1978). Gilles de la Tourette syndrome after long-term chlorpromazine therapy. *Neurology, 28,* 1064-1066.

Kuhn, J., Janouschek, H., Raptis, M., Rex, S., Lenartz, D., Neuner, I., …Vernaleken, I. (2012). In vivo evidence of deep brain stimulation-induced dopaminergic modulation in Tourette's syndrome. *Biol Psychiatry, 71,* e11-e13.

Kushner, H.I. (1999). *A Cursing Brain?: The Histories of Tourette Syndrome.* Cambridge, Mass: Harvard University Press.

Kwak, C., Dat Vuong, G., & Jankovic, J. (2003). Premonitory sensory phenomenon in Tourette's syndrome. *Mov Disord, 18,* 1530-1533.

Leckman, J.F., Goodman, W.K., Anderson, G.M., Riddle, M.A., Chappell, P.B., McSwiggan-Hardin, M.T., Price, L.H. (1995). Cerebrospinal fluid biogenic amines in obsessive-compulsive disorder, Tourette's syndrome, and healthy controls. *Neuropsychopharmacology, 12,* 73-86.

Leckman, J.F. (2002). Tourette's syndrome. *Lancet, 360,* 1577-1586.

Leckman, J.F., Bloch, M.H., Smith, M.E., Larabi, D., & Hampson, M. (2010). Neurobiological substrates of Tourette's disorder. *J Child Adolesc Psychopharmacol, 20,* 237-247.

Lichter, D.G., & Cummings, J.L. (2001). Introduction and Overview. In D.G. Lichter & J.L. Cummings (Eds), *Frontal-subcortical circuits in psychiatric and neurological disorders* (pp. 1-43). New York, NY: the Guilford Press.

Lichter, D.G. (2011). Substance use disorder in adult Tourette syndrome: frequency, profile and co-morbidities. *Mind and Brain, The Journal of Psychiatry, 2(1),* 9-15.

Lin, H., Katsovich, L., Ghebremichael, M., Findley, D.B., Grantz, H., Lombroso, P.J., …Leckman, J.F. (2007). Psychosocial stress predicts future symptom severities in children and adolescents with Tourette syndrome and/or obsessive-compulsive disorder. *J Child Psychol Psychiatry, 48,* 157-166.

Liu, H., Dong, F., Meng, Z., et al. (2010). Evaluation of Tourette's syndrome by (99m)Tc-TRODAT-1 SPECT/CT imaging. *Ann Nucl Med 24,* 515-521.

Lookingland, K.J. & Moore, K.E. (2005). Functional neuroanatomy of hypothalamic dopaminergic neuroendocrine systems. In: S.B. Dunnett, M. Bentivoglio, A. Bjorklund, T. Hokfelt (Eds.), *Handbook of Chemical Neuroanatomy, Volume 21, Dopamine* (p. 435-524). Amsterdam: Elsevier.

Malison, R.T., McDougle, C.J., van Dyck, C.H., Scahill, L., Baldwin, R.M., Seibyl, J.P., Innis, R.B. (1995). [123I]beta-CIT SPECT imaging of striatal dopamine transporter binding in Tourette's disorder. *Am J Psychiatry 152,* 1359-1361.

McCairn, K.W., Bronfeld, M., Belelovsky, K., and Bar-Gad, I. (2009). The neurophysiological correlates of motor tics following focal striatal disinhibition. *Brain, 132,* 2125-2138.

Mena, I., Miranda, M., & Hernandez, M. (2004). Dopamine transporter imaging in Tourette syndrome: evaluation by neuroSPECT of Trodat-1-Tc99m. *Mov Disord 19,* 1282.

Mink, J.W. (2001). Basal ganglia dysfunction in Tourette's syndrome: a new hypothesis. *Pediatr Neurol, 25,* 190-198.

Minzer, K., Lee, O., Hong, J.J., & Singer, H.S. (2004). Increased prefrontal D2 protein in Tourette syndrome: a postmortem analysis of frontal cortex and striatum. *J Neurol Sci, 219,* 55-61.

Mora, F., Segovia, G., Del Arco, A., de Blas, M., & Garrido, P. (2012). Stress, neurotransmitters, corticosterone and body-brain integration. *Brain Res, 1476,* 71-85.

Moriarty, J., Costa, D.C., Schmitz, B., Trimble, M.R., Ell, P.J., & Robertson, M.M. (1995). Brain perfusion abnormalities in Gilles de la Tourette's syndrome. *Br J Psychiatry, 167,* 249-254.

Muller-Vahl, K.R., Berding, G., Kolbe, H., Meyer, G.J., Hundeshagen, H., Dengler, R., …Emrich, H.M. (2000). Dopamine D2 receptor imaging in Gilles de le Tourette syndrome. *Acta Neurol Scand, 101,* 165-171.

O'Rourke, J.A., Scharf, J.M., Yu., D., & Pauls, D.L. (2009). The genetics of Tourette syndrome: a review. *J Psychosom Res, 67,* 533-545.

Orth, M., Amann, B., Robertson, M.M., & Rothwell, J.C. (2005). Excitability of motor cortex inhibitory circuits in Tourette syndrome before and after single dose nicotine. *Brain, 128,* 1292-1300.

Orth, M. & Rothwell, J.C. (2009). Motor cortex excitability and comorbidity in Gilles de la Tourette syndrome. *J Neurol Neurosurg Psychiatry, 80,* 29-34.

Pan, J.-T., Lookingland, K.J., & Moore, K.E. (1995). Differential effects of corticotropin-releasing hormone on central dopaminergic and noradrenergic neurons. *J Biomed Sci, 2,* 50-56.

Plessen, K.J., Bansal, R., & Peterson, B.S. (2009). Imaging evidence for anatomical disturbances and neuroplastic compensation in persons with Tourette syndrome. *J Psychosom Res, 67,* 559-573.

Porta, M., Sassi, M., Cavallazzi, M., Fornari, M., Brambilla, A., & Servello, D. (2008). Tourette's syndrome and the role of tetrabenazine: review and personal experience. *Clin Drug Investig, 28,* 443-459.

Price, R.A., Leckman, J.F., Pauls, D.L., Cohen, D.J., & Kidd, K.K. (1986). Gilles de la Tourette's syndrome: tics and central nervous system stimulants in twins and nontwins. *Neurology, 36,* 232-237.

Pruessner, J.C., Champagne, F., Meaney, M.J., & Dagher, A. (2004). Dopamine release in response to a psychological stress in humans and its relationship to early life maternal care: a positron emission tomography study using [11C]raclopride. *J Neurosci, 24,* 2825-2831.

Rabey, J.M., Oberman, Z., Graff, E., & Korczyn, A.D. (1995). Decreased dopamine uptake into platelet storage granules in Gilles de la Tourette disease. *Biol Psychiatry 38,* 112-115.

Roussos, P., Giakoumaki, S.G., & Bitsios, P. (2009). Tolcapone effects on gating, working memory, and mood interact with the synonymous catechol-O-methyltransferase rs4818/g polymorphism. *Biol Psychiatry, 66,* 997-1004.

Serra-Mestres, J., Ring, H.A., Costa, D.C., Gacinovic, S., Walker, Z., Lees, A.J., Trimble, M.R. (2004). Dopamine transporter binding in Gilles de la Tourette syndrome: a [^{123}I]FP-CIT/SPECT study. *Acta Psychiatr Scand 109,* 140-146.

Shapiro, A.K., & Shapiro, E. (1968). Treatment of Gilles de la Tourette's syndrome with haloperidol. *Brit J Psychiatry, 114,* 345-350.

Silva, R.R., Munoz, D. M., Barickman, J., & Friedhoff, A.J. (1995). Environmental factors and related fluctuation of symptoms in children and adolescents with Tourette's disorder. *J Child Psychol Psychiatry, 36,* 305-312.

Singer, H.S., Butler, I.J., Tune, L.E., et al. (1982). Dopaminergic dysfunction in Tourette syndrome. *Ann Neurol, 12,* 361-366.

Singer, H.S., Hanh, I.H., Moran, T. H. (1991). Abnormal dopamine uptake sites in postmortem striatum from patients with Tourette's syndrome. *Ann Neurol, 30,* 558-562.

Singer, H.S., Szymanski, S., Giuliano, J., Yokoi, F., Dogan, A.S., Brasic, J.R., …Wong, D.F. (2002). Elevated intrasyaptic dopamine release in Tourette's syndrome measured by PET. *Am J Psychiatry, 159,* 1329-1336.

Singer, H.S., & Minzer, K. (2003). Neurobiology of Tourette syndrome: concepts of neuroanatomical localization and neurochemical abnormalities. *Brain Dev, 25(Suppl),* S70-S84.

Singer, H.S. (2010). Treatment of tics and Tourette syndrome. *Curr Treat Options Neurol, 12,* 539-561.

Singer, H.S. (2013). The Neurochemistry of Tourette syndrome. In D. Martino & J.F. Leckman (Eds), *Tourette Syndrome* (pp. 276-300). New York, NY:Oxford University Press.

Stamenkovic, M., Schindler, S.D., Asenbaum, S., Neumeister, A., Willeit, M., Willinger, U., Kasper, S. (2001). No change in striatal dopamine re-uptake site density in psychotropic drug naïve and in currently treated Tourette's disorder patients: a [^{123}I]-beta-CIT SPECT-study. *Eur Neuropsychopharmacol 11,* 69-74.

Steeves, T.D., Ko, J.H., Kideckel, D.M., Rusjan, P, Houle, S., Sandor, P., Strafella, A.P. (2010). Extrastriatal dopaminergic dysfunction in Tourette syndrome. *Ann Neurol 67,* 170-181.

Sutherland Owens, A.N., Miguel, E.C., & Swerdlow, N.R. (2011). Sensory gating scales and premonitory urges in Tourette syndrome. *TheScientificWorldJournal, 11,* 736-741.

Sweet, R.D., Bruun, R., Shapiro, E., & Shapiro, A.K. (1974). Presynaptic catecholamine antagonists as treatment for Tourette syndrome. Effects of alpha methyl para tyrosine and tetrabenazine. *Arch Gen Psychiatry, 31,* 857-861.

Swerdlow, N.R., Karban, B., Ploum, Y., Sharp, R., Geyer, M.A., & Eastvold, A. (2001). Tactile prepuff inhibition of startle in children with Tourette's syndrome: in search of an fMRI-friendly startle paradigm. *Biol Psychiatry, 50,* 578-585.

Swerdlow, N.R. & Sutherland, A.N. (2005). Using animal models to develop therapeutics for Tourette Syndrome. *Pharmacol Ther, 108,* 281-293.

Swerdlow, N.R., Bongiovanni, M.J., Tochen, L., & Schoemaker, J.M. (2006a). Separable noradrenergic and dopaminergic regulation of prepulse inhibition in rats: implications for predictive validity and Tourette syndrome. *Psychopharmacology (Berl), 186,* 246-254.

Swerdlow, N.R., Krupin, A.S., Bongiovanni, M.J., Shoemaker, J.M., Goins, J.C., & Hammer, R.P. (2006b). Heritable differences in the dopaminergic regulation of behavior in rats: relationship to D2-like receptor G-protein function. *Neuropsychopharmacology, 31,* 721-729.

Swerdlow, N.R. (2013). Update: studies of prepulse inhibition of startle, with particular relevance to the pathophysiology or treatment of Tourette syndrome. *Neurosci Biobehav Rev, 37(6),* 1150-1156.

Tokimura, H., Di Lazzaro, V., Tokimura, Y., Oliviero, A., Profice, P., Insola, A., & Rothwell, J.C. (2000). Short latency inhibition of human hand motor cortex by somatosensory input from the hand. *J Physiol, 523(Pt 2),* 503-513.

Turjanski, N., Sawle, G.V., Playford, E.D., Weeks, R., Lammerstma, A.A., Lees, A.J., & Brooks, D.J. (1994). PET studies of the presynaptic and postsynaptic dopaminergic system in Tourette's syndrome. *J Neurol Neurosurg Psychiatry, 57,* 688-692.

Vernaleken, I., Kuhn, J., Lenartz, D., Raptis, M., Huff, W., Janouschek, H., Sturm, V. (2009). Bithalamical deep brain stimulation in Tourette syndrome is associated with reduction in dopaminergic transmission. *Biol Psychiatry, 66,* e15-e17.

Wichmann, T., Bergman, H., DeLong, M.R. (1994). The primate subthalamic nucleus. I. Functional properties in intact animals. *J Neurophysiol, 72,* 494-506.

Wong, D.F., Brasic, J.R., Singer, H.S., Schretlen, D.J., Kuwabara, H., Zhou, Y., Grace, A.A. (2008). Mechanisms of dopaminergic and serotonergic neurotransmission in Tourette syndrome: clues from an *in vivo* neurochemistry study with PET. *Neuropsychopharmacology, 33,* 1239-1251.

Worbe, Y., Gerardin, E., Hartmann, A., Valabregue, R., Tremblay, L, Vidailhet. M. Lehericy, S. (2010). Distinct structural changes underpin clinical phenotypes in patients with Gilles de la Tourette syndrome. *Brain, 133,* 3649-3660.

Yeh, C.B., Lee, C.S., Ma, K.H., Lee, M-S., Chang, C-J., & Huang, W-S. (2007). Phasic dysfunction of dopamine transmission in Tourette's syndrome evaluated with 99mTc TRODAT-1 imaging. *Psychiatry Res, 156,* 75-82.

Yoon, D.Y., Gause, C.D., Leckman, J.F., and Singer, H.S. (2007a). Frontal dopaminergic abnormality in Tourette syndrome: A postmortem analysis. *J Neurol Sci, 255,* 50-56.

Yoon, D.Y., Rippel, C.A., Kobets, A.J., Morris, C.M., Lee, J.E., Williams, P.N., & Singer, H.S. (2007b). Dopaminergic polymorphisms in Tourette syndrome: association with the DAT gene (SLC6A3). *Am J Med Genet B Neuropsychiatr Genet, 144,* 605-610.

Zebardast, N., Crowley, M.J., Bloch, M.H., Mayes, L.C., Vander Wyk, B., Leckman, J.F., Swain, J.E. (2013). Brain mechanisms for prepulse inhibition in adults with Tourette syndrome: Initial findings. *Psychiatry Res, 214,* 33-41.

Index

A

D

E

F

G

H

N

O

P

Q

R

S

T

U

V

W